Trauma

Editors

YORAM G. WEISS
MICHA Y. SHAMIR

ANESTHESIOLOGY CLINICS

www.anesthesiology.theclinics.com

Consulting Editor
LEE A. FLEISHER

March 2013 • Volume 31 • Number 1

ELSEVIER

1600 John F. Kennedy Boulevard • Suite 1800 • Philadelphia, Pennsylvania, 19103-2899

http://www.theclinics.com

ANESTHESIOLOGY CLINICS Volume 31, Number 1
March 2013 ISSN 1932-2275, ISBN-13: 978-1-4557-5062-7

Editor: Pamela Hetherington

Anesthesiology Clinics (ISSN 1932-2275) is published quarterly by Elsevier Inc., 360 Park Avenue South, New York, NY 10010-1710. Months of issue are March, June, September, and December. Periodicals postage paid at New York, NY and at additional mailing offices. Subscription prices are $154.00 per year (US student/resident), $313.00 per year (US individuals), $383.00 per year (Canadian individuals), $516.00 per year (US institutions), $639.00 per year (Canadian institutions), $216.00 per year (Canadian and foreign student/resident), $434.00 per year (foreign individuals), and $639.00 per year (foreign institutions). To receive student and resident rate, orders must be accompanied by name of affiliated institution, date of term, and the *signature* of program/residency coordinator on institutions letterhead. Orders will be billed at individual rate until proof of status is received. Foreign air speed delivery is included in all *Clinics'* subscription prices. All prices are subject to change without notice. POSTMASTER: Send address changes to *Anesthesiology Clinics,* Elsevier Health Sciences Division, Subscription Customer Service, 3251 Riverport Lane, Maryland Heights, MO 63043. Customer Service (orders, claims, online, change of address): Elsevier Health Sciences Division, Subscription Customer Service, 3251 Riverport Lane, Maryland Heights, MO 63043. Tel:1-800-654-2452 (U.S. and Canada); 314-447-8871 (outside U.S. and Canada). Fax: 314-447-8029. E-mail: journalscustomerservice-usa@elsevier.com (for print support); journalsonlinesupport-usa@elsevier.com (for online support).

Reprints. For copies of 100 or more of articles in this publication, please contact the Commercial Reprints Department, Elsevier Inc., 360 Park Avenue South, New York, NY 10010-1710. Tel.: 212-633-3812; Fax: 212-462-1935; E-mail: reprints@elsevier.com.

Anesthesiology Clinics, is also published in Spanish by McGraw-Hill Inter-americana Editores S. A., P.O. Box 5-237, 06500 Mexico D. F., Mexico.

Anesthesiology Clinics, is covered in *MEDLINE/PubMed (Index Medicus), Current Contents/Clinical Medicine, Excerpta Medica, ISI/BIOMED*, and *Chemical Abstracts*.

Printed in the United States of America.

Contributors

CONSULTING EDITOR

LEE A. FLEISHER, MD, FACC
Robert D. Dripps Professor and Chair of Anesthesiology and Critical Care, Professor of Medicine, Perelman School of Medicine, University of Pennsylvania School of Medicine, Philadelphia, Pennsylvania

EDITORS

YORAM G. WEISS, MD, MBA, FCCM
Associate Professor, Department of Anesthesia, Hadassah Hebrew University Medical Center, Jerusalem, Israel; Adjunct Associate Professor, Department of Anesthesia and Critical Care Medicine, University of Pennsylvania School of Medicine, Philadelphia, Pennsylvania

MICHA Y. SHAMIR, MD
Department of Anesthesia, Hadassah Hebrew University Medical Center, Jerusalem, Israel

AUTHORS

MICHAEL AZIZ, MD
Associate Professor, Department of Anesthesiology & Perioperative Medicine, Oregon Health & Science University, Portland, Oregon

MAGDALENA BAKOWITZ, MD, MPH
Fellow in Cardiothoracic Anesthesiology, Hospital of the University of Pennsylvania, Philadelphia, Pennsylvania

SHAWN E. BANKS, MD
Attending Anesthesiologist, Assistant Professor of Clinical Anesthesiology, Ryder Trauma Center, University of Miami Miller School of Medicine, Miami, Florida

DIMITRY BARANOV, MD
Department of Anesthesiology and Critical Care, Hospital of University of Pennsylvania, Philadelphia, Pennsylvania

EREZ BEN-MENACHEM, MBCHB, MBA, FANZCA
Department of Anesthesiology, Sheba Medical Center, Tel Aviv University, Tel Hashomer, Israel

HAIM BERKENSTADT, MD
The Israel Center for Medical Simulation (MSR); Department of Anesthesiology; Sackler Faculty of Medicine, Sheba Medical Center, Tel Aviv University, Tel Hashomer, Israel

ROMAN DUDARYK, MD
Assistant Professor of Clinical Anesthesiology, Divisions of Trauma Anesthesia and Critical Care Medicine, Department of Anesthesiology, Perioperative Medicine and Pain Management, Ryder Trauma Center, Jackson Memorial Hospital, University of Miami Miller School of Medicine, Miami, Florida

SHARON EINAV, MD
Director of Surgical Critical Care, Shaare Zedek Medical Centre, Senior Lecturer in Anesthesiology and Critical Care Medicine, Hebrew University School of Medicine, Jerusalem, Israel

SAMUEL M. GALVAGNO Jr, DO, PhD
Division of Trauma Anesthesiology (Program in Trauma, R Adams Cowley Shock Trauma Center); Division of Adult Critical Care Medicine, Assistant Professor, Department of Anesthesiology, Faculty, Shock Trauma Anesthesia Organized Research Center (STAR ORC), R Adams Cowley Shock Trauma Center, University of Maryland School of Medicine, Baltimore, Maryland

OLIVER GROTTKE, MD, PhD, MPH
Anesthesiologist, Department of Anesthesiology, RWTH Aachen University Hospital, Aachen, Germany

JERROLD H. LEVY, MD, FAHA, FCCM
Professor and Deputy Chair for Research, Emory University School of Medicine, Atlanta, Georgia

MICHAEL C. LEWIS, MD
Senior Associate Dean for Graduate Medical Education, Professor of Clinical Anesthesiology, University of Miami Miller School of Medicine, Miami, Florida

COLIN F. MACKENZIE, MBChB, FRCA, FCCM
Clinical Professor, Department of Anesthesiology, Faculty, Shock Trauma Anesthesia Organized Research Center (STAR ORC) and Charles McMathias Jr., National Study Center for Trauma and Emergency Medical Systems, University of Maryland School of Medicine, Baltimore, Maryland

MAUREEN McCUNN, MD, MIPP, FCCM
Assistant Professor of Anesthesiology and Critical Care, Hospital of the University of Pennsylvania, Philadelphia, Pennsylvania

RICHARD R. McNEER, MD, PhD
Division of Trauma Anesthesiology, Assistant Professor, Department of Anesthesiology, University of Miami Miller School of Medicine, Miami; Assistant Professor (Secondary Appointment), Department of Biomedical Engineering, College of Engineering, University of Miami, Coral Gables, Florida

TIMOTHY E. MOREY, MD
Professor, Associate Chair for Research, Department of Anesthesiology, University of Florida, Gainesville, Florida

MASAHIRO MURAKAWA, MD
Professor and Chair, Department of Anesthesiology, Fukushima Medical University School of Medicine, Fukushima City, Fukushima, Japan

PATRICK J. NELIGAN, MD
Department of Anaesthesia and Intensive Care, Galway University Hospitals, Galway, Ireland

ERNESTO A. PRETTO Jr, MD, MPH
Professor and Chief, Division of Transplant and Vascular Anesthesia, Department of Anesthesiology, Perioperative Medicine and Pain Management, Jackson Memorial Hospital, University of Miami Miller School of Medicine, Miami, Florida

MARK J. RICE, MD
Associate Professor, Section Chief, Liver Transplantation and General Surgery Sections, Department of Anesthesiology, University of Florida, Gainesville, Florida

KRISTEN CAREY ROCK, MD
Resident in Anesthesia and Critical Care Medicine, Hospital of the University of Pennsylvania, Philadelphia, Pennsylvania

ROLF ROSSAINT, MD
Professor and Head of the Department of Anesthesiology, Department of Anesthesiology, RWTH Aachen University Hospital, Aachen, Germany

HEN Y. SELA, MD
Director, Allen Hospital MFM Ultrasound & Consult Services, Division of Maternal Fetal Medicine, Department of Obstetrics and Gynecology, Columbia University Medical Center, New York, New York

DANIEL SIMON, MD
Trauma Unit, Sheba Medical Center, Tel Aviv University, Tel Hashomer, Israel

DONAT R. SPAHN, MD, FRCA
Professor and Head of the Institute of Anesthesiology, University of Zurich, Zurich, Switzerland

OLIVER M. THEUSINGER, MD
Staff Member, Institute of Anesthesiology, University Zurich, University Hospital Zurich, Zurich, Switzerland

ALBERT J. VARON, MD, MHPE, FCCM
Division of Trauma Anesthesiology, Professor and Vice Chair for Education, Department of Anesthesiology, University of Miami Miller School of Medicine; Chief of Anesthesiology, Ryder Trauma Center at Jackson Memorial Hospital, Miami, Florida

CAROLYN F. WEINIGER, MBChB
Senior Lecturer, Department of Anesthesiology and Critical Care Medicine, Hadassah Hebrew University Medical Center, Jerusalem, Israel

CHRISTIAN ZENTAI, MD
Anesthesiologist, Department of Anesthesiology, RWTH Aachen University Hospital, Aachen, Germany

AMITAI ZIV, MD, MHA
The Israel Center for Medical Simulation (MSR); Sackler Faculty of Medicine, Sheba Medical Center, Tel Aviv University, Tel Hashomer, Israel

Contents

Foreword **xiii**

Lee A. Fleisher

Preface: Postmarketing Pharmaceutical Product Pitfalls in Trauma Care **xv**

Yoram G. Weiss and Micha Y. Shamir

New and Future Resuscitation Fluids for Trauma Patients Using Hemoglobin and Hypertonic Saline **1**

Samuel M. Galvagno Jr and Colin F. Mackenzie

Hemoglobin-based oxygen carriers (HBOC) and hypertonic saline solutions (HSS) are used for resuscitation of trauma patients with hemorrhagic shock. In this review, the clinical application, dosing, administration, and side effects of these solutions are discussed. Although HBOC and HSS are not ideal resuscitation fluids, until rapidly thawed universal donor frozen blood and blood component therapy becomes widely available in North America, these fluids should to be considered immediately after injury and throughout the spectrum of care for patients with hemorrhagic shock, until blood and blood components become available.

Trauma and Aggressive Homeostasis Management **21**

Patrick J. Neligan and Dimitry Baranov

Homeostasis refers to the capacity of the human body to maintain a stable constant state by means of continuous dynamic equilibrium adjustments controlled by a medley of interconnected regulatory mechanisms. Patients who sustain tissue injury, such as trauma or surgery, undergo a well-understood reproducible metabolic and neuroendocrine stress response. This review discusses 3 issues that concern homeostasis in the acute care of trauma patients directly related to the stress response: hyperglycemia, lactic acidosis, and hypothermia. There is significant reason to question the "conventional wisdom" relating to current approaches to restoring homeostasis in critically ill and trauma patients.

Nonsurgical Techniques to Control Massive Bleeding **41**

Christian Zentai, Oliver Grottke, Donat R. Spahn, and Rolf Rossaint

Significant advancements in nonsurgical and surgical approaches to control bleeding in severely injured patients have also improved the treatment of critical trauma-related coagulopathy. Nonsurgical procedures such as angiographic embolization are progressively considered to terminate arterial bleeding from pelvic fractures. The disturbance of coagulation may aggravate bleeding and hamper surgical procedures. The administration of coagulation factors and factor concentrates may be useful for correcting systemic coagulopathy and reducing the need for fresh frozen plasma, platelet, and red blood cell transfusions, which are associated with various

adverse outcomes. In this review, nonsurgical management of critical trauma bleeding is discussed.

Point of Care Devices for Assessing Bleeding and Coagulation in the Trauma Patient **55**

Oliver M. Theusinger and Jerrold H. Levy

Severe trauma is associated with bleeding, coagulopathy, and transfusion of blood and blood products, all contributing to higher rates of morbidity and mortality. The aim of this review is to focus on point-of-care devices to monitor coagulation in trauma. Close monitoring of bleeding and coagulation as well as platelet function in trauma patients allows goal-directed transfusion and an optimization of the patient's coagulation, reduces the exposure to blood products, reduces costs, and probably improves clinical outcome. Noninvasive hemoglobin measurements are not to be used in trauma patients due to a lack in specificity and sensitivity.

Advances in the Management of the Critically Injured Patient in the Operating Room **67**

Kristen Carey Rock, Magdalena Bakowitz, and Maureen McCunn

Care of trauma patients continues to improve through better understanding of optimal timing of operating room (OR) interventions, improved monitoring for patients with head injury and hemodynamic compromise, optimization of volume status, and use of appropriate vasoactive agents. Investigation of the pathophysiology of trauma patients as they progress to the chronic phase continues to advance interventions in the ICU and the OR. This article is an evidence-based update of anesthetic considerations for these patients, including management of intracranial pressure, cardiac monitoring, management of the damage control abdomen, fluid and hemodynamic management, and control of coagulopathies.

Resuscitation in a Multiple Casualty Event **85**

Roman Dudaryk and Ernesto A. Pretto Jr

A major weakness in the emergency medical response to multiple casualty events continues to be the resuscitation component, which should consist of the systematic application of basic, advanced, and prolonged life support and definitive care within 24 hours. There have been major advances in emergency medical care over the last decade, including the feasibility of point-of-care ultrasound to aid in rapid assessment of injuries in the field, damage control resuscitation, and resuscitative surgery protocols, delivered by small trauma/resuscitation teams equipped with regional anesthesia capability for rapid deployment. Widespread adoption of these best practices may improve the delivery of resuscitative care in future multiple casualty events.

Anesthesia in an Austere Setting: Lessons Learned from the Haiti Relief Operation **107**

Timothy E. Morey and Mark J. Rice

The practice of medicine to care for injured patients after an earthquake can challenge physicians. The great need requires an open mind to develop anesthetic plans around locally available resources. A focus on monitored anesthetic care and regional anesthesia is frequently practiced and beneficial to patients. Anesthesiologists will serve as leaders to organize perioperative surgical services and provide input into the ethical triage of patients. The physicians should be mentally and physically prepared to enter into service in this disorganized zone of service to provide care.

Anesthesia Department Preparedness for a Multiple-Casualty Incident: Lessons Learned from the Fukushima Earthquake and the Japanese Nuclear Power Disaster **117**

Masahiro Murakawa

In the Great East Japan Earthquake, which occurred on March 11, 2011, many lives were lost in the accompanying giant tsunami. Fukushima prefecture was widely contaminated with radioactive substances emitted by the accident at the nuclear power plant. Only a few trauma and emergency patients were brought to our hospital by ambulance, and an unexpectedly small number of emergency surgeries performed. There were patients with radiation-induced sickness and injury, but no cases of severe exposure requiring surgery or intensive care. As a logistic support hospital, we should prepare for and simulate these cases to respond to any such future occurrence.

Trauma in the Elderly: Considerations for Anesthetic Management **127**

Shawn E. Banks and Michael C. Lewis

The volume of geriatric trauma patients is expected to increase significantly in coming years. Recognition of severe injuries may be delayed because they are less likely to mount classic symptoms of hemodynamic instability. Head injuries of any severity may place geriatric patients at increased risk of mortality, but there are currently no geriatric-specific treatment recommendations that differ from usual adult guidelines. Our understanding of best practices in geriatric trauma and anesthesia care continues to expand, as it does in all other areas of medicine.

Management and Outcomes of Trauma During Pregnancy **141**

Sharon Einav, Hen Y. Sela, and Carolyn F. Weiniger

Approximately 1% to 4% of pregnant women are evaluated in emergency/delivery room because of traumatic injury, yet there are few educational strategies targeted toward prevention/management of maternal trauma. Use of illicit drugs and alcohol, domestic abuse, and depression contribute to maternal trauma; thus a high index of suspicion should be maintained when treating injured young women. Treating the mother appropriately is beneficial for both the mother and the fetus. Fetal viability should be assessed after maternal stabilization. Pregnancy-related morbidity occurs in approximately 25% of cases and may include placental abruption, uterine rupture, preterm delivery, and the need for cesarean delivery.

Use of Video-assisted Intubation Devices in the Management of Patients with Trauma **157**

Michael Aziz

Patients with trauma may have airways that are difficult to manage. Patients with blunt trauma are at increased risk of unrecognized cervical spine injury, especially patients with head trauma. Manual in-line stabilization reduces cervical motion and should be applied whenever a cervical collar is removed. All airway interventions cause some degree of cervical spine motion. Flexible fiberoptic intubation causes the least cervical motion of all intubation approaches, and rigid video laryngoscopy provides a good laryngeal view and eases intubation difficulty. In emergency medicine departments, video laryngoscopy use is growing and observational data suggest an improved success rate compared with direct laryngoscopy.

Training in Trauma Management: The Role of Simulation-Based Medical Education **167**

Haim Berkenstadt, Erez Ben-Menachem, Daniel Simon, and Amitai Ziv

Simulation-based medical education (SBME) offers a safe and "mistake-forgiving" environment to teach and train medical professionals. The diverse range of medical-simulation modalities enables trainees to acquire and practice an array of tasks and skills. SBME offers the field of trauma training multiple opportunities to enhance the effectiveness of the education provided in this challenging domain. Further research is needed to better learn the role of simulation-based learning in trauma management and education.

Pitfalls of Hemodynamic Monitoring in Patients with Trauma **179**

Richard R. McNeer and Albert J. Varon

This article provides an update for the anesthesiology community on the mechanisms and limitations of common modalities used to assess the early hemodynamic status in patients with trauma. Figures are provided to illustrate important concepts through the use of computer simulation and real-world examples. This article is of value to anesthesiologists whose practice includes management of hemorrhagic shock.

Index **195**

ANESTHESIOLOGY CLINICS

FORTHCOMING ISSUES

June 2013
Cardiac Anesthesia
Colleen Koch, MD, *Editor*

September 2013
Obstetric and Gynecologic Anesthesia
Robert Gaiser, *Editor*

December 2013
Transplantation
Claus Niemann, *Editor*

RECENT ISSUES

December 2012
Thoracic Anesthesia
Peter Slinger, MD, FRCPC, *Editor*

September 2012
Postanesthesia Care Unit
Scott A. Falk, MD, *Editor*

June 2012
Neurosurgical Anesthesia
Ansgar M. Brambrink, MD, PhD and
Jeffrey R. Kirsch, MD, *Editors*

RELATED INTEREST

Chest Surgery Clinics, February 2012 (Volume 22, Issue 1)
Current Management Guidelines in Thoracic Surgery
M. Blair Marshall, *Editor*

Foreword

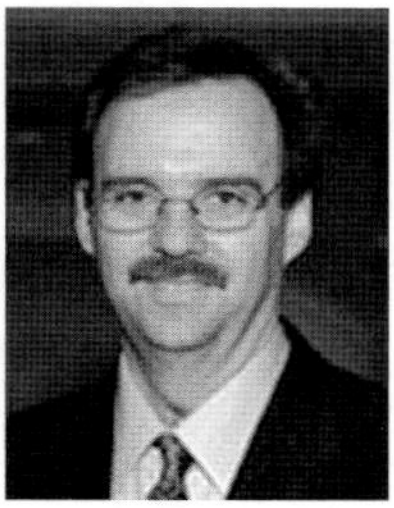

Lee A. Fleisher, MD, FACC
Consulting Editor

Trauma is a major cause of morbidity and mortality worldwide. The role of the anesthesiologist in trauma care is critical and an increasing number of departments are developing special programs in trauma education and fellowships. The need to create such programs has resulted in the development of new knowledge of how best to care for these patients. In this issue of *Anesthesiology Clinics of North America*, the editors have assembled a group of articles that detail many of these advances, including lessons learned from recent disasters. They have also focused on special vulnerable populations. Finally, they have provided information on training in trauma. As most hospital-based anesthesiologists care for trauma patients, the information provided in this issue should be helpful in providing the best and most up-to-date practices.

As guest editors for this issue, we are fortunate to have Yoram Weiss, MD and Micha Shamir, MD. Dr Weiss is the chairman of the Department of Anesthesiology at the Hadassah Hebrew University Medical Center. He received his medical degree from the Israel Institute of Technology–Technion, Haifa, Israel in 1990, following which he trained in Anesthesiology and Critical Care Medicine at Hadassah and the University of Pennsylvania. Dr Weiss has research interests focusing on advanced physiologic monitoring as well as the 2 most severe forms of respiratory failure and infection: acute respiratory distress syndrome and sepsis. Dr Shamir received his medical degree from the Hebrew University–Hadassah School of Medicine and is currently a Lecturer in Anesthesiology on their faculty and Director of the Hadassah Resuscitation School and Service. His major areas of special interest include the care of victims of multiple casualty events, early detection of hypovolemia, and resuscitation practice and teaching. They have assembled a stellar international group of authors who provide

Anesthesiology Clin 31 (2013) xiii–xiv
http://dx.doi.org/10.1016/j.anclin.2012.11.008 **anesthesiology.theclinics.com**
1932-2275/13/$ – see front matter

important information for the anesthesiologist to understand all of the recent advances in trauma anesthesia care.

Lee A. Fleisher, MD, FACC
Perelman School of Medicine
University of Pennsylvania School of Medicine
3400 Spruce Street, Dulles 680
Philadelphia, PA 19104, USA

E-mail address:
lee.fleisher@uphs.upenn.edu

Preface

Postmarketing Pharmaceutical Product Pitfalls in Trauma Care

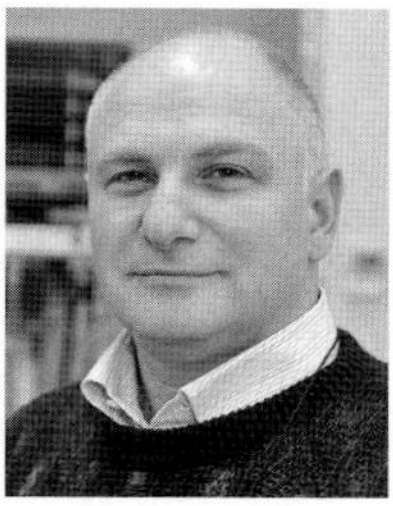

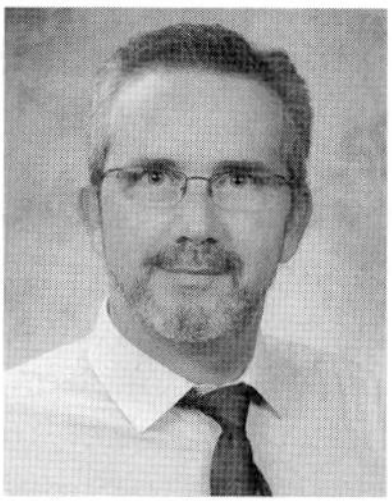

Yoram G. Weiss, MD, MBA, FCCM   Micha Y. Shamir, MD
Editors

Implementing novel therapies into daily medical practice requires thorough research before regulatory approval and thereafter awareness of cumulative postmarketing medical knowledge. This editorial addresses 2 postmarketing controversies affecting trauma treatment: the retraction of published articles regarding hydroxyethyl starch (HES) and the "back-door" (off-label use) introduction of recombinant factor VIIa (rFVIIa) for intractable hemorrhage in nonhemophiliacs.

In this issue, Galvagno et al, did not address the use of HES for fluid resuscitation in their review. This comes as no surprise because the routine use of HES has been recently revisited. In 2010, a group of medical journal editors retracted 88 articles published by Dr Joachim Boldt, a leading investigator in many publications studying the use of HES.[1] A recent review on the use of HES concluded that "a shadow is cast on a bulk of literature on HES safety and efficacy."[2] Furthermore, the authors also noted that there is great concern due to the lack of safety data on new IV solutions using HES 130/0.4. These solutions were approved based on equivalence studies, which focused on elective surgeries—associated acute hypovolemia. These studies used other synthetic colloids as comparators, had small sample sizes, and were not suitable for assessing safety. It was concluded that "there is no convincing evidence that third-generation HES 130/0.4 is safe in surgical, emergency, or intensive care patients despite publication of numerous clinical studies."[3]

A recent Cochrane meta-analysis reviewed randomized controlled trials comparing colloids to crystalloids used for volume replacement.[4] The authors found no evidence that resuscitation with colloids reduced mortality compared to crystalloids in postoperative patients or those suffering from trauma or burns. The authors questioned the use of these colloids in these patient groups considering lack of proven effect on mortality and increased cost.

Anesthesiology Clin 31 (2013) xv–xviii
http://dx.doi.org/10.1016/j.anclin.2012.11.006   **anesthesiology.theclinics.com**
1932-2275/13/$ – see front matter

A recently published study shed additional light on the safety and efficacy of HES for volume resuscitation.[5] In this study, 7000 intensive care unit patients, including some suffering from multiple trauma and traumatic brain injury, were randomly assigned to receive either 6% HES (130/0.4) or 0.9% sodium chloride (saline) as the sole intravenous fluid until intensive care unit discharge or death. No significant difference in 90-day mortality was found between the 2 groups. However, more patients in the HES group required renal-replacement therapy. This study provides additional support to concerns regarding possible adverse kidney effects (acute kidney injury and risk for renal replacement therapy) when using HES for volume resuscitation.[2]

The role of rFVIIa in the management of uncontrolled bleeding is addressed in the review, "Nonsurgical Techniques to Control Massive Bleeding," by Zentai et al. This is a case where specific guidelines for a specific disease, namely Hemophilia A/B, were generalized to recommendations encompassing a larger population suffering from a different disease, namely, traumatic hemorrhage, based on relative small studies and case reports. rFVIIa (NovoSeven, Novo Nordisk, Bagsværd, Denmark) was approved in March 1999 by the FDA for the management of patients with hemophilia.[6,7] Seven months later, in the November 1999 issue of *The Lancet*, Kenet et al, published the first description of off-label use of rFVIIa to control traumatic bleeding in a nonhemophilic patient.[8] This has led to an eruption of publications describing the off-label use of rFVIIa in nonhemophiliacs. In 2005 a review article summarizing the preclinical studies used as the scientific basis for rFVIIa use in nonhemophiliacs was able to identify only 10 relevant articles.[9] On the other hand, at the same time, numerous case reports and small case series describing the off-label use of rFVIIa were published. It was estimated that by the end of 2004 approximately 4500 patients were treated with rFVIIa for off-label indications, in the United States only.[7] By the end of 2008 this number skyrocketed to almost 74,000, a 143-fold increase in off-label use of rFVIIa, as opposed to the 3.8-fold increase use for hemophilia A or B patients.[10] At this time, rFVIIa became an integral part of the treatment for significant hemorrhage, almost a "must." As most studies did not present a risk associated with its use, it was considered a safe drug. However, part of the medical community was concerned about the efficacy and safety of this very expensive drug for bleeding in nonhemophiliacs.

In 2005 Boffard et al, published the largest randomized controlled trial on the use of rFVIIa in trauma (301 patients).[11] This study failed to demonstrate a decrease in mortality in patients suffering from penetrating or blunt trauma being treated with rFVIIa. In patients suffering from blunt trauma treated with rFVIIa, they showed a 2.6 reduction in blood units transfused and a reduced occurrence of acute respiratory distress syndrome. A similar frequency and severity of adverse events were found between the treatment groups. Nevertheless, the indiscriminate use of rFVIIa caused the Food and Drug Administration (FDA) to conduct its own inquiry that was published in 2006 and was based on the FDA's Adverse Event Reporting System database.[7] This report identified 185 arterial or venous thromboembolic adverse events, mostly in patients receiving the drug for off-label indications.

Where are we in 2013, following 13 years of off-label use? Yank et al, analyzed the existing data in a meta-analysis that included studies that compared the use of rFVIIa for 5 off-label indications: intracerebral hemorrhage, cardiac surgery, trauma, liver transplantation, and prostatectomy.[12] A total of 62 higher scientific level reports were identified with a total of 3965 patients (2283 treated, 1682 controls). Off-label use of rFVIIa for intracerebral hemorrhage and cardiac surgery did not reduce mortality but increased the risk for thromboembolism. For body trauma, there was no increased risk for thromboembolism but also no difference in mortality. For the remaining indications, the available evidence was too limited.

A more recent Cochrane review analyzed the results of 29 studies.[13] Sixteen of the trials were prospective (1361 patients, 729 received rFVIIa). A reduction in blood loss and blood transfusion was found, yet mortality did not differ. There was a trend against rFVIIa attributed to increased thromboembolic adverse events. Thirteen trials (2929 patients, 1878 received rFVIIa) examined the therapeutic use of rFVIIa. No statistically significant decrease in mortality or increase in thromboembolic complications was noted. However, when all trials were pooled together to examine the risk of thromboembolic events, a significant increase in total arterial events was observed (RR 1.45).

In their *British Journal of Anesthesia* editorial, Spahn et al, asked. "...where do we stand in May 2005? Are we obliged to give rFVIIa to patients with major bleeding to avoid accusation of substandard treatment or is rFVIIa treatment not indicated, owing to the lack of high level scientific evidence, lack of approval by any health authority, the potential of serious side-effects and its high cost?"[14] In 2011, Avron and Kesselheim answer this question in their *Annals of Internal Medicine* editorial: "Although off-label prescribing by physicians is not illegal, physicians who persist in such use (i.e. prescribing rFVIIa–YGW MYS) in the face of clear evidence of inutility and harm could be subject to civil action by the affected patients or their heirs."[6]

Yoram G. Weiss, MD, MBA, FCCM
Department of Anesthesia
Hadassah Hebrew University Medical Center
Jerusalem, Israel

Micha Y. Shamir, MD
Department of Anesthesia
Hadassah Hebrew University Medical Center
Jerusalem, Israel

E-mail address:
weiss@hadassah.org.il (Y.G. Weiss)

REFERENCES

1. Editors-in-Chief statement regarding published clinical trials conducted without IRB approval by Joachim Boldt. Minerva Anestesiol 2011;77:562–3. Available at. www.ncbi.nlm.nih.gov/pubmed/21540815.
2. Reinhart K, Takala J. Hydroxyethyl starches: What do we still know? Anesth Analg 2011;112:507–11.
3. Hartog CS, Kohl M, Reinhart K. A systematic review of third-generation hydroxyethyl starch (HES 130/0.4) in resuscitation: safety not adequately addressed. Anesth Analg 2011;112(3):635–45.
4. Perel P, Roberts I. Colloids versus crystalloids for fluid resuscitation in critically ill patients. Cochrane Database Syst Rev 2012;(6):CD000567.
5. Myburgh JA, Finfer S, Bellomo R, et al. Hydroxyethyl starch or saline for fluid resuscitation in intensive care. N Engl J Med 2012;367:1901–11.
6. Avorn J, Kesselheim A. A hemorrhage of off-label use. Ann Intern Med 2011; 154(8):566–7.
7. O'Connell KA, Wood JJ, Wise RP, et al. Thromboembolic adverse events after use of recombinant human coagulation factor VIIa. JAMA 2006;295(3):293–8.
8. Kenet G, Walden R, Eldad A, et al. Treatment of traumatic bleeding with recombinant factor VIIa. Lancet 1999;354(9193):1879.

9. Schreiber MA, Holcomb JB, Rojkjaer R. Preclinical trauma studies of recombinant factor VIIa. Crit Care 2005;9(Suppl 5):S25–8.
10. Logan AC, Yank V, Stafford RS. Off-label use of recombinant factor VIIa in U.S. hospitals: Analysis of hospital records. Ann Intern Med 2011;154:516–22.
11. Boffard KD, Riou B, Warren B, et al. Recombinant factor VIIa as adjunctive therapy for bleeding control in severely injured trauma patients: Two parallel randomized, placebo-controlled, double-blind clinical trials. J Trauma 2005; 59(1):8–18.
12. Yank V, Tuohy CV, Logan AC. Systematic review: Benefits and harms of in-hospital use of recombinant factor VIIa for off-label indications. Ann Intern Med 2011; 154(8):529–40.
13. Simpson E, Lin Y, Stanworth S, et al. Recombinant factor VIIa for the prevention and treatment of bleeding in patients without haemophilia. Cochrane Database Syst Rev 2012;14:3:CD005011.
14. Spahn DR, Tucci MA, Makris M. Is recombinant FVIIa the magic bullet in the treatment of major bleeding? Br J Anaesth 2005;94(5):553–5.

New and Future Resuscitation Fluids for Trauma Patients Using Hemoglobin and Hypertonic Saline

Samuel M. Galvagno Jr, DO, PhD[a,b],
Colin F. Mackenzie, MBChB, FRCA, FCCM[c,*]

KEYWORDS

• Trauma • Resuscitation • Hemoglobin-based oxygen carriers (HBOC)
• Hypertonic saline solutions (HSS) • Frozen blood • Frozen plasma and platelets
• Coagulopathy of trauma • Inflammatory response

KEY POINTS

- Hemoglobin-based oxygen carriers (HBOC) and hypertonic saline solutions (HSS) are used for resuscitation of trauma patients with hemorrhagic shock.
- HBOC and HSS are not ideal resuscitation fluids, but have advantages when blood is unavailable or refused. Until regulatory authorities approve use of rapidly thawed universal donor frozen blood and blood component therapy in North America, HBOC and HSS should be considered immediately after injury and throughout the spectrum of care for patients with hemorrhagic shock, until blood and blood components can be transfused.
- HBOC and HSS could be useful in the prehospital environment, military conflicts, disasters, and in the developing world, and in other situations where blood is not readily accessible.
- Neither resuscitation fluid is without risk, but should be used when the benefits outweigh such risks.

Disclosure: Dr Mackenzie acknowledges receiving funding as an ad hoc consultant, as chair of a symposium on HBOC-210 (Hemopure) and as a Site PI on the Phase III HEM-0115 Trial but has no equity interests in Biopure Corporation or in its successor OPK Biotech. Dr Galvagno has no disclosures to report.

[a] Division of Trauma Anesthesiology (Program in Trauma, R Adams Cowley Shock Trauma Center), Department of Anesthesiology, Shock Trauma Anesthesia Organized Research Center (STAR ORC), University of Maryland School of Medicine, T1R83, 22 South Greene Street, Baltimore, MD 21201, USA; [b] Division of Adult Critical Care Medicine, Department of Anesthesiology, Shock Trauma Anesthesia Organized Research Center (STAR ORC), R Adams Cowley Shock Trauma Center, University of Maryland School of Medicine, T1R83, 22 South Greene Street, Baltimore, MD 21201, USA; [c] Department of Anesthesiology, Shock Trauma Anesthesia Organized Research Center (STAR ORC) and Charles McMathias Jr, National Study Center for Trauma and Emergency Medical Systems, University of Maryland School of Medicine, 110 S.Paca Street, Baltimore, MD 21201, USA
* Corresponding author. 419 Redwood Street, 2nd Floor STAR ORC, Baltimore, MD 21201.
E-mail address: cmack003@gmail.com

Anesthesiology Clin 31 (2013) 1–19
http://dx.doi.org/10.1016/j.anclin.2012.10.004 **anesthesiology.theclinics.com**

INTRODUCTION

Major hemorrhage is the most frequent avoidable cause of early mortality in combat casualties,[1] and even in the civilian setting; among those who survive at least 15 minutes into advanced trauma care, but go on to die of bleeding, half are dead within 2 hours.[2] One of the most important advances in trauma transfusion medicine in the last decade has been the recognition of the acute coagulopathy of trauma and the need to supply coagulation factors (such as plasma) and platelets in near-equivalence ratio with red cells.[3] In the military setting, where fresh whole blood may be available as a walking blood bank, prescreened donors need to be identified, prepped, and bled. This process requires a minimum of 60 minutes. Moreover, although large numbers of units of packed red cells (pRBC) can be provided on arrival in a civilian trauma center or military combat support hospital, equivalent proportions of platelets and plasma typically require a minimum of 20 minutes lead time to be thawed or otherwise processed. Significant advances have been made in rapidly processing frozen or freeze-dried blood, plasma, and platelets for use in the blood bank of the military combat support hospital for the Netherlands Military in Afghanistan, with potential future application in the United States. Nevertheless, alternative resuscitative fluids are often required during the acute stage of resuscitation when blood component therapy may not be available, and tissue perfusion must be maintained. In this review, 2 resuscitative solutions are discussed: hemoglobin-based oxygen carriers (HBOC) and hypertonic saline solutions (HSS). Clinical applications, mechanisms, dosing, and side effects are discussed.

CURRENT CONCEPTS IN TRAUMA RESUSCITATION

Early infusion of fresh whole blood, cryoprecipitate, and fresh frozen plasma (FFP) is necessary because delay to surgical intervention has been reported to increase mortality in patients with intra-abdominal hemorrhage.[4] Increasing the ratio of FFP to pRBC improves survival in combat casualties,[5–10] and in coagulopathic patients, early platelet transfusion is beneficial. Decreasing blood and blood component loss from vascular injuries is the primary initial resuscitation management using rapid application of tourniquets, pressure bandages, and clotting gels until definitive vascular surgical control can be achieved.[11–13] Decreasing the transfusion requirement in trauma patients is important, because pRBC are associated with infection, multiorgan failure, and mortality.[14–17] At the R Adams Cowley Shock Trauma Center (STC) of the University of Maryland, more than 8000 trauma patients are admitted each year. Approximately 2% to 3% receive universal donor blood immediately on arrival, 3% to 5% receive a massive transfusion (variously defined as >4 units of pRBC in 4 hours, >10 units of pRBC in 6 hours or >10 units of pRBC in 24 hours), and 8% of STC trauma patients receive blood during their hospitalization; transfusion of 2 to 3 units of pRBC is the most common mode of administration.[18]

RESUSCITATION CAPABILITY GAP

Before casualties with blood loss in both military and civilian settings reach advanced care, there is a need for a universally compatible, intravenous oxygen-carrying solution with reduced risk of disease transmission and long-term storage capability for field use. Military battlefield casualties,[19] disaster scenarios,[20] blood incompatibility and shortages, and religious objection[21] represent additional situations in which an oxygen-carrying solution can address this medical need. Natural and man-made disasters, lack of a mature and widespread blood bank system in most of the developing world, and the threat of terrorism heighten the urgency for an alternative oxygen-carrying solution to blood that can allow survival until the casualty is transported to the available blood supply. There are 47,000,000 Americans who live more than 1 hour from a trauma center[22] and most ambulances do not carry blood.[23] The mortality rate of trauma patients with prehospital shock who do not receive blood until arrival at the hospital is 17% to 54%[24–27] and mortality increases with time and distance to definitive care. Rural settings account for only 20% of the population but 60% of trauma deaths because of longer transport times and lack of the facilities available in trauma centers, such as blood, during care en route.[28] In addition, stored pRBC are sometimes incompatible for in-hospital use because of inadequate inventory, immunologic states such as autoimmune hemolytic anemia, and certain religious groups do not accept transfusion.[21,23,24] Allogeneic pRBC transfusions may provoke adverse immunoinflammatory responses in high-risk patients.[16,29]

OXYGEN-CARRYING SOLUTIONS

The term oxygen-carrying solution includes blood (fresh, stored, frozen, and lyophilized) and cell-free HBOC, cell-free hemoglobin solutions encapsulated in artificial cells, and perfluorocarbon solutions. Perfluorocarbons have been discredited by their inability to carry clinically significant quantities of oxygen, even with high inspired oxygen.[30] Similarly, encapsulated (in artificial liposomes) hemoglobin oxygen carriers have major immune effects that have prevented their use in clinical trials.[31] Genetically produced HBOC have research interest as a tool to probe toxicity, but their clinical use is currently restricted by their exorbitant cost and an inability to produce large quantities sufficient to provide supplies for an appropriately powered clinical trial. HBOC have only 2 functions: carrying and delivering oxygen and augmenting blood volume. The ideal features of an HBOC resuscitation fluid are shown in **Box 1**.

RATIONALE FOR HBOC USE

There are many reasons why an HBOC is useful as a prehospital resuscitation fluid. More than two-thirds of the world does not have adequate blood supplies.[32] There may be a lack or shortage of compatible blood, the means to collect and process blood, and the means to keep blood refrigerated and have it available at all times for all those requiring transfusion. Blood shortages are expected to occur during mass casualty events, military operations, natural disasters, or terrorist attacks. HBOCs lack the numerous and complex antigens of the pRBC membrane, so are universally compatible, and can be readily administered to patients in shock. HBOC's

Box 1
Ideal and equivalent features of an HBOC resuscitation fluid

Increases oxygen carriage and tissue oxygen delivery equivalent to whole blood

Treats hypovolemia, restores perfusion, but no pressure increase greater than the equivalent colloid volume

Safe, with toxicities equivalent to pRBCs

Efficacious for all age groups and acute anemia management pathologies

Long shelf life, minimal or no processing, no refrigeration, no disease transmission, and low cost universal donor status (due to removal of red cell wall antibodies in processing) avoids the need for crossmatching. The stability of HBOC-201 (Hemopure, OPK Biotech LLC, Cambridge, MA) at ambient temperature (2–30°C), its prolonged shelf life of 3 years, and a hemoglobin concentration equivalent to whole blood make HBOC-201 an ideal choice for field use and for stockpiling, especially in rural areas distant from blood bank facilities. When compatible blood is not available or needs to be conserved because of rare red cell types in recipients, HBOCs can function as a fluid for intentional hemodilution to conserve red cells, or can be used in tandem with other conservation techniques under the rubric of bloodless surgery. In a recent large animal study of hemorrhagic shock, a combination of PEGylated HBOC and HSS (Aftershock, Prolong Pharmaceuticals Inc, Monmouth Junction, NJ) showed a trend toward improved short-term survival, and the addition of HSS ameliorated the increase in blood pressure and decrease in cardiac output normally seen when HBOC is administered alone.[33] In addition, HBOCs have benefits in extending the useful life of donor organs awaiting transplant.

HBOC fluids have no cells, so the rheology in hemorrhagic shock is optimized, and oxygen delivery can be enhanced to reverse ischemia in tissues beyond arteriolar stenosis, and inaccessible to red cells. Furthermore, due to concerns about infectious and immunosuppressive risks of allogeneic blood, and current convergence of blood quantities donated in comparison with those consumed, HBOCs are a practicable means of supporting demand in the face of diminishing blood supplies, especially as a worldwide shortage of safe and viable allogeneic donor blood is projected.[34–36]

CELL-FREE HBOCS

The biochemical, physiologic, and logistical characteristics of the 2 currently available HBOCs that have undergone phase III clinical trials are listed in **Table 1**.

HBOC-201 (Hemopure) is approved by regulatory authorities for human use in South Africa and in Russia, and was used in the largest phase III clinical trial (HEM-0115) of any HBOC[37] (n = 350 subjects randomized to HBOC-201) and has been administered to more than 800 humans in 22 completed clinical trials including

Table 1
Comparison of HBOCs in clinical trials with red cells

Feature	Hemopure/HBOC-201 (OPK Biotech)	Hemospan/MP4 (Sangart)	Red Blood Cells
Hemoglobin source	Bovine	Human	Human
Type of modification	Glutaraldehyde polymerization	Polyethylene glycol conjugation	Not applicable
Average molecular weight (kDa)	64–500	90	Not applicable
Hemoglobin level (g/dL)	13	4.2	13
Volume (mL)	250	250 or 500	
O_2 pressure at 50% oxygen saturation (mm Hg)	40	5–6	26–27
Oncotic pressure (mm Hg)	25	49	25
Viscosity (cP)	1.3	2.2–2.5	5–10
Half-life	19 h	43–66 h	31 d
Shelf life	<3 y (at 2–30°C)	<3 y (frozen)	42 d (at 4°C) <6 h (at 21°C)

4 advanced pRBC controlled trials in cardiac, vascular, general noncardiac, and orthopedic surgery,[38] and for compassionate use in more than 70 patients up to September 2012.[20] HBOC-201 has not received approval by the US Food and Drug Administration (FDA) other than under the Code of Federal Regulations Title 21 Parts 312 and 316 (Expanded access to investigational drugs for treatment use).[39] The FDA cited serious adverse events as the cause of failure to obtain approval after the HEM-0115 trial. These events were the result of a combination of comorbidities in compromised elderly patients, and various clinical mismanagement issues including initial hemodilution with crystalloids, followed by overdosing with HBOC-201 resulting in heart failure. In addition, there was a failure to maintain plasma hemoglobin levels consistent with the 19-hour half-life of HBOC-201. The half-life of pRBCs is 22 to 33 days, so management of acute anemia is more readily sustained.

Dosing and Monitoring

Intravenous dosing of HBOC-201 should not consider hematocrit (as HBOCs are acellular) but total hemoglobin (= red cell + plasma hemoglobin [from HBOC-201]) and maintain this greater than 5 g/dL by continuous slow (2–6 hours) infusion of consecutive units of HBOC-201. Redosing should not wait until total hemoglobin decreases, rather continuous HBOC-201 infusion should be repeated after 12 to 18 hours to ensure oxygen carriage is maintained.

Safety and Efficacy

Total hemoglobin concentration in HEM-0115 patients randomized to HBOC-201 (containing 13 g/dL hemoglobin) was lower than in patients randomized to pRBC (containing 32–36 g/dL of hemoglobin), affecting overall efficacy and safety results.[40] Because patients randomized to HBOC-201 were maintained at a lower hemoglobin level than those randomized to pRBCs, HBOC patients had a persistent anemia and lower ongoing oxygen-carrying capacity that did not exist in patients randomized to pRBC. Total hemoglobin concentration in patients randomized to HBOC-201 versus pRBC was less, which affected overall FDA efficacy and safety results.[37] Alternatively, if an intrinsic toxicity was responsible for the safety imbalance, a positive correlation between adverse events and increasing dose would be expected in only the HBOC group, which as **Fig. 1** shows, was not the case. Despite this hemoglobin concentration difference, there was a 96% transfusion avoidance for 24 hours in those randomized to HBOC-201, allowing adequate time to sustain field resuscitation and allow transport to facilities with blood for transfusion. There were no adverse event differences between those receiving 3 units of pRBC or less or equivalent amounts of HBOC-201 (see **Fig. 1**; **Fig. 2**). Within 1 week, there was 67% transfusion avoidance, making HBOC-201 a practical alternative when blood is unlikely to ever become available, because erythropoesis due to the iron load after HBOC-201 infusion restores total hemoglobin concentration within 7 to 10 days. A further analysis of HEM-0115 data showed an acceptable safety profile in younger acute trauma populations, especially in settings where rapid access to safe blood transfusions is unavailable.[41] In South Africa, there have been no issues regarding management of blood pressure, myocardial infarction, renal effects, mortality, and adverse events/serious adverse events in more than 480 patients (including trauma and elective surgery patients) treated with HBOC-201.[42] A prehospital trauma patient resuscitation clinical trial with HBOC-201 has received regulatory and ethical approval to begin shortly in Victoria, Australia. The trial design and setting differ from the PolyHeme trial (see later discussion) in that there are longer prehospital transport times, the trial includes more robust enrollment criteria (Shock Index $\geq$1), and younger patients (<55 years of age).

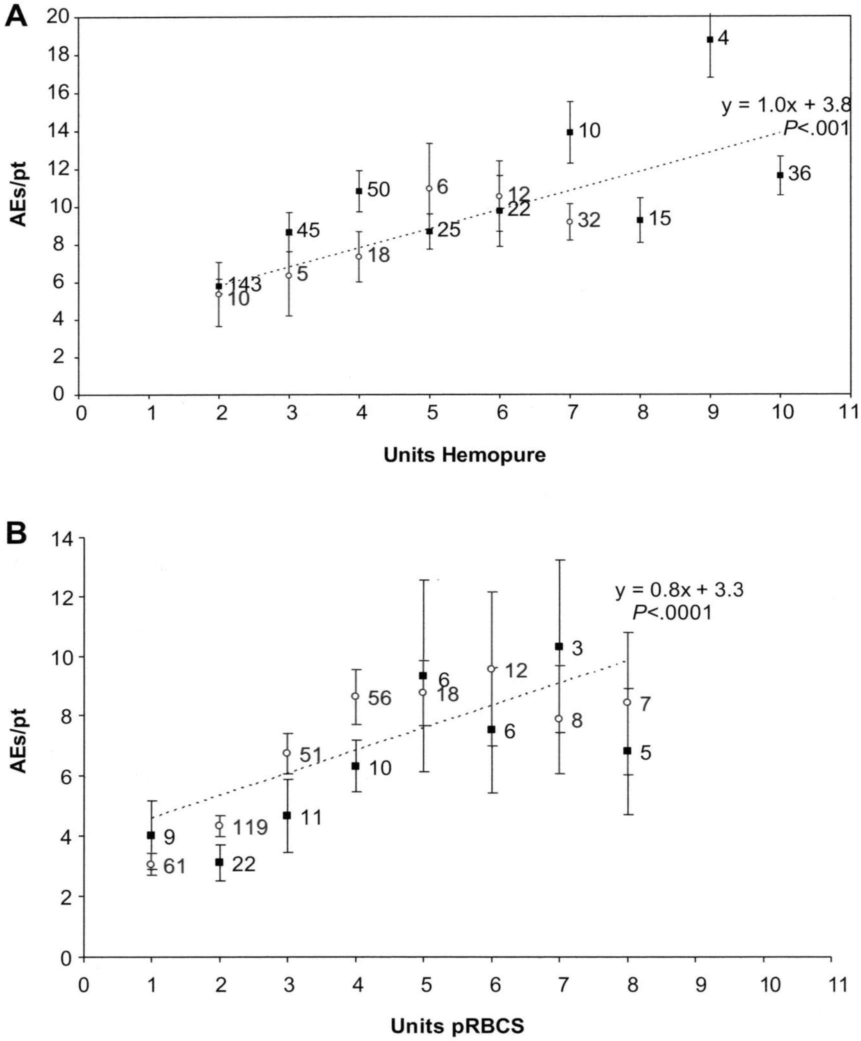

Fig. 1. (*A*) Regression analysis of the relationship between adverse events (AEs)/patient (pt) and dose (in units) of Hemopure received in study HEM-0115 (*black filled squares*) and study HEM-0114 (*blue open circles*). (*B*) AEs/pt as a function of dose of pRBCs: Regression analysis of the relationship between AEs/pt and dose (in units) of pRBCs received in study HEM-0115 (*black filled squares*) and study HEM-0114 (*blue open circles*). The correlation between the dose of pRBCs and incidence of AEs in an acutely anemic population is driven by the patient's clinical need and the patient's underlying comorbidities. Similar correlations are observed between increasing doses of pRBCs or Hemopure and increasing rates of FDA-defined AEs/patient.

Administration of HBOC-201 ceases on trauma center admission unlike the PolyHeme trial.

MP4OX (MalPEG-hemoglobin) is a polyethylene glycol (PEG)-conjugated hemoglobin, and is being tested as a volume-expansion hemodilution product. MP4OX has

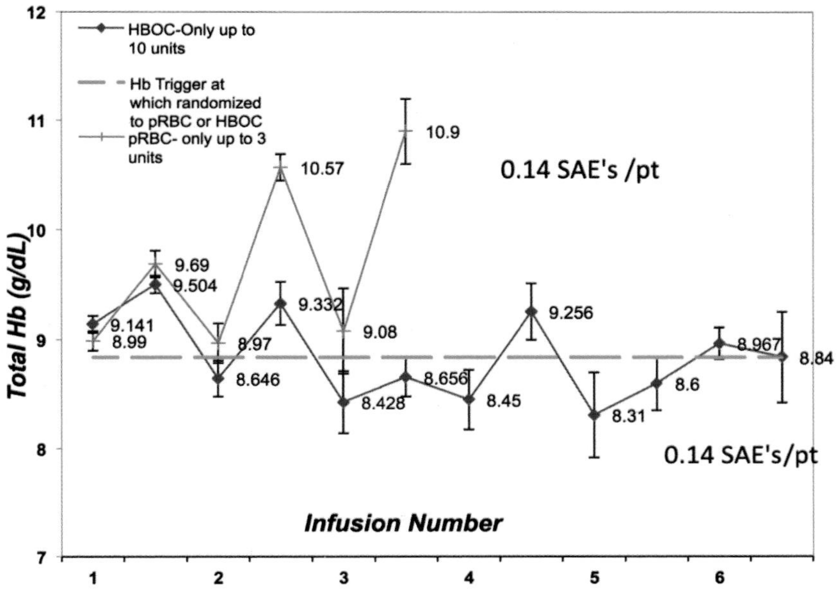

Fig. 2. Effects of dosing HBOC-201 alone up to 10 units and pRBC alone up to 3 units on total hemoglobin (Hb) in HEM-0115 trial. Incidence of serious adverse events/patient (pt) was 0.14/pt in both groups. Mann-Whitney estimator of safety noninferiority (MW), derived from the results of an independent review of each case report and medical records by at least 2 physician reviews of a 27-member independent Safety Endpoint Evaluation Committee. MW 0.519, 95% confidence interval [CI] 0.481–0.558.

a low hemoglobin concentration, requires refrigeration, cannot be stored for prolonged periods at higher than room temperature, and is not approved by any regulatory body. This molecule is characterized by high oxygen affinity that limits oxygen release in arterioles and has decreased rates of oxidation, with low hemoglobin concentration and increased oncotic pressure. These characteristics suggest that MP4OX might preserve functional capillary density in anemic and shock states and reduce the incidence of hypertension and other adverse events. Six clinical trials in elective surgery, chronic critical limb ischemia, and prevention of hypotension are either underway or already completed. The safety results of a phase II trial in orthopedic surgery[34,43–47] showed an imbalance in cardiac and vascular events, including bradycardia and increased blood pressure, gastrointestinal events including nausea, cardiac rhythm changes, and pancreatic enzymatic activity (lipase and amylase) with greater frequency after administration of MP4OX than placebo (Ringer acetate). The small increases in mean arterial pressure seen in clinical trials may be attributable to MP4OX's hyperoncotic volume-expansion properties rather than nitric oxide scavenging.

Current testing (http://clinicaltrials.gov/ct/show/NCT00420277?order=1) will determine if MP4OX can improve perfusion and oxygenation of ischemic tissues in trauma patients in hemorrhagic shock with lactic acidosis (serum lactate level >−5 mmol/L) within 2 hours of arrival at the study hospital and within 4 hours of traumatic injury. Two dose levels 250 mL and 500 mL are being compared with isotonic Ringer lactate solution to reduce lactic acidosis. Secondary outcomes include SOFA (sequential organ failure assessment) score, renal replacement, and vasopressor use. Adverse effects and mortality outcome will be evaluated up to day 28.

PolyHeme, a polymerized HBOC successfully used in the management of trauma patients,[23] completed a phase III clinical trial involving administration in a prehospital setting and during the initial 12 hours of hospitalization in patients with major trauma. PolyHeme failed to achieve its dual primary end point of superiority/noninferiority of mortality outcome (compared with expected mortality in a rural setting with longer transit times to hospital and availability of blood).[40] PolyHeme is now no longer being produced, nor is it available.

Side Effects Associated with HBOC

There is no consensus on the underlying mechanisms of the toxicities and side effects of existing HBOCs. Adverse events associated with HBOC administration include gastrointestinal effects, nausea and vomiting, diarrhea, abdominal pain, and bloating (binding of nitrous oxide to gastrointestinal intestine tissues is the proposed cause), skin rashes, jaundice without increased bilirubin levels (due to metabolism of free hemoglobin), fever, and interference with laboratory assays because of high concentrations of plasma hemoglobin causing anomalies such as increase in lipase levels and interference with tests for liver enzymes, bilirubin, and amylase. Inaccurate results in the presence of HBOCs may be avoided by use of different analytic devices. Clinicians should be aware that methemoglobinemia can be a problem, especially at low red cell hemoglobin concentrations, when methemoglobin reductase (in the red cell wall) levels are low. Side effects can be mitigated (eg, by nitric oxide donor, β-blocker or calcium channel blocker, or changing the infusion rate for blood pressure, use of diuretics to reduce volume effects, methylene blue infusion or the use of ascorbic acid to reduce methemoglobin, and anticholinergics for gastrointestinal discomfort). Current HBOCs elicit serious adverse events (as defined by the FDA) including increased blood pressure, myocardial infarction, stroke, hemostatic effects (platelet aggregation), and renal toxicity. HBOC-201, however, is metabolized through the liver and reticuloendothelial system[48] and MP4OX has chemically cross-linked hemoglobin chains resulting in molecules 128 kDa or larger that are not readily filtered by the glomerulus, thus greatly increasing the half-life. Risks are not uniform across all populations. Probable differences occur by patient age, disease process, and other important factors. It is possible that improved benefit-to-risk ratios for HBOC use occur in populations of younger age and with minimal comorbidities.[49]

One of the major challenges for the development of HBOCs is their vasoactive properties. Soluble hemoglobin, unlike hemoglobin in RBCs, interacts with nitric oxide (NO) to form methemoglobin and *S*-nitrosohemoglobin (by interaction with heme thiol) and nitrosylhemoglobin (via interaction with heme iron). NO is a potent endothelial vasorelaxant that inhibits the conversion of proendothelin to the vasoconstrictor endothelin. In the prevailing theory on vasoactive properties, NO sequestration by hemoglobin is responsible for vasoconstriction. Alternative theories suggest that too much oxygen is delivered causing an autoregulatory vasoconstrictor reflex. Yet another theory argues that oxidation of soluble hemoglobin can result in heme loss, free radical formation, loss of reactive iron, and oxidation of lipids. Such reaction and products result in endothelial stress causing vasoconstriction.[50]

A recent meta-analysis concluded that there was no role for any of the HBOCs currently in clinical development and proposed that an HBOC class effect is responsible for myocardial infarction and increased mortality.[51] However, the meta-analysis is seriously flawed, and the statistical tools and methods used inappropriately combined dissimilar studies, as described in a series of letters to the Editor.[52–55] The proposed HBOC cardiotoxic class effect has been disproved for HBOC-201 (**Fig. 3**).[56–58] Statistical significance for a mortality class effect in the meta-analysis derives solely from

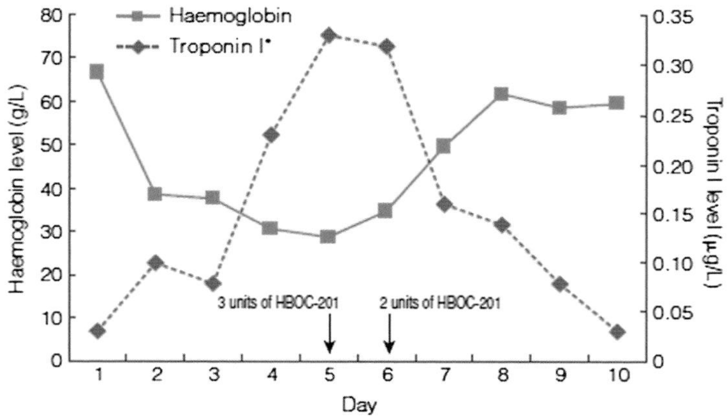

Fig. 3. Haemoglobin and troponin I levels of a woman who has treated with a haemoglobin-based oxygen carrier (HBOC) following severe trauma. * Troponin I levels were measured using the Architect i2000 immunoassy analyser (Abbott Diagnostics, Abbott Park, Ill, USA). (*From* Fitzgerald M, Chan J, Ross A. A synthetic haemoglobin-based oxygen carrier and the reversal of cardiac hypoxia secondary to severe anemia following trauma. Med J 2011;194:472.)

1 HBOC (Hemassist), withdrawn some 15 years earlier. Meta-analysis methodology evaluates the effects of multiple trials, and does not speculate on the mechanism of action or the risk-to-benefit ratio of any single product. The risk/benefit ratio of such a clinical situation in which blood is limited, not available, or not an option must weigh the risks associated with HBOC against the risk of death.[59] The benefits of HBOC over pRBC are summarized in **Box 2**.

Box 2
HBOC benefits over blood

- Ready to use with no planning, and no equipment, no blood collection or blood processing laboratories, and no cost
- No donor recruitment, no collection (personnel/equipment), no blood transport, and no distribution
- No pretransfusion preparation, limited blood hemovigilance, and limited paperwork
- No processing and no separation of components
- No waste as HBOC is 30 to 50 times longer than blood until expiration date. Long HBOC shelf life allows stockpiling for battlefield readiness, disasters, managing post partum hemorrhage in remote areas, in emergency service ambulances, and helicopters
- Some HBOCs need no refrigeration, hence availability in two-thirds of the developing world with inadequate blood bank facilities
- Universally compatible, could replace uncrossmatched blood use. No transfusion errors as no crossmatching
- Immediately offloads oxygen, no 2,3-diphosphoglycerate (DPG)–dependent tissue oxygen off-loading
- May be used by Jehovah's Witnesses
- Provides oxygenation when blood not an option, eg, autoimmune hemolytic anemia
- Extends the useful life of donor organs awaiting transplant

FROZEN AND LYOPHILIZED BLOOD AND COMPONENT THERAPY

Frozen blood components of universal donor red cells, plasma, and platelets have been used by the Netherlands Military Blood Bank since August 2006 and more than 400 patients have been transfused with more than 2500 units of components stored frozen for up to 10 years.[60] The system includes inventory frozen at −80°C, which is available immediately after thawing and washing. This has enabled the Netherlands military to abandon the walking blood bank. The process allows improved control over ice crystal morphology during freezing, in the absence of cryoprotectant agents such as glycerol, and enables dry thawing of 500-mL blood samples in 2 minutes. There is 100% recovery of cells with less than 3% hemolysis and ATP and 2,3-DPG values similar to fresh samples and unchanged blood typing on thawing. This approach may improve the availability of rare phenotypes and result in improved and more rapid processing of frozen blood. Freeze-dried (lyophilized) red cells are also prepared in single units that are easily transported and ready for use on rehydration. Lyophilized plasma is being tested by the US Military because it requires less processing time (about 5 minutes vs 20 minutes or more for FFP processing) and is safer to handle because the plasma bags are not subjected to the low temperatures currently necessary. Cryopreserved platelets (CPP) consist of human platelets preserved in dimethyl sulfoxide that are frozen at −80°C and stored at −65°C. Frozen platelets have a longer shelf life and can be thawed within 2 minutes of casualties arriving at a combat support hospital. Although CPPs are used by the Netherland Military, phase I, II, and III studies are required by the FDA before this platelet product can be considered for use in United States. The shelf life of deep frozen and freeze-dried blood and blood components is increased relative to that of conventional storage formats (**Table 2**). In the future, after FDA approval, civilian trauma centers in the United States may be the earliest adopters of this military technology.

HSS: CLINICAL APPLICATIONS

In 1980, the beneficial effects of an accidental infusion of 100 mL of 7.5% hypertonic saline to an obtunded and hypotensive Brazilian patient stimulated a renewed interest in HSS as a potential resuscitation fluid for the critically ill.[61] Over the past several decades, there has been extensive clinical experience involving the use of HSS for volume support in trauma patients.[62] HSS has several theoretical and practical advantages over traditional isotonic crystalloids,[63] and an expanding body of work in both animal and human subjects suggests numerous physiologic benefits.[64] In this section, the discussion is limited to the use of HSS for traumatic hemorrhagic shock, even

Table 2
Comparison of the shelf life of blood components stored as standard liquids and deep frozen

	Red Cells	Plasma	Platelets
Standard Liquid Stored			
Temperature (°C)	4	−30	22
Shelf life	42 d	1 y	5 d
Deep Frozen			
Temperature (°C)	−80	−80	−80
Shelf life (y)	10	7	2

Courtesy of Lacey Johnson. Frozen blood products: taking blood to the front line. Research Development, Australian Red Cross Blood Service, Sydney.

though HSS has also been shown to be effective for patients with raised intracranial pressure,[65–68] burns,[69] and other types of shock.[70,71]

HSS facilitates a near instantaneous mobilization of fluids from intracellular to extracellular compartments through an osmotic gradient (**Fig. 4**). Physiologic transcapillary refill is rapidly augmented with movement from the tissues into the vascular space to promote tissue blood flow.[64] Redistribution of fluid, caused by a higher intravascular colloid osmotic pressure, leads to plasma expansion with a resultant increase in mean arterial pressure.[72,73] When a large-molecular-weight hyperoncotic colloid is added to HSS (ie, dextran 70), translocated fluid remains in the intravascular space for prolonged periods of time.[64] The main effects of administration of HSS are reduced pulmonary and systemic vascular resistance, expansion of interstitial and plasma volumes, and increased cardiac output.[62] Additional cardiovascular responses include natriuresis, restoration of membrane potentials, prevention of cellular edema, improved microcirculation, and a smaller volume of fluid required for resuscitation.[62,63,72,74]

HSS is associated with other salutary physiologic effects (**Table 3**). The immune-modulating properties of HSS have been well established in animal models, but the benefit of this property in clinical practice remains unclear.[75] Hypertonicity has been shown to impede the oxidative burst, degranulation, and release of various inflammatory molecules from polymorphonuclear neutrophils.[74–78] HSS has also been experimentally associated with lower rates of bacterial translocation,[79] attenuation of pulmonary inflammation and shock-induced acute lung injury,[80,81] enhancement of host defenses,[82,83] attenuation of postshock gut injury,[81,84] decreased apoptosis,[82] and prevention of end organ damage after hemorrhagic shock.[85] However, the results of experimental animal studies have not been completely replicated in humans, and at the doses commonly delivered in clinical practice, it is unclear if complications related to immune dysfunction in hemorrhagic shock can be significantly reduced with HSS.[75]

In most controlled human clinical trials conducted to date, HSS has not been shown to be associated with a statistically significant survival advantage compared with isotonic fluids.[86] Interpretation of clinical trials has been difficult because of heterogeneous patient populations, underpowered studies, timing of fluid administration, type of HSS used, and additional colloid additives used in conjunction with HSS.[87] HSS has been shown to restore hemodynamics without complications.[63,72] In a few of the

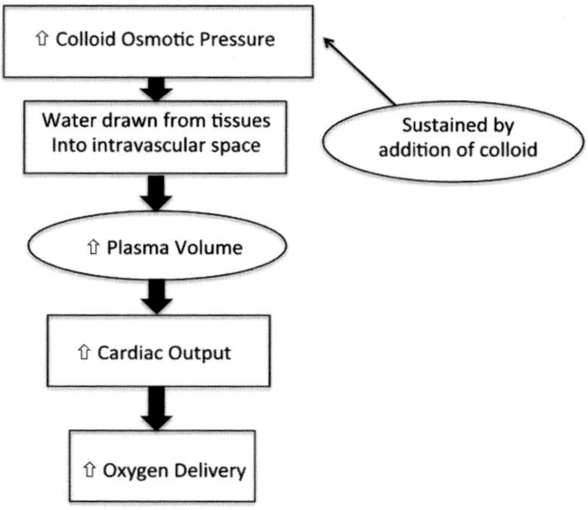

Fig. 4. Hemodynamic response to administration of HSS.

Table 3
Summary of the molecular benefits of HSS and proposed mechanisms in studies of hemorrhagic shock and under conditions associated with a systemic inflammatory response

Benefit	Mechanism
Antiinflammatory effect in humans requiring femoral reaming and intramedullary nailing[103]	Antiinflammatory effect; attenuation of polymorphonuclear leukocytes
Restores T-cell function[a,83]	Enhanced T-cell proliferation, mediated by macrophage migration inhibitory factor
Improves intestinal microcirculation[a,104]	Selective vasodilation of precapillary arterioles, even at low mean arterial pressures
Attenuates gut injury[a,81]	Downregulation of inducible nitric oxide synthase (iNOS)
Enhances host defenses[a,82]	Increases tolllike receptors (TLR4 expression)
Limits human neutrophil activation[76]	Reduced neutrophil activity in a hypertonic environment
Prevention of polymorphonuclear leukocyte activation[77]	Suppression of cell function by HSS through cyclic adenosine monophosphate signaling, when HSS are given early
Limits shock-induced acute lung injury[a,80]	Prevention of gut injury and neutrophil activation
Reduces pulmonary inflammation[a,105]	Attenuation of oxidative stress, neutrophil degranulation, and proinflammatory mediator synthesis
Reduced bacterial translocation[a,79]	Reversal of immunosuppression (CD4+ and CD8+ lymphocytes)
Improves intestinal mucosa barrier function and prevents lung injury[a,84]	Less intestinal bacterial overgrowth and preservation of intestinal barrier function
Decreases systemic inflammatory response[a,85]	Preservation of splanchnic perfusion; prevention of inflammatory mediator release
Promotes a more balanced inflammatory response[106]	Inhibition of neutrophil and monocyte activation

[a] In vitro or experimental animal study.

controlled trials comparing HSS with isotonic fluids, subsets of patients with low systolic blood pressure (<70 mm Hg)[88] and penetrating injuries to the torso requiring surgery[89] had a statistically significant survival advantage when HSS was administered. In 2 case-controlled studies, HSS was associated with a trend toward decreased mortality in patients with low Glasgow Coma Scale scores (<8)[90] and a decreased incidence of postoperative infections in patients undergoing major spinal surgery.[91] In a randomized controlled trial including patients with blunt trauma and hypotension, HSS was associated with improved survival without acute respiratory distress syndrome in a subset of patients requiring more than 10 units of packed red blood cells in the first 24 hours (hazard ratio [HR] 2.18; 95% confidence interval [CI] 1.09–4.36).[92]

Although HSS has not been definitively shown to improve outcomes in trauma patients, this solution may be a viable alternative to consider for resuscitation, especially considering the accumulating evidence that colloids such as hydroxyethyl starch may be harmful in critically ill patients.[93,94] In a recent trial in which patients with septic shock were randomized to Ringer lactate or hydroxyethyl starch, patients in the starch group were more likely to die (relative risk [RR] 1.17; 95% CI 1.01–1.36) or require renal replacement therapy (RR 1.35; 95% CI 1.01–1.80; $P = .04$).[93] Even though the study population consisted of patients with septic, not hemorrhagic shock, the investigators expressed concern about the long-term toxic effects of hydroxyethyl starch, such as deposition in the kidney, liver, and bone marrow, with potential inflammatory and toxic effects, even when lower-molecular-weight formulations of hydroxyethyl starch are used.[93] In another retrospective trial of 2225 critically ill trauma patients, the use of hetastarch was found to be statistically significantly associated with acute kidney injury (RR 1.73; 95% CI 1.30–2.28) and increased mortality (RR 1.84; 95% CI 1.48–2.29).[94] Hence, given the cost of other colloids such as 5% albumin (average cost USD $222.00), and in view of the accumulating evidence of beneficial effects, HSS should be considered as an option for resuscitation when blood component therapy is not readily available.

Dosing and Monitoring

In most controlled HSS trials, boluses of 250 mL of 5%, 6%, or 7.5% HSS with dextran 70 have been used.[62,72] More than 300 studies in animals and humans have been published using HSS with NaCl concentrations ranging from 3%[85] to 7.5%, and usually combined with 6% or 10% dextran 70 or hetastarch.[62] The most commonly used HSS formulation in humans has been 7.5% NaCl/6% dextran 70.[62,95] Most animal studies have used a fixed dose of 4 to 6 mL/kg HSS of various concentrations for hemorrhagic shock.[62]

At our institution, solutions of either 3% or 5% HSS without dextran are commonly used; doses up to 4 to 6 mL/kg have been safely used with these concentrations. A usual intraoperative dose of HSS at our trauma center is 5 mL/kg of 3% NaCl, repeated as necessary. We recommend regular and diligent monitoring of serum sodium, potassium, and creatinine levels; serum sodium should be measured at least every 6 to 8 hours. Central venous lines are generally recommended for administration, although in several prehospital studies, peripherally administered HSS was not found to be associated with regional vascular complications.[26,96] Volume and rate of administration are factors that ought to be considered if HSS is administered peripherally[63]; vigilance is imperative.

Side Effects

A principal concern with the administration of HSS is the theoretical risk of inducing osmotic demyelination syndrome (ODS). However, only 1 case of ODS has ever been reported in patients receiving HSS for trauma resuscitation.[72,97] Metabolic acidosis is a concern with repeated administration because of the high chloride content in HSS, with a resultant decrease in the strong ion difference. HSS preparations buffered with acetate are available to mitigate this potential complication. Hypokalemia is a common electrolyte disorder encountered after repeated doses of HSS. Potassium levels typically decrease during initial administration, then increase over time.[72] Hypernatremia is inevitable with repeated administration of HSS. After a bolus of 4 to 5 mL/kg, serum sodium levels may transiently increase 12 to 15 mEq/L.[64] At our institution, when sodium levels reach 155 mEq/L, we withhold administration of HSS, although in many studies, plasma sodium levels have transiently exceeded 160 mEq/L without deleterious effects.[64] Theoretical concerns about renal failure with HSS have not been substantiated by most of the literature[64]; however, several reports of dextran-induced renal failure have been published.[98,99] The occurrence of dextran-associated anaphylactoid reactions has been well known since the 1960s.[100,101] Allergic reactions induced by dextran preparations are caused by dextran-reactive antibodies, and are historically more prevalent when high-molecular-weight (MW >100,000) or highly branched preparations are used.[64] A newer, low-molecular-weight (MW 1000) preparation, dextran 1, when preadministered before HSS containing dextran is given, has been reported to significantly lower the incidence of dextran-associated anaphylaxis.[102]

SUMMARY

Stabilization of trauma patients in shock requires aggressive hemorrhage control and restoration of tissue perfusion. HBOC and HSS both have physiologic and logistical advantages over standard isotonic crystalloids. Both of these fluid preparations may help bridge critical gaps when blood component therapy is not available, buying time to facilitate definitive surgical hemorrhage control. HBOC and HSS could be useful in the prehospital environment, military conflicts, disasters, and in the developing world, and in other situations where blood is not readily accessible. HBOC could potentially replace the standard 2 to 3 unit pRBC transfusions that 20% to 35% of all transfused patients admitted to trauma centers receive.[18] Future resuscitation fluids may contain combinations of both HBOC and HSS. Naturally, the risks associated with HBOC and HSS must always be weighed against the risk of complications and death. Neither resuscitation fluid is without risk. Future use of rapidly thawed universal donor frozen blood and blood component therapy will revolutionize the initial resuscitation of trauma patients, reduce the coagulopathy of trauma, minimize the need for blood and blood exposure, reduce the cost of trauma care, and increase survival. However, until this technology becomes widely available, HBOC and HSS may be considered for the resuscitation of patients in hemorrhagic shock.

REFERENCES

1. Bellamy R. The causes of death in conventional land warfare. Mil Med 1984;149:55–62.
2. Dutton D, Stansbury L, Leone S, et al. Trauma mortality in mature trauma systems: are we doing better? An analysis of trauma mortality patterns, 1997-2008. J Trauma 2010;69(3):620–6.
3. Borgman M, Spinella P, Perkins J, et al. The ratio of blood products transfused affects mortality in patients receiving massive blood transfusions at a combat support hospital. J Trauma 2007;63(4):805–13.
4. Clarke J, Trooskin S, Doshi P, et al. Time to laparotomy for intra-abdominal bleeding from trauma does affect survival for delays up to 90 minutes. J Trauma 2002;52(3):420–5.
5. de Biasi AR, Stansbury LG, Dutton RP, et al. Blood product use in trauma resuscitation: plasma deficit versus plasma ratio as predictors of mortality in trauma. Transfusion 2011;51(9):1925–32.
6. Spinella P, Perkins J, Grathwohl K, et al. Effect of plasma and red blood cell transfusion on survival in patients with combat related traumatic injuries. J Trauma 2008;64(Suppl 2):S69–77.
7. Ketchum L, Hess J, Hippala S. Indications for early fresh frozen plasma, cryoprecipitate, and platelet transfusion in trauma. J Trauma 2006;60(Suppl 6):S51–8.
8. Gonzalez E, Moore F, Holcomb J, et al. Fresh frozen plasma should be given earlier to patients requiring massive transfusion. J Trauma 2007;62(1):112–9.
9. Cinat M, Wallace W, Nastanski F, et al. Improved survival following massive blood transfusion in patients who have undergone trauma. Arch Surg 1999;134(9):964–8.

10. Perkins J, Schreiber M, Wade C, et al. Early versus late recombinant factor VIIa in combat trauma patients requiring massive transfusion. J Trauma 2007;62(5): 1095–9.
11. White J, Stannard A, Burkhardt G, et al. The epidemiology of vascular injury in the wars in Iraq and Afghanistan. Ann Surg 2011;253(6):1184–9.
12. Starnes B, Beekley A, Sebesta J, et al. Extremity vascular injuries on the battlefield: tips for surgeons deploying to war. J Trauma 2006;60(2):432–42.
13. Woodward E, Clouse W, Eliason J, et al. Penetrating femoropopliteal injury during modern warfare: experience of the Balad Vascular Registry. J Vasc Surg 2008;47(6):1259–64.
14. Claridge J, Sawyer R, Schulman A, et al. Blood transfusions correlate with infections in trauma patients in a dose-dependent manner. Am Surg 2002;68(7): 566–72.
15. Sauaia A, Moore F, Moore E, et al. Early predictors of postinjury multiple organ failure. Arch Surg 1994;129(1):39–45.
16. Moore F, Moore E, Sauaia A. Blood transfusion. An independent risk factor for postinjury multiple organ failure. Arch Surg 1997;132(6):620–4.
17. Malone D, Dunne J, Putnam JTA, et al. Blood transfusion, independent of shock severity, is associated with worse outcome in trauma. J Trauma 2003;54(5): 898–905.
18. Como J, Dutton R, Scalea T, et al. Blood transfusion rates in the care of acute trauma. Transfusion 2004;44(6):809–13.
19. Moore E, Cheng A, Moore H, et al. Hemoglobin-based oxygen carriers in trauma care: scientific rationale for the US multicenter prehospital trial. World J Surg 2006;30(7):1247–57.
20. Reid T. Hb-based oxygen carriers: are we there yet? Transfusion 2003;43(2): 280–7.
21. Mackenzie C, Moon-Massat P, Shander A, et al. When blood is not an option: factors affecting survival after use of a hemoglobin-based oxygen carrier in 54 patients with life-threatening anemia. Anesth Analg 2010;110(3):685–93.
22. Branas C, MacKenzie E, Williams J, et al. Access to trauma centers in the United States. JAMA 2005;293(1):2626–33.
23. Gould S, Moore E, Hoyt D, et al. The life-sustaining capacity of human polymerized hemoglobin when red cells might be unavailable. J Am Coll Surg 2002; 195(4):445–52.
24. Heckbert S, Vedder N, Hoffman W, et al. Outcome after hemorrhagic shock in trauma patients. J Trauma 1998;45(3):545–9.
25. Sloan E, Koenigsberg M, Gens D, et al. Diaspirin cross-linked hemoglobin (DCLHb) in the treatment of severe traumatic hemorrhagic shock. A randomized controlled efficacy trial. JAMA 1999;282(19):1857–64.
26. Mattox K, Maningas P, Moore E, et al. Prehospital hypertonic saline/dextran infusion for post-traumatic hypotension: the U.S.A. multicenter trial. Ann Surg 1991; 213(5):482–91.
27. Bickell W, Wall M, Pepe P, et al. Immediate versus delayed fluid resuscitation for hypotensive patients with penetrating torso injuries. N Engl J Med 1994;331(17): 1105–9.
28. Landro L. The informed patient: a dangerous gap in trauma care; systems to transfer patients to best-equipped hospitals fall short in most states. Wall Street Journal October 3, 2007.
29. Silliman C, Moore E, Johnson J, et al. Transfusion of the injured patient: proceed with caution. Shock 2004;21(4):291–9.

30. Stowell C, Levin J, Spiess B, et al. Progress in the development of RBC substitutes. Transfusion 2001;41(2):287–99.
31. Rudolph A, Cliff R, Spargo B, et al. Transient changes in the mononuclear phagocytes system following administration of blood substitutes, liposome-encapsulated hemoglobin. Biomaterials 1994;15(10):796–804.
32. Klein H, Spahn D, Carson J. Red blood cell transfusion in clinical practice. Lancet 2007;370(9585):415–26.
33. Leong B, Reynolds P, Tiba M, et al. Effects of a combination hemoglobin based oxygen carrier-hypertonic saline solution on oxygen transport in the treatment of hemorrhagic shock. Resuscitation 2011;82:937–43.
34. Vandergriff K, Young M, Keipert P, et al. The safety profile of Hemospan: a new oxygen therapeutic designed using maleimide poly(ethylene) glycol conjugation to human hemoglobin. Transfus Altern Transfus Med 2008;9: 213–25.
35. Zou S, Musavi F, Notari E, et al. Donor deferral and resulting donor loss at the American Red Cross Blood Services, 2001 through 2006. Transfusion 2008; 48(12):2531–9.
36. Vamvakas E, Taswell H. Epidemiology of blood transfusion. Transfusion 1994; 34(6):464–70.
37. Jahr J, Mackenzie C, Pearce L, et al. HBOC-201 as an alternative to blood transfusion: efficacy and safety evaluation in a multicenter phase III trial in elective orthopedic surgery. J Trauma 2008;64(6):1484–97.
38. Gawryl M, Moon-Massat P, Pearce L. Chapter 37. In: Winslow R, editor. Blood substitutes. London: Academic Press; 2006. p. 437–50.
39. US Food and Drug Administration. Code of Federal Regulations Title 21, parts 312 and 316. Expanded access to investigational drugs for treatment use. 74FR40900. 2009.
40. Silverman T, Weiskopf R. Hemoglobin-based oxygen carriers current status and future directions. Anesthesiology 2009;111(5):946–63.
41. Freilich D, Pearce L, Pitman A, et al. HBOC-201 vasoactivity in a phase III clinical trial in orthopedic surgery subjects—extrapolation of potential risk for acute trauma trials. J Trauma 2009;66(2):365–76.
42. Levien L. South Africa: clinical experience with hemopure. ISBT Sci Ser 2006;1: 167–73.
43. Winslow R. Red cell substitutes. Semin Hematol 2007;44:51–9.
44. Olofsson C, Ahl T, Johansson T, et al. A multicenter clinical study of the safety and activity of maleimide-polyethylene glycol-modified hemoglobin (Hemospan) in patients undergoing major orthopedic surgery. Anesthesiology 2006;105(6): 1153–63.
45. Olofsson O, Nygards E, Ponzer S, et al. A randomized, single-blind, increasing dose safety trial of an oxygen-carrying plasma expander (Hemospan) administered to orthopaedic surgery patients with spinal anaesthesia. Transfus Med 2008;18(1):28–39.
46. van der Linden P, Gazdizik TS, Jahoda D, et al. A double-blind, randomized, multicenter study of MP4OX for treatment of perioperative hypotension in patients undergoing primary hip arthroplasty under spinal anesthesia. Anesth Analg 2011;112(4):759–73.
47. Olofsson C, Gorecki A, Dirksen R, et al. Evaluation of MP4OX for prevention of perioperative hypotension in patients undergoing primary hip arthroplasty with spinal anesthesia: a randomized, double-blind, multicenter study. Anesthesiology 2011;114(5):1048–63.

48. Beuzard Y, Lubin B, Rosa J. Sickle cell disease and thalassemia: new trends in therapy, vol. 234. Montrogue (France): Colloque INSERM/John Libbey Eurotext; 1995.
49. Dietz N, Joyner M, Warner M. Blood substitutes: fluids, drugs, or miracle solutions? Anesth Analg 1996;82(2):390–405.
50. Alayash A. Hemoglobin-based blood substitutes: oxygen carriers, pressor agents or oxidants? Nat Biotechnol 1999;17:545–9.
51. Natanson S, Kern S, Lurie P, et al. Cell-free hemoglobin-based blood substitutes and risk of myocardial infarction and death: a meta-analysis. JAMA 2008; 299(12):2304–12.
52. Levien L, Hodgson R, James M. Hemoglobin-based blood substitutes and risk of myocardial infarction and death [letter]. JAMA 2008;300:1295.
53. Keipert P, Olofsson C, Winslow R. Hemoglobin-based blood substitutes and risk of myocardial infarction and death [letter]. JAMA 2008;300:1295–6.
54. Shander A, Javidroozi M, Thompson G. Hemoglobin-based blood substitutes and risk of myocardial infarction and death [letter]. JAMA 2008;300:1296–7.
55. Sauaia A, Moore E, Banerjee A. Hemoglobin-based blood substitutes and risk of myocardial infarction and death [letter]. JAMA 2008;300:1297.
56. Hekkert MTL, Dube G, Regar E, et al. Preoxygenated hemoglobin-based oxygen carrier HBOC-201 annihilates myocardial ischemia during brief coronary artery occlusion in pigs. Am J Physiol Heart Circ Physiol 2010;298(3):H1103–13.
57. Meliga E, Vranckx P, Regar E, et al. Proof-of-concept trial to evaluate haemoglobin based oxygen therapeutics in elective percutaneous coronary revascularisation. Rationale, protocol design and haemodynamic results. EuroIntervention 2008;4(1):99–107.
58. Fitzgerald M, Chan J, Ross A. A synthetic haemoglobin-based oxygen carrier and the reversal of cardiac hypoxia secondary to severe anemia following trauma. Med J Aust 2011;194:471–3.
59. Mackenzie C. Hemoglobin-based oxygen carriers: is the benefit worth the risk? Br J Hosp Med (Lond) 2009;70(1):26–30.
60. Lelkens CCM, Koning JG, de Kort IBG, et al. Experiences with frozen blood products in the Netherlands military. Transfus Apher Sci 2006;34(3):289–98.
61. Velasco IT, Pontieri V, Rocha e Silva M Jr, et al. Hyperosmotic NaCl and severe hemorrhagic shock. Am J Physiol 1980;239:H664–73.
62. Kramer G. Hypertonic resuscitation: physiological mechanisms and recommendations for trauma care. J Trauma 2003;54:S89–99.
63. Patanwala A, Amini A, Erstad B. Use of hypertonic saline injection in trauma. Am J Health Syst Pharm 2010;67:1920–8.
64. Dubick M, Bruttig S, Wade C. Issues of concern regarding the use of hypertonic/hyperoncotic fluid resuscitation of hemorrhagic hypotension. Shock 2006;25(4): 321–8.
65. Ropper A. Hyperosmolar therapy for raised intracranial pressure. N Engl J Med 2012;367:746–52.
66. Bratton S, Chestnut R, Ghajar J, et al. II. Hyperosmolar therapy. J Neurotrauma 2007;24(Suppl 1):S14–20.
67. Rockswold G, Solid C, Paredes-Andrade E, et al. Hypertonic saline and its effect on intracranial pressure, cerebral perfusion pressure, and brain tissue oxygen. Neurosurgery 2009;65:1035–42.
68. Pinto F, Capone-Neto A, Prist R, et al. Volume replacement with lactated Ringer's or 3% hypertonic saline solution during combined experimental hemorrhagic shock and traumatic brain injury. J Trauma 2006;60:758–64.

69. Belba M, Petrela E, Belba G. Comparison of hypertonic vs isotonic fluids during resuscitation of severely burned patients. Am J Emerg Med 2009;27: 1091–6.
70. Standvik G. Hypertonic saline in critical care: a review of the literature and guidelines for use in hypotensive states and raised intracranial pressure. Anaesthesia 2009;64:990–1003.
71. Oliveira R, Velasco I, Soriano FG. Clinical review: hypertonic saline resuscitation in sepsis. Crit Care 2002;6:418–23.
72. Banks C, Furyk J. Review article: hypertonic saline use in the emergency department. Emerg Med Australas 2008;20:294–305.
73. Galvagno S. Emergency pathophysiology. Jackson (WY): Teton NewMedia; 2004.
74. Tyagi R, Donaldson K, Loftus C, et al. Hypertonic saline: a clinical review. Neurosurg Rev 2007;30:277–90.
75. Kolsen-Petersen J. Immune effect of hypertonic saline: fact or fiction? Acta Anaesthesiol Scand 2004;48:667–78.
76. Deitch E, Shi H, Feketeova E, et al. Hypertonic saline resuscitation limits neutrophil activation after trauma-hemorrhagic shock. Shock 2003;19(4):328–33.
77. Hashiguchi N, Lum L, Romeril E, et al. Hypertonic saline resuscitation: efficacy may require early treatment in severely injured patients. J Trauma 2007;62:299–306.
78. Pascual J, Khwaja K, Chaudhury P, et al. Hypertonic saline and the microcirculation. J Trauma 2003;54:S133–40.
79. Hirsh M, Dyugovskaya L, Bashenko Y, et al. Reduced rate of bacterial translocation and improved variables of natural killer cell and T-cell activity in rats surviving controlled hemorrhagic shock and treated with hypertonic saline. Crit Care Med 2002;30:861–7.
80. Homma H, Deitch E, Feketeova E, et al. Small volume resuscitation with hypertonic saline is more effective in ameliorating trauma-hemorrhagic shock-induced lung injury, neutrophil activation and red blood cell dysfunction than pancreatic protease inhibition. J Trauma 2005;59:266–72.
81. Deree J, de Campos T, Shenvi E, et al. Hypertonic saline and pentoxyfylline attenuates gut injury and hemorrhagic shock: the kinder, gentler resuscitation. J Trauma 2007;62:818–28.
82. Chen L, Su M, Chen P, et al. Hypertonic saline enhances host defense and reduces apopotosis in burn mice by increasing toll-like receptors. Shock 2011;35(1):59–66.
83. Yoon Y, Choi S, Hong Y, et al. Effect of hypertonic saline and macrophage migration inhibitory factor in restoration of T cell dysfunction. J Korean Surg Soc 2011; 81(4):229–34.
84. Shi H, Deitch E, Xu D, et al. Hypertonic saline improves intestinal mucosa barrier function and lung injury after trauma-hemorrhagic shock. Shock 2002;17(6): 496–501.
85. Vincenzi R, Cepeda L, Pirani W, et al. Small volume resuscitation with 3% hypertonic saline decrease inflammatory response and attenuates end organ damage after controlled hemorrhagic shock. Am J Surg 2009;198:407–14.
86. Bunn F, Roberts I, Tasker R, et al. Hyeprtonic versus near isotonic crystalloid for fluid resuscitation in critically ill patients (Assessed as up to date, October 15, 2007). Cochrane Database Syst Rev 2007;(3):CD002045.
87. Rotstein O. Novel strategies for immunomodulation after trauma: revisiting hypertonic saline as a resuscitation strategy for hemorrhagic shock. J Trauma 2000;49:580–3.

88. Younes R, Aun F, Ching C, et al. Prognostic factors to predict outcome following the administration of hypertonic/hyperoncotic solution in hypovolemic patients. Shock 1997;7(2):79–83.
89. Wade C, Grady J, Kramer G. Efficacy of hypertonic saline dextran fluid resuscitation for patients with hypotension from penetrating trauma. J Trauma 2003; 54(Suppl 5):S144–8.
90. DuBose J, Kobayashi L, Lozaornio A, et al. Clinical experience using 5% hypertonic saline as a safe alternative fluid for trauma. J Trauma 2010;68:1172–7.
91. Charalambous M, Swoboda S, Lipsett P. Perioperative hypertonic saline may reduce postoperative infections and lower mortality rates. Surg Infect (Larchmt) 2008;9:67–74.
92. Bulger E, Jurkovich G, Nathens A, et al. Hypertonic resuscitation of hypovolemic shock after blunt trauma. Arch Surg 2008;143(2):139–48.
93. Perner A, Haase N, Guttormsen A, et al. Hydroxyethyl starch 130/0.4 versus Ringer's acetate in severe sepsis. N Engl J Med 2012;367(2):124–34.
94. Lissauer M, Chi A, Kramer M, et al. Association of 6% hetastarch resuscitation with adverse outcomes in critically ill trauma patients. Am J Surg 2011;202(1): 53–8.
95. Coimbra R. 3% and 5% hypertonic saline. J Trauma 2011;70(5):S25–6.
96. Marko N. Hyperosmolar therapy for intracranial hypertension: time to dispel antiquated myths. Am J Respir Crit Care Med 2012;185(5):467–78.
97. Schimetta W, Schochl H, Kroll W, et al. Safety of hypertonic hyperoncotic solutions–a survey from Austria. Wien Klin Wochenschr 2002;114(3):89–95.
98. Moran M, Kapsner C. Acute renal failure associated with elevated plasma oncotic pressure. N Engl J Med 1987;317:150–3.
99. Chertow G, Mason P, Vaage-Nilsen O, et al. On the relative safety of parenteral iron formulations. Nephrol Dial Transplant 2004;19(6):1571–5.
100. Department of Health and Human Services. Topic III: Prophylaxis of dextran-induced anaphylactoid reactions (DIAR) by dextran 1 pre-administration. Gaithersburg (MD): Food and Drug Administration, Blood Products Advisory Committee; 2005.
101. Hedin H, Richter W, Ring J. Dextran-induced anaphylactoid reactions in man: role of dextran reactive antibodies. Int Arch Allergy Appl Immunol 1976; 52(1–4):145–59.
102. Ljungstrom K, Renck H, Hedin H, et al. Prevention of dextran-induced anaphylactic reactions by hapten inhibition. I. A Scandinavian multicenter study on the effects of 10 mL dextran 1, 15% administered before dextran 70 or dextran 40. Acta Chir Scand 1983;149(4):341–8.
103. Agudelo J, Flierl M, Smith W, et al. Influence of preoperative 7.5% hypertonic saline on neutrophil activation after reamed intramedullary nailing of femur shaft fractures: a prospective randomized pilot study. J Orthop Trauma 2012;26:86–91.
104. Zakaria E, Tsakadze N, Garrison R. Hypertonic saline resuscitation improves intestinal microcirculation in a rat model of hemorrhagic shock. Surgery 2006; 140:579–88.
105. Deree J, Martins J, Leedom A, et al. Hypertonic saline and pentoxifylline reduces hemorrhagic shock resuscitation-induced pulmonary inflammation through attenuation of neutrophil degranulation and proinflammatory mediator synthesis. J Trauma 2007;62:104–11.
106. Rizoli S, Rhind S, Shek P, et al. The immunomodulatory effects of hypertonic saline resuscitation in patients sustaining traumatic hemorrhagic shock. Ann Surg 2006;243:47–57.

Trauma and Aggressive Homeostasis Management

Patrick J. Neligan, MD[a,*], Dimitry Baranov, MD[b]

KEYWORDS

• Inflammation • Homeostasis • Lactic acidosis • Hyperglycemia • Glycemic control • Hypothermia • Cooling • Brain injury

KEY POINTS

- Trauma injury should be seen as a part of the well-defined paradigm of stress response associated with acute depletion of physiologic reserve.
- Many of the observed homeostatic upsets associated with trauma can be explained as part of this process and should not be considered pathologic.
- Stress hyperglycemia is a necessary component of this paradigm, and enthusiasm for tight glycemic control in hemorrhagic shock (HS) and traumatic brain injury (TBI) should be tempered by evidence of hypoglycemia and adverse outcomes.
- Lactic acidosis is quantitatively associated with adverse outcomes, and failure to clear (or continued production of) lactate is a bad prognostic sign. However, lactate is not always quantitatively associated with volume depletion, and it must be used cautiously as an end point of resuscitation.
- Overresuscitation is associated with abdominal compartment syndrome and coagulopathy.
- Coagulopathy is also associated with accidental hypothermia, and emerging data on damage control resuscitation and antifibrinolytic therapy suggest a changing paradigm of trauma therapy.
- Accidental hypothermia is associated with adverse outcomes in trauma; it is multifactorial in origin and is, at least partially, associated with limited physiologic reserve.
- Therapeutic hypothermia has been used successfully in cardiac surgery and after cardiac arrest; there are limited data to support this intervention in TBI.

INTRODUCTION

Homeostasis refers to the capacity of the human body to maintain a stable constant state by means of continuous dynamic equilibrium adjustments controlled by a medley of interconnected regulatory mechanisms. The concept dates from the foundations of

[a] Department of Anaesthesia and Intensive Care, Galway University Hospitals, Newcastle Road, Galway, Ireland; [b] Department of Anesthesiology and Critical Care, Hospital of University of Pennsylvania, 3400 Spruce Street, Philadelphia, PA 19107, USA
* Corresponding author.
E-mail address: Patrick.neligan@hse.ie

Anesthesiology Clin 31 (2013) 21–39
http://dx.doi.org/10.1016/j.anclin.2012.10.007 anesthesiology.theclinics.com

scientific medicine, specifically the work of Claude Bernard (1813–1878). Multiple systems exist in the body to test and control any deviation from the normal range in vital functions. The autonomic nervous system is a good example of such a system. It self-regulates to maintain a variety of physiologic and metabolic variables in the state of equilibrium, despite a staggering range of variations in the level of human activities and externalities.

Patients who sustain tissue injury, such as trauma or surgery, undergo a well-understood reproducible metabolic and neuroendocrine stress response. The ability of the body to deal with stress is known as physiologic reserve, which is the excess capacity that exists in organ systems to deal with injury; it allows the body to restore homeostasis. The cardiovascular system, lungs, kidneys, and liver have enormous functional reserve. Aging and chronic illness deplete the physiologic reserve. Critical illness is a state in which physiologic reserve is inadequate to maintain life and exogenous organ support is required.

This review discusses 3 issues that concern homeostasis in the acute care of trauma patients directly related to the stress response: hyperglycemia, lactic acidosis, and hypothermia. Recently, there has been a resurgence of interest in investigating the effects of aggressive thermal and glycemic control and volume resuscitation on outcomes in critically ill and trauma patients. There is significant reason to question the "conventional wisdom" relating to current approaches to restoring homeostasis in this patient population.

HYPERGLYCEMIA AND TRAUMA

Trauma and tissue injury is associated with organism-wide changes in metabolism and neurohormonal function that are often referred to as "stress" response. These alterations are characterized by enhanced release of pituitary hormones, increased sympathoadrenal activity, pancreatic hypersecretion, and activation of inflammation. The last of these is manifest by proliferation of leukocytes and adhesion molecules, complement activation, and cytokine release. As part of this response, there is a dramatic increase in blood glucose levels, due to enhanced glycogenolysis and gluconeogenesis. This increase is a homeostatic mechanism to mobilize substrate, principally from the liver and skeletal muscle, to restore function, fight infection, and repair damaged tissue. Key to this response is the presence of white cells in the damaged tissues. These cells phagocytose cellular debris, secrete growth factors, and catalyze the synthesis of collagen. White cells are obligate glucose users. Hence, in the setting of significant tissue damage, glucose liberation and metabolism increase exponentially. In order for glucose to penetrate damaged tissue, a significant concentration gradient is required.

Hyperglycemia is facilitated by a dramatic increase in secretion of proglycemic factors: cortisol, growth hormone, epinephrine, and glucagon. Epinephrine, in particular, is responsible for many of the metabolic perturbations seen in trauma. Epinephrine induces vasoconstriction in the midline and vasodilatation in skeletal muscle, and it increases heart rate and thus the cardiac output. Epinephrine induces glycogenolyis, lipolysis, and increased lactate production, independent of the cellular redox state.[1] This process has been termed "aerobic glycolysis." Lactate is reconstructed to glucose, providing a continuous source of glucose for white cells. Simultaneous increase in insulin production leads to increased peripheral glucose uptake.[2]

Hyperglycemia should be considered a "normal" response to tissue injury. However, there seems to be a ceiling glycemic level above which hyperglycemia is associated with adverse outcomes,[3] and this has led to significant interest in "tight glycemic control" in perioperative medicine and critical care. There are many advocates for the extension of this principle to all critically ill populations.[4] Should blood glucose levels be tightly controlled in trauma patients?

It is important to differentiate association and causality. Currently, no data exists to implicate stress hyperglycemia and adverse outcomes in trauma; however, substantial data are available in other clinical and laboratory conditions.[5–7] Hyperglycemia can directly affect fluid balance, by inducing diuresis, leading to dehydration. Hyperglycemia can induce immune dysfunction, by promoting inflammation because of induced abnormalities of white cell function,[8,9] and these include granulocyte adhesion, chemotaxis, phagocytosis, respiratory burst and superoxide formation, and intracellular killing.[7] Hyperglycemia negatively affects wound healing.[10] However, these data are from patients with diabetes, not from those with stress hyperglycemia: immune suppression may result from the disease—one of absolute or relative insulin deficiency, rather than the glucose level.

In the clinical arena there is accumulating data that hyperglycemia, and poor control of diabetes, results in worse outcomes from myocardial ischemia and stroke.[5,11–13] In the trauma population, a series of studies have associated the magnitude of hyperglycemia with adverse outcomes.[13–20] In addition, difficulty in controlling blood glucose with insulin was associated with adverse outcomes.[21] Two very separate conclusions can be derived from these data: hyperglycemia causes adverse outcomes and it is a surrogate marker of severity of illness, including inadequacy of physiologic reserve. In the latter hypothesis, stress hyerglycemia is analogous to stress hypoalbuminemia—the magnitude of change from homeostatic norm indicates the degree of injury.[22]

In view of the association between adverse outcomes and hyperglycemia, it has been proposed that aggressive glycemic control may improve outcomes. Analogously, intensive insulin therapy may be used to achieve glycemic control.

Insulin has significant antiinflammatory properties.[23] It has powerful antioxidant activity. Insulin suppresses several proinflammatory transcription factors (nuclear factor-κB, EBR, and AP-1 [activating protein 1]) and reduces the quantity of circulating cytokines. Takebayashi and colleagues[24] found that treatment of type 2 diabetes with insulin for 2 weeks reduced the levels of C-reactive protein and chemotactic protein-1. Stentz and colleagues[25] demonstrated that treatment of severe hyperglycemia with insulin led to a marked reduction in the levels of inflammatory mediators. In an endotoxin rat of sepsis, insulin suppressed interleukin (IL)-1B, IL-6, Macrophage migration inhibitory factor, and tumor necrosis factor-α.[23] In a rat model of thermal injury treated with insulin, there was a similar reduction in inflammatory mediators.[26]

Obese patients with insulin-resistant type 2 diabetes have larger infarcts than nondiabetic patients. In a rat model of myocardial ischemia, the introduction of insulin into the reperfusion fluid reduced the infarct size by 50%.[27] A similar effect was seen in humans given insulin, tissue plasminogen activator, and heparin.[28]

Insulin seems to be cardioprotective in the presence of ischemia.[27,29] Insulin therapy in perioperative patients, and, in particular, patients who have undergone cardiothoracic surgery, was associated with a significant reduction in the risk of death.[30] Enthusiasm for insulin therapy, rather than glycemic control, must be tempered by the knowledge that increased insulin administration is positively associated with death in the intensive care unit (ICU) regardless of the prevailing blood glucose level.[31] In addition, it remains unclear whether these data may be applicable in other clinical situations.

Does intensive insulin therapy improve outcomes in perioperative and critically ill patients? Zerr and colleagues[32] and Furnari and colleagues,[33] demonstrated that meticulous control of blood glucose levels significantly reduces the incidence of deep sternal wound infections. They also demonstrated a significant reduction in perioperative mortality in diabetic patients undergoing cardiac surgery who were managed with intensive insulin therapy.[34]

The case for intensive insulin therapy was advanced significantly by the work of Van den Berghe and colleagues.[35] This was a prospective randomized unblinded clinical trial of 1548 patients admitted into the surgical ICU of a single academic medical center. Patients were randomized into 2 groups. The first group, the conventional therapy group, received an insulin drip if the blood glucose level exceeded 215 mg/dL, and the level was adjusted to maintain the blood glucose level in the range 180 to 200 mg/dL. The second group received "intensive insulin therapy": an insulin drip was started if the blood glucose level exceeded 100 mg/dL, and the level was adjusted to maintain the blood glucose level in the range 80 to 100 mg/dL. All patients were given dextrose on day 1 and received nutrition on day 2. Most of the patients enrolled into this study had undergone cardiothoracic surgery (974). There were only 68 trauma patients. Overall, intensive insulin therapy resulted in an absolute risk reduction of death of 3.4% (4.6% vs 8.0% $P<.04$), a number needed to treat of 30. Subgroup analysis suggested that this mortality difference accrued principally to patients with prolonged ICU stays. In effect, this referred to patients who were critically ill rather than those who had undergone a standard perioperative stress response. Subsequent data suggested that the mechanism of benefit was endothelial protection and reduced hepatocyte mitochondrial damage.[36,37] Given the small number of patients who had been involved in trauma, it is unlikely that Van den Berghe's data can be applied to that patient population.

A single-center cohort study of intensive insulin therapy, versus recent historic controls, found a significant reduction in hospital mortality, ICU length of stay, and blood transfusion.[38]

A question that arose was whether the clinical benefit was a result of glucose control or was due to the effect of insulin. Van den Berghe and colleagues[35,39] concluded that glycemic control was more important than insulin dose. Indeed, increasing insulin dose was related to increased incidence of renal failure in their study.[35] Finney and colleagues[31] showed that increased insulin administration is positively associated with death in the ICU regardless of the prevailing blood glucose level.

The Leuven group followed their initial report with a study of intensive insulin therapy in the medical ICU.[40] A total of 1200 patients were enrolled in the study. There was no statistically significant difference in mortality outcomes (37.3% in the intensive insulin therapy group vs 40.0% in the conventional therapy group [$P = .33$]). Subgroup analysis suggested that patients who stayed in the ICU for more than 3 days benefited from insulin therapy, although it is difficult to interpret the utility of these data.

Taken together, a question that remains about the 2 studies by the group at Leuven is whether or not one should be skeptical of clinical trials stopped early: the study was unblinded and there were multiple interim analyses.[41] Moreover, Hawthorne effects cannot be discounted: perhaps the patients received more nursing attention as a result of fear of hypoglycemia. The issue of hypoglycemia cannot be ignored: a German multicenter study (Visep) of intensive insulin therapy in patients with severe sepsis was stopped early because of a significant excess risk of severe hypoglycemia without any evidence of improved survival.[42] Similar data were published in the Glucontrol study.[43] Finally, the NICE-SUGAR study demonstrated that for a general ICU population, tight glycemic control may actually worsen outcomes, principally associated with hypoglycemia.[44] However, this result disproves neither the hypothesis that hyperglycemia is harmful nor that there is a relative insulin deficiency in critical illness; it merely shows that the glycemic limits proposed by Van den Berghe's group is unlikely to benefit a general population of ICU patients. In medium term, until better tools become available to dynamically and safely monitor blood glucose levels, tight limits, such as those that have been proposed by the Leuven group, cannot be recommended.

It has long been observed that hyperglycemia is associated with worsened outcomes in patients with brain injury.[45] However, this association may be the consequence of the magnitude of the stress response rather than of the glucose itself.[46]

Data exist in animal models of stroke that hyperglycemia in the presence of cerebral ischemia may be detrimental.[47] Hyperglycemia may worsen prognosis as a result of increased brain tissue acidosis, accumulation of extracellular glutamate, increased blood–brain barrier permeability, and increased formation of cerebral edema. A consensus exists among neuroscientists that hyperglycemia leads to localized tissues acidosis[48] and that this in turn may increase the risk of ischemia in the penumbra.[49] Consequently, clinicians have used observational data, animal studies,[47] and human studies in different fields[50,51] to justify tight glycemic control in this patient population.

The brain depends on glucose as its main source of energy, thus a significant blood to brain glucose gradient is required to maintain tissue integrity and prevent ischemic injury. Interstitial glucose levels decrease dramatically during brain ischemia. Cerebral microdialysis directly measures brain glucose and lactate levels.[52] Vespa and colleagues[53] have shown that the cerebral microdialysis glucose levels of 0.2 mmol/L or less during intensive glucose control is an independent predictor of bad outcome in a patient with TBI. Low microdialysis glucose levels were associated with a net increase in microdialysis glutamate and lactate/pyruvate levels. Strong and colleagues[54] have reported similar findings: there is complete disappearance of glucose from brain dialysate in a patient with TBI receiving insulin. Oddo and colleagues[55] demonstrated a powerful relationship between falling blood and microdialysate glucose levels, escalating insulin doses, and the likelihood of brain energy crisis and adverse outcome. These data have been replicated by Vespa and colleagues.[56] Hence, care must be taken to avoid hypoglycemia in patients with TBI receiving intravenous insulin. The margin between beneficial and detrimental effects seems to be narrow. Tight glycemic control in the range of 80 to 115 mg/dL cannot be recommended.[57]

In summary, current data do not support intensive insulin therapy in trauma patients.

LACTATE, TISSUE ACIDOSIS, AND TRAUMA

Volume replacement with crystalloid remains the mainstay of therapy before and after source control in trauma. The objective of resuscitation is to restore homeostasis and maintain tissue perfusion. This objective is based on the "golden hour" hypothesis that arose from observed improvements in outcomes with the introduction of trauma centers in the United States in the 1970s and 1980s. One of the greatest challenges for trauma surgeons, emergency medicine physicians, and anesthesiologists has been to determine the most effective and most easily available end points to direct resuscitative efforts.[58] Unfortunately, conventional clinical and laboratory signs, such as heart rate, blood pressure, and hemoglobin, may be misleading in trauma patients.[58]

As early as the 1980s it was observed that hypothermia, coagulopathy, and acidosis constituted a "triad of death" in trauma patients.[59] The mechanism of acidosis is presumed to be oxygen debt as a consequence of hypoperfusion due to hypovolemia and anaerobic glycolysis. The anion implicated in this acidosis is lactate. Lactate is a strong ion, whose pK_a is 3.6. Consequently, lactic acid is fully dissociated along all values of physiologic pH. The extent to which acidosis, per se, injures the body is unclear. Acidosis has a negative inotropic effect, induces vasoplegia, alters the shape of the oxyhemoglobin dissociation curve, and is widely thought to reduce the effectiveness of vasopressors. In addition, acidosis may reduce splanchnic perfusion, including glomerular filtration rate.

The capability to measure serum lactate levels was not universally available, and a surrogate method, the base deficit,[60] was used for many years. Care should be taken when using this tool, and inferences about its validity should be placed in the context of quantitative acid-base chemistry.[61–64] In the setting of acute trauma, there may be multiple acidifying and alkalinizing processes occurring simultaneously depending on the volume and nature of intravenous fluids.[65] A "normal" base deficit or excess may hide potentially dangerous acid-base disturbances.[65] An elevated base deficit is more significant if caused by lactate rather than ketones or chloride, particularly if hyperchloremia is associated with fluid resuscitation.[66]

Unsurprisingly, base deficit does not reliably reflect lactate in the emergency setting.[63,67,68] Clearly, the direct measurement of lactate levels is more important, if available, assuming that acidosis due to lactate has prognostic indications and reversal of the acidosis improves outcomes, which remains controversial, as is discussed later.[69–72]

Lactic acidosis (with an associated base deficit) on admission to the emergency room is a marker of severity of illness.[73,74] The magnitude of acidosis and the degree of elevation of serum lactate levels correlates well with patient outcomes.[59,71,75] Indeed, the speed of clearance of lactate from circulation is also a known prognostic indicator.[71,76–78] Conventional medical school teaching describes lactate as the byproduct of glycolytic activity that occurs in presence of hypoxemia. The inevitable assumption made by traumatologists was that increasing oxygen delivery would increase tissue perfusion and reduce lactate levels. This assumption led to the current era of highly aggressive crystalloid resuscitation for patients to "wash out lactate." This approach is widely adopted despite lack of evidence that fluid resuscitation clears lactate and the emergence of abdominal compartment syndrome as a consequence of overenthusiastic resuscitation.[79] For example, in the study by McNelis and colleagues,[77] nonsurvivors in the ICU took significantly longer to clear lactate. However, there was no difference in oxygen delivery and consumption parameters between survivors and nonsurvivors.[77] This observation indicates that although admission lactate and lactate clearance may be independent predictors of mortality, the mechanism of hyperlactemia may not necessarily be hypoperfusion. In addition, lactate, itself may be harmless.[1,72,80]

Lactate is an important intermediate in the process of wound healing and repair. There is a strong association between collagen synthesis and lactate levels. Oxygen levels have little impact on wound lactate levels[1]; in fact, wound lactate levels remain remarkably stable over a large range of Pa_{O_2} from hypoxemia to hyperoxia.[1] The explanation for this seems to be the "Warburg effect": rapidly proliferating cells seem to be heavily reliant on glycolysis, independent of the tissue O_2 level. Leukocytes, as discussed above, are centrally involved in inflammation and wound healing. Leukocytes contain few mitochondria. These cells are highly metabolically active and undergo significant glycolytic activity to produce superoxides that are essential to wound immunity (the "oxidative burst"). This process is oxygen dependent—the greater the amount of oxygen delivered, the greater is the amount of lactate produced as a consequence of the oxidative burst. Lactate enhances collagen production and deposition and angiogenesis.[81] Lactate is a direct vasodilator and may actually increase wound oxygen tension.

There is emerging evidence that lactic acidosis in trauma and critical illness may not be due to hypoxemia but due to epinephrine-driven aerobic glycolysis.[80,82] This glycolysis results from cyclic-AMP-medicated Na^+K^+ ATPase activity that is driven by beta-adrenoceptor activation.[83] Administration of β-adrenergic agents increases tissue lactate levels, whereas administration of antiadrenergic agents reduces tissue lactate levels.[80]

High-quality goal-directed studies of lactate as an end point of resuscitation in trauma are unavailable. However, some inferences can be learned from data using lactate as a marker in sepsis. Lactate clearance has been proposed as an end point of resuscitation, and this refers to the expected decrease in lactate levels associated with the onset of resuscitation. The assumption is that lactate reflects low perfusion; once perfusion is improved by fluids, pressors, and blood products, lactate levels should decrease. If lactate levels fail to decrease, in response to these measures, lactate may not reflect global perfusion and a more sinister cause may be evident. Consequently, patients who fail to clear lactate have worse outcomes, and lactate in this situation does not seem to correlate with SvO_2 (mixed venous oxygen saturation).[84] Among 166 patients, 15 (9%) had lactate nonclearance. Mortality was 60% for these patients versus 19% for those with lactate clearance ($P<.001$). Lactate nonclearance independently predicted death (odds ratio, 4.9; confidence interval, 1.5–15.9). Importantly, 79% of patients with lactate nonclearance had concomitant central venous oxygen saturation ($ScvO_2$) of 70% or greater.[84] This discordance between $ScvO_2$ and lactate suggests that in patients who fail to clear lactate, global oxygen delivery may not be a good therapeutic option.

Nguyen and colleagues[78] demonstrated, in a cohort of patients with septic shock over 1 year, that the ability to clear lactate was associated with improved outcomes. There was an approximately 11% decreased likelihood of mortality for each 10% increase in lactate clearance.

Jones and colleagues[85] evaluated lactate clearance and $ScvO_2$ as goals of early sepsis resuscitation, in a multicenter randomized noninferiority trial of 300 patients. To be admitted to the trial patients had to be in septic shock or have lactate levels greater than 4 mmol/L. Lactate clearance was defined by the equation $[(lactate_{initial} - lactate_{delayed})/lactate_{initial}] \times 100\%$, where $lactate_{initial}$ was the measurement at the start of the resuscitation and $lactate_{delayed}$ was measured after a minimum of 2 hours after resuscitation was initiated. A 10% reduction in [lactate] was the resuscitation goal. There were no differences in treatments during the initial 72 hours of hospitalization—fluids, antibiotics, and vasopressors. The mortality rate in the $ScvO_2$ group was 23% versus 17% the lactate clearance group. This study suggests that lactate clearance is a reasonable end point of early resuscitation, compared with $ScvO_2$.

Jansen and colleagues[86] evaluated lactate-guided therapy in 317 patients. Patients with serum lactate levels greater than 3 mmol/L were randomized to reduce lactate levels by 20% over 3 hours. The control group was resuscitated to the following end points: heart rate less than 100 beats/min, mean arterial pressure at or above 60 mm Hg, central venous pressure 8 to 12 mm Hg (12–15 mm Hg in mechanically ventilated patients), urinary output more than 0.5 mL/kg/h, arterial oxygen saturation (Sao_2) at or above 92%, and hemoglobin levels at or above 7.0 g/dL. SvO_2 could be used at the discretion of the intensivist. The lactate clearance group was resuscitated using both lactate and $ScvO_2$ in addition to the other end points. The aim of this strategy was to optimize global perfusion, assuming that this would be reflected by both indices.

Although, based on intention- to-treat analysis, in-hospital mortality did not reach statistically significant difference between the groups; outcomes were improved in the lactate-guided group once adjustments were made for predefined risk factors. In addition, patients had better Sequential Organ Failure Assessment (SOFA) scores, weaned from pressors earlier, and had shorter duration of mechanical ventilation if resuscitated based on lactate clearance. Where the indices did not correlate—$ScvO_2$ was normal, but lactate levels failed to correct by at least 20% during a 2-hour time interval—microvascular dysfunction was assumed and vasodilator therapy (nitroglycerin) was administered. Curiously, the lactate levels were not different between the groups. Patients in the lactate group received more fluid (on an average 500 mL) over the first 8 hours but less over the next 64 hours. Patients in the lactate group received more vasodilators at all stages. This observation weakens the case for lactate as an independent goal of resuscitation, as it is an insensitive indicator of global oxygen delivery and consumption.

Let us return to the issue of hyperglycemia, lactic acidosis, and brain injury. As already stated, it is widely believed that hyperglycemia predisposes to ischemic brain damage as a consequence of increased anaerobic glycolysis, lactate production, and tissue acidosis.[87] The major problem with this hypothesis is that the brain is glucose dependent and glycolysis supplies energy for metabolism during hypoxemia. In addition, lactate may be a source of energy during the postischemic state. Thus we have the "glucose paradox of cerebral ischemia"—increased energy delivery seems to be associated with worsened outcomes.[88] However, association does not prove causality: a significant problem with all studies on lactate and hyperglycemia.

Elevated blood glucose and lactate levels are associated with stress; stress is associated with increase in blood corticosteroid levels. An alternative hypothesis suggests that elevated serum cortisol levels may be related to brain injury.[88] This hypothesis results from several observations in animal studies that the timing of hyperglycemia before and after ischemic brain injuries significantly changes outcomes. The application of corticosteroid inhibitors reduced the severity of brain injuries, whereas the application of steroid increased the severity of brain injuries.[88]

In summary, in trauma and critical illness, increased lactate levels may result from a medley of processes unrelated to oxygen delivery and hypoxemia. The assumption that elevated serum lactate levels is a marker of tissue hypoperfusion rather of inflammation has led to an approach to resuscitation (ie, aggressive fluid administration until lactate clears) that may result in significant hypervolemia. Indeed, in the setting of acute severe trauma, an elevated serum lactate level represents a homeostatic mechanism and prolonged lactate clearance represents prolonged hyperadrenergic activity.

HYPOTHERMIA AND TRAUMA

Trauma patients routinely present to the emergency room and operating room in a state of mild-to-moderate hypothermia, which results from many environmental and iatrogenic factors such as exposure, large volumes of unwarmed resuscitative fluids and blood products, anesthetic agents, intoxication with alcohol or drugs, and the temperature of the interior of the ambulance.[89] In addition, the capacity of the patient to produce heat internally may be severely limited in trauma patients because of the impairment of thermoregulatory mechanisms and reduced oxygen delivery to tissues in hypovolemic shock. In cardiac surgery and after cardiac arrest, induced hypothermia is neuroprotective and modulates the immune response and apoptosis, and this is considered beneficial.[90] Is hypothermia a foe or friend of trauma patients?

It has been well established that accidental hypothermia even in uninjured patients is a significant risk factor for mortality.[91] Multiple clinical retrospective studies have demonstrated the association of exposure hypothermia with a poor outcome in severe trauma. Up to 50% of trauma patients are hypothermic on arrival to the hospital, and this increases the risk of multiorgan failure.[92] For rural trauma patients, hypothermia, below 36°C, is associated with increased mortality.[93] Accordingly, the American College of Surgeons Advanced Trauma Life Support Program recommends prevention, prompt detection, and treatment of hypothermia in patients with trauma and HS. This recommendation is based on the hypothesis that because hypothermia is associated with a higher risk of mortality in trauma patients, prevention of hypothermia or gentle rewarming will lead to improved outcomes. Again, this may be a case of conclusions derived from epidemiology rather than pathophysiology.

Historically, induced hypothermia has been used to protect organs, in particular the brain, in cardiac surgery, neurosurgery, and transplant surgery. Hypothermia has been used, on and off, for more than 60 years, since it first had been suggested as a therapeutic option for the management of patients with head injury.[94] More recently, mild-to-moderate induced hypothermia has been shown to have a significant neuroprotective effect in multiple laboratory and clinical models of ischemic injury and TBI. Patients with cardiac arrest who have been resuscitated have been shown to benefit greatly from prolonged induced hypothermia.[95–97] Numerous laboratory studies have also indicated that induced mild hypothermia improves survival in laboratory animals after a traumatic HS. These data seemingly conflict with a well-established belief that hypothermia has deleterious impact on the morbidity and mortality of major trauma patients. Does hypothermia independently increase patient risk in HS and severe trauma, or is it a consequence of these injuries? Do hypothermic trauma patients need to be actively rewarmed, or is there some beneficial protective/therapeutic effect in allowing and even inducing certain degree of hypothermia in some of these patients?

To resolve these conflicts, the reader must understand the role of hypothermia in trauma patients and the different types of hypothermia that exist.

Hypothermia can be accidental or induced. Major trauma is typically associated with accidental hypothermia, whereas induced hypothermia is used for preventive or therapeutic purposes. Accidental hypothermia is characteristically uncontrolled. Induced hypothermia, conversely, is well controlled and easily monitored. Induced hypothermia can be protective-preservative (preinsult and intrainsult) or resuscitative (postinsult).[98] For example, protective hypothermia has been universally used in cardiac surgery for brain protection; the protective effects in this setting are well established. The use of therapeutic hypothermia as an adjunct to resuscitation was first proposed in the 1950s, but it has only recently been validated in patients with out-of-hospital cardiac arrest who have been resuscitated.[99,100]

Hypothermia is also often classified according to arbitrary chosen ranges in body temperature as mild (34°C –36°C), moderate (30°C –33°C), or deep hypothermia (<30°C). In the setting of resuscitation, mild induced hypothermia is typically used. Poor outcomes in major trauma patients are usually associated with deeper degrees of accidental hypothermia. All trauma patients are not the same, and an understanding of hypothermia in major trauma requires separation of the patients into 2 distinct groups: those whose main injury is a TBI and those whose main treatment challenge is hypovolemic shock/HS.

LABORATORY STUDIES OF HYPOTHERMIA IN HEMORRHAGIC SHOCK MODEL

The successful use of hypothermia for organ and brain protection against hypoperfusion–ischemic injuries in cardiac surgery and organ transplantation led to interest in the use of therapeutic and resuscitative hypothermia for HS.[101] HS has been implicated in ischemic injury of vital organs because of hypoperfusion and is associated with high mortality rates in trauma patients. The reduction in metabolic rate associated with moderate hypothermia could potentially alleviate the degree of ischemia in HS.[102] In addition, mild hypothermia can reduce postischemic oxidative damage during the resuscitative phase in the treatment of HS. This fact is supported by laboratory data. Mild hypothermia induced during HS or during the fluid resuscitation phase improved survival of experimental animals in the models of uncontrolled HS, volume-controlled HS,[103,104] pressure-controlled HS,[105] and prolonged HS combined with significant tissue trauma[106] compared with normothermic resuscitation. Wu and colleagues[106] created a clinically relevant animal outcome model of HS with extensive tissue damage, which included intensive care environment similar to that found in clinical situation. The mechanism by which hypothermia improved survival in these animals could not be determined.

Conversely, other studies found in experimental and clinical models of hypothermia that during HS and resuscitative phase vital organs and systems were adversely affected. The adverse effects of hypothermia on individual vital functions may explain why hypothermia may contribute to mortality and morbidity in clinical observational studies, while being useful in laboratory experiments, in which the adverse effects of hypothermia could be well controlled and easily monitored. For example, Mizushima and colleagues[107] demonstrated that hypothermia depressed cardiac function and hepatic blood flow in an HS model. Active rewarming during resuscitation improved cardiac function and hepatic blood flow, compared with animals that were allowed to remain hypothermic.[107] Interestingly, the hypothermia-rewarming group of animals had improved parameters compared with the control group, in which normothermia was maintained during and after injury.[107]

Coagulopathy is part of the "triad of death" associated with trauma. It is widely believed that hypothermia-induced coagulopathy is a significant contributing factor to adverse outcomes in trauma.[108] There is a strong association between hypothermia, blood loss, and impaired hemostasis in these patients.[109,110] Hypothermia, below 34°C to 33°C, directly impairs clotting enzyme activity[111–113] and platelet function.[113,114] It has been suggested that hypothermia and resuscitative hemodilution and acidosis may have a synergistic impact on coagulation.[111,115] This fact may explain the absence of association between induced hypothermia and bleeding in laboratory experiments,[116] and in clinical studies of head injury, in which fluid administration was restricted.[117] It has led to a renewed interest in damage control resuscitation,[108] associated with permissive hypotension; aggressive treatment of coagulopathy; particularly with antifibrinolytic drugs[118,119]; and avoidance of acidosis. Indeed, only time, experience, and extensive research will tell if adverse outcomes associated with hypothermia and coagulopathy result more from resuscitative efforts than from the disease process.[120] The CRASH-2 trial[121] was an international multicenter trial of tranexamic acid versus placebo within 8 hours of injury. A total of 20,000 patients at risk for bleeding were recruited. The investigators demonstrated a modest, although significant, mortality benefit with this agent (14.5% vs 16.0%; $P = .0035$). The risk of death due to bleeding was significantly reduced (44.9% vs 5.7%; $P = .0077$). Death was associated with advancing age, low Glasgow Coma Score, and lower systolic blood pressure on admission.

Another mechanism by which hypothermia may worsen outcomes in trauma patients is immunosuppression. Mild hypothermia may reduce the expression of heat shock protein, impair granulocyte recruitment, and alter cytokine balance.[122,123]

CLINICAL STUDIES OF HYPOTHERMIA IN PATIENTS WITH TRAUMA AND HS

There is a strong correlation between the magnitude of tissue injury and the degree of hypothermia.[124,125] In earlier observational retrospective studies,[126–128] investigators found that hypothermia was associated with a higher mortality, greater need for transfusion, longer hospital stay, acidosis, and higher injury severity scores. Later studies confirmed that hypothermia, independent of severity of injury and shock, was associated with increased risk of death.[129–131] Again, association does not prove causality.

Gentilello and colleagues[132] studied the effect of rapid rewarming versus standard rewarming in moderately severe injured patients with admission hypothermia. This study showed that continuous arteriovenous (rapid) rewarming reduced fluid and blood product requirements, reduced length of ICU stay, and improved short-term, but not long-term, survival. This remains the only published prospective randomized controlled clinical trial of management of hypothermia in trauma patients. It is not known whether or not hypothermia per se increases mortality or whether it is simply an indicator of depleted physiologic reserve in patients with greater injury severity or greater baseline risk.[101]

The current consensus in the literature and among traumatologists indicates that hypothermia in patients with HS should be prevented and promptly treated until new evidence emerges to the contrary.

HYPOTHERMIA IN TRAUMATIC BRAIN INJURY (TBI)

Multiple animal studies demonstrated beneficial effects of mild-to-moderate induced hypothermia on mortality and neurologic outcomes and brain physiologic parameters after severe TBI. This demonstration resulted in a series of randomized controlled trials of induced hypothermia in TBI. The data were disappointing. For example, Clifton and colleagues[133] showed no neurologic benefit from hypothermia in TBI; there were greater complication rates associated with hypothermia versus normothermia. Similarly, a multicenter Japanese study of mild hypothermia in TBI demonstrated significantly more complications, such as pneumonia and meningitis in hypothermia group.[134] Two meta-analyses on the use of hypothermia for the treatment of TBI, published in the same year, came out with conflicting results.[135,136] A 2009 Cochrane meta-analysis failed to detect an outcome benefit from induced hypothermia in higher-quality trials.[137] This result conflicted with that of a contemporaneous systematic review by Fox and colleagues.[138]

When the literature on hypothermia is evaluated, the duration of hypothermia seems to be important: outcomes are improved when hypothermia is used early and for a prolonged period (at least 72 hours, associated with stabilization of intracranial pressure for at least 24 hours), with slower rewarming.[138,139]

Two randomized clinical trials,[140,141] which included 396 and 215 patients, demonstrated improved outcomes in patients with severe TBI with raised intracranial pressure when treated with prolonged (5 days) mild hypothermia. More recently, the National Acute Brain Injury Study: Hypothermia II (NABIS: H II) failed to demonstrate a benefit from early mild hypothermia ($<35.0^\circ C$) in patients with brain injury[142]; it is likely, however, that this smaller study was underpowered to detect an outcome difference.

In conclusion, data are insufficient to recommend routine induced hypothermia in TBI. Only those patients who have raised intracranial pressure are likely to benefit. Hypothermia should be maintained for no less than 48 hours, and the rate of rewarming needs to be not faster than over 24 hours.

REFERENCES

1. Gladden LB. Lactate metabolism: a new paradigm for the third millennium. J Physiol 2004;558:5–30.
2. Lang CH, Obih JC, Bagby GJ, et al. Increased glucose uptake by intestinal mucosa and muscularis in hypermetabolic sepsis. Am J Physiol 1991;261: G287–94.
3. Langouche L, Van den BG. Glucose metabolism and insulin therapy. Crit Care Clin 2006;22:119–29, vii.
4. Gropper MA. Evidence-based management of critically ill patients: analysis and implementation. Anesth Analg 2004;99:566–72.
5. Capes SE, Hunt D, Malmberg K, et al. Stress hyperglycaemia and increased risk of death after myocardial infarction in patients with and without diabetes: a systematic overview. Lancet 2000;355:773–8.
6. Umpierrez GE, Isaacs SD, Bazargan N, et al. Hyperglycemia: an independent marker of in-hospital mortality in patients with undiagnosed diabetes. J Clin Endocrinol Metab 2002;87:978–82.
7. Montori VM, Bistrian BR, McMahon MM. Hyperglycemia in acutely ill patients. JAMA 2002;288:2167–9.
8. Guha M, Bai W, Nadler JL, et al. Molecular mechanisms of tumor necrosis factor alpha gene expression in monocytic cells via hyperglycemia-induced oxidant stress-dependent and-independent pathways. J Biol Chem 2000;275: 17728–39.
9. Sampson MJ, Davies IR, Brown JC, et al. Monocyte and neutrophil adhesion molecule expression during acute hyperglycemia and after antioxidant treatment in type 2 diabetes and control patients. Arterioscler Thromb Vasc Biol 2002;22:1187–93.
10. Lin LH, Hopf HW. Paradigm of the injury-repair continuum during critical illness. Crit Care Med 2003;31:S493–5.
11. Wahab NN, Cowden EA, Pearce NJ, et al. Is blood glucose an independent predictor of mortality in acute myocardial infarction in the thrombolytic era? J Am Coll Cardiol 2002;40:1748–54.
12. Iwakura K, Ito H, Ikushima M, et al. Association between hyperglycemia and the no-reflow phenomenon in patients with acute myocardial infarction. J Am Coll Cardiol 2003;41:1–7.
13. O'Neill PA, Davies I, Fullerton KJ, et al. Stress hormone and blood glucose response following acute stroke in the elderly. Stroke 1991;22:842–7.
14. Yendamuri S, Fulda GJ, Tinkoff GH. Admission hyperglycemia as a prognostic indicator in trauma. J Trauma 2003;55:33–8.
15. Laird AM, Miller PR, Kilgo PD, et al. Relationship of early hyperglycemia to mortality in trauma patients. J Trauma 2004;56:1058–62.
16. Sung J, Bochicchio GV, Joshi M, et al. Admission hyperglycemia is predictive of outcome in critically ill trauma patients. J Trauma 2005;59:80–3.
17. Bochicchio GV, Sung J, Joshi M, et al. Persistent hyperglycemia is predictive of outcome in critically ill trauma patients. J Trauma 2005;58:921–4.
18. Bochicchio GV, Salzano L, Joshi M, et al. Admission preoperative glucose is predictive of morbidity and mortality in trauma patients who require immediate operative intervention. Am Surg 2005;71:171–4.
19. Vogelzang M, Nijboer JM, van dH I, et al. Hyperglycemia has a stronger relation with outcome in trauma patients than in other critically ill patients. J Trauma 2006;60:873–7.

20. Desai D, March R, Watters JM. Hyperglycemia after trauma increases with age. J Trauma 1989;29:719–23.
21. Gale SC, Sicoutris C, Reilly PM, et al. Poor glycemic control is associated with increased mortality in critically ill trauma patients. Am Surg 2007;73:454–60.
22. Sung J, Bochicchio GV, Joshi M, et al. Admission serum albumin is predictive of outcome in critically ill trauma patients. Am Surg 2004;70:1099–102.
23. Jeschke MG, Klein D, Bolder U, et al. Insulin attenuates the systemic inflammatory response in endotoxemic rats. Endocrinology 2004;145:4084–93.
24. Takebayashi K, Aso Y, Inukai T. Initiation of insulin therapy reduces serum concentrations of high-sensitivity C-reactive protein in patients with type 2 diabetes. Metabolism 2004;53:693–9.
25. Stentz FB, Umpierrez GE, Cuervo R, et al. Proinflammatory cytokines, markers of cardiovascular risks, oxidative stress, and lipid peroxidation in patients with hyperglycemic crises. Diabetes 2004;53:2079–86.
26. Jeschke MG, Einspanier R, Klein D, et al. Insulin attenuates the systemic inflammatory response to thermal trauma. Mol Med 2002;8:443–50.
27. Jonassen AK, Sack MN, Mjos OD, et al. Myocardial protection by insulin at reperfusion requires early administration and is mediated via Akt and p70s6 kinase cell-survival signaling. Circ Res 2001;89:1191–8.
28. Chaudhuri A, Janicke D, Wilson MF, et al. anti-inflammatory and profibrinolytic effect of insulin in acute ST-segment-elevation myocardial infarction. Circulation 2004;109:849–54.
29. Lazar HL, Chipkin SR, Fitzgerald CA, et al. Tight glycemic control in diabetic coronary artery bypass graft patients improves perioperative outcomes and decreases recurrent ischemic events. Circulation 2004;109:1497–502.
30. Van den BG, Wouters P, Weekers F, et al. Intensive insulin therapy in the critically ill patients. N Engl J Med 2001;345:1359–67.
31. Finney SJ, Zekveld C, Elia A, et al. Glucose control and mortality in critically ill patients. JAMA 2003;290:2041–7.
32. Zerr KJ, Furnary AP, Grunkemeier GL, et al. Glucose control lowers the risk of wound infection in diabetics after open heart operations. Ann Thorac Surg 1997;63:356–61.
33. Furnary AP, Zerr KJ, Grunkemeier GL, et al. Continuous intravenous insulin infusion reduces the incidence of deep sternal wound infection in diabetic patients after cardiac surgical procedures. Ann Thorac Surg 1999;67:352–60.
34. Furnary AP, Gao G, Grunkemeier GL, et al. Continuous insulin infusion reduces mortality in patients with diabetes undergoing coronary artery bypass grafting. J Thorac Cardiovasc Surg 2003;125:1007–21.
35. Van den Berghe G, Wouters PJ, Bouillon R, et al. Outcome benefit of intensive insulin therapy in the critically ill: insulin dose versus glycemic control. Crit Care Med 2003;31:359–66.
36. Langouche L, Vanhorebeek I, Vlasselaers D, et al. Intensive insulin therapy protects the endothelium of critically ill patients. J Clin Invest 2005;115: 2277–86.
37. Vanhorebeek I, De Vos R, Mesotten D, et al. Protection of hepatocyte mitochondrial ultrastructure and function by strict blood glucose control with insulin in critically ill patients. Lancet 2005;365:53–9.
38. Krinsley JS. Effect of an intensive glucose management protocol on the mortality of critically ill adult patients. Mayo Clin Proc 2004;79:992–1000.
39. Van den Berghe G. How does blood glucose control with insulin save lives in intensive care? J Clin Invest 2004;114:1187–95.

40. Van den Berghe G, Wilmer A, Hermans G, et al. Intensive insulin therapy in the medical ICU. N Engl J Med 2006;354:449–61.
41. Montori VM, Devereaux PJ, Adhikari NKJ, et al. Randomized trials stopped early for benefit: a systematic review. JAMA 2005;294:2203–9.
42. Brunkhorst FM, Engel C, Bloos F, et al. Intensive insulin therapy and pentastarch resuscitation in severe sepsis (visep study). N Engl J Med 2008;358:125–39.
43. Preiser JC, Devos P, Ruiz-Santana S, et al. A prospective randomised multicentre controlled trial on tight glucose control by intensive insulin therapy in adult intensive care units: the Glucontrol study. Intensive Care Med 2009;35: 1738–48.
44. NICE-SUGAR Study Investigators, Finfer S, Chittock DR, et al. Intensive versus conventional glucose control in critically ill patients. N Engl J Med 2009;360: 1283–97.
45. Jeremitsky E, Omert LA, Dunham CM, et al. The impact of hyperglycemia on patients with severe brain injury. J Trauma 2005;58:47–50.
46. Yang SY, Zhang S, Wang ML. Clinical significance of admission hyperglycemia and factors related to it in patients with acute severe head injury. Surg Neurol 1995;44:373–7.
47. Garg R, Chaudhuri A, Munschauer F, et al. Hyperglycemia, insulin, and acute ischemic stroke: a mechanistic justification for a trial of insulin infusion therapy. Stroke 2006;37:267–73.
48. Wagner KR, Kleinholz M, de Court-Myers GM, et al. Hyperglycemic versus normoglycemic stroke: topography of brain metabolites, intracellular pH, and infarct size. J Cereb Blood Flow Metab 1992;12:213–22.
49. Anderson RE, Tan WK, Martin HS, et al. Effects of glucose and PaO_2 modulation on cortical intracellular acidosis, NADH redox state, and infarction in the ischemic penumbra ò editorial comment. Stroke 1999;30:160–70.
50. Van den BG, Wouters P, Weekers F, et al. Intensive insulin therapy in the surgical intensive care unit. N Engl J Med 2001;345:1359–67.
51. Malmberg K, Ryden L, Efendic S, et al. Randomized trial of insulin-glucose infusion followed by subcutaneous insulin treatment in diabetic patients with acute myocardial infarction (DIGAMI study): effects on mortality at 1 year. J Am Coll Cardiol 1995;26:57–65.
52. Goodman JC, Valadka AB, Gopinath SP, et al. Extracellular lactate and glucose alterations in the brain after head injury measured by microdialysis. Crit Care Med 1999;27:1965–73.
53. Vespa P, Boonyaputthikul R, McArthur DL, et al. Intensive insulin therapy reduces microdialysis glucose values without altering glucose utilization or improving the lactate/pyruvate ratio after traumatic brain injury. Crit Care Med 2006;34:850–6.
54. Strong AJ, Boutelle MG, Vespa PM, et al. Treatment of critical care patients with substantial acute ischemic or traumatic brain injury. Crit Care Med 2005;33: 2147–9.
55. Oddo M, Schmidt JM, Carrera E, et al. Impact of tight glycemic control on cerebral glucose metabolism after severe brain injury: a microdialysis study. Crit Care Med 2008;36:3233–8.
56. Vespa P, McArthur DL, Stein N, et al. Tight glycemic control increases metabolic distress in traumatic brain injury: a randomized controlled within-subjects trial. Crit Care Med 2012;40:1923–9.
57. Magnoni S, Tedesco C, Carbonara M, et al. Relationship between systemic glucose and cerebral glucose is preserved in patients with severe traumatic

brain injury, but glucose delivery to the brain may become limited when oxidative metabolism is impaired: implications for glycemic control. Crit Care Med 2012;40:1785–91.
58. Dabrowski GP, Steinberg SM, Ferrara JJ, et al. A critical assessment of endpoints of shock resuscitation. Surg Clin North Am 2000;80:825–44.
59. Eddy VA, Morris JA Jr, Cullinane DC. Hypothermia, coagulopathy, and acidosis. Surg Clin North Am 2000;80:845–54.
60. Runciman WB, Skowronski GA. Pathophysiology of haemorrhagic shock. Anaesth Intensive Care 1984;12:193–205.
61. Schlichtig R, Grogono AW, Severinghaus JW. Current Status of acid-base quantitation in physiology and medicine. Anesthesiol Clin North Am 1998;16: 211–33.
62. Fencl V, Leith DE. Stewart's quantitative acid-base chemistry: applications in biology and medicine. Respir Physiol 1993;91:1–16.
63. Brill SA, Stewart TR, Brundage SI, et al. Base deficit does not predict mortality when secondary to hyperchloremic acidosis. Shock 2002;17:459–62.
64. Stewart PA. Modern quantitative acid-base chemistry. Can J Physiol Pharmacol 1983;61:1444–61.
65. Fencl V, Jabor A, Kazda A, et al. Diagnosis of metabolic acid-base disturbances in critically ill patients. Am J Respir Crit Care Med 2000;162:2246–51.
66. Gunnerson K, Saul M, He S, et al. Lactate versus non-lactate metabolic acidosis: a retrospective outcome evaluation of critically ill patients. Crit Care 2006;10:R22.
67. Kaplan LJ, Kellum JA. Initial pH, base deficit, lactate, anion gap, strong ion difference, and strong ion gap predict outcome from major vascular injury. Crit Care Med 2004;32:1120–4.
68. Martin MJ, FitzSullivan E, Salim A, et al. Discordance between lactate and base deficit in the surgical intensive care unit: which one do you trust? Am J Surg 2006;191:625–30.
69. Pal JD, Victorino GP, Twomey P, et al. Admission serum lactate levels do not predict mortality in the acutely injured patient. J Trauma 2006;60:583–7.
70. Aslar AK, Kuzu MA, Elhan AH, et al. Admission lactate level and the APACHE II score are the most useful predictors of prognosis following torso trauma. Injury 2004;35:746–52.
71. Husain FA, Martin MJ, Mullenix PS, et al. Serum lactate and base deficit as predictors of mortality and morbidity. Am J Surg 2003;185:485–91.
72. James JH, Luchette FA, McCarter FD, et al. Lactate is an unreliable indicator of tissue hypoxia in injury or sepsis. Lancet 1999;354:505–8.
73. Mikkelsen ME, Miltiades AN, Gaieski DF, et al. Serum lactate is associated with mortality in severe sepsis independent of organ failure and shock. Crit Care Med 2009;37:1670–7.
74. Lee SW, Hong YS, Park DW, et al. Lactic acidosis not hyperlactatemia as a predictor of in hospital mortality in septic emergency patients. Emerg Med J 2008;25:659–65.
75. Vitek V, Cowley RA. Blood lactate in the prognosis of various forms of shock. Ann Surg 1971;173:308–13.
76. Abramson D, Scalea TM, Hitchcock R, et al. Lactate clearance and survival following injury. J Trauma 1993;35:584–8.
77. McNelis J, Marini CP, Jurkiewicz A, et al. Prolonged lactate clearance is associated with increased mortality in the surgical intensive care unit. Am J Surg 2001; 182:481–5.

78. Nguyen HB, Rivers EP, Knoblich BP, et al. Early lactate clearance is associated with improved outcome in severe sepsis and septic shock. Crit Care Med 2004; 32:1637–42.
79. Balogh Z, McKinley BA, Cocanour CS, et al. Supranormal trauma resuscitation causes more cases of abdominal compartment syndrome. Arch Surg 2003;138: 637–42.
80. Luchette FA, Jenkins WA, Friend LA, et al. Hypoxia is not the sole cause of lactate production during shock. J Trauma 2002;52:415–9.
81. Constant JS, Feng JJ, Zabel DD, et al. Lactate elicits vascular endothelial growth factor from macrophages: a possible alternative to hypoxia. Wound Repair Regen 2000;8:353–60.
82. James JH, Wagner KR, King JK, et al. Stimulation of both aerobic glycolysis and Na(+)-K(+)-ATPase activity in skeletal muscle by epinephrine or amylin. Am J Physiol 1999;277:E176–86.
83. Clausen T. Na+-K+ pump regulation and skeletal muscle contractility. Physiol Rev 2003;83:1269–324.
84. Arnold RC, Shapiro NI, Jones AE, et al. Multicenter study of early lactate clearance as a determinant of survival in patients with presumed sepsis. Shock 2009; 32:35–9.
85. Jones AE, Shapiro NI, Trzeciak S, et al. Lactate clearance vs central venous oxygen saturation as goals of early sepsis therapy: a randomized clinical trial. JAMA 2010;303:739–46.
86. Jansen TC, van Bommel J, Schoonderbeek FJ, et al. Early lactate-guided therapy in intensive care unit patients: a multicenter, open-label, randomized controlled trial. Am J Respir Crit Care Med 2010;182:752–61.
87. Schurr A. Lactate, glucose and energy metabolism in the ischemic brain (Review). Int J Mol Med 2002;10:131–6.
88. Payne RS, Tseng MT, Schurr A. The glucose paradox of cerebral ischemia: evidence for corticosterone involvement. Brain Res 2003;971:9–17.
89. Lapostolle F, Sebbah JL, Couvreur J, et al. Risk factors for onset of hypothermia in trauma victims: the HypoTraum study. Crit Care 2012;16:R142.
90. Frink M, Flohe S, van GM, et al. Facts and fiction: the impact of hypothermia on molecular mechanisms following major challenge. Mediators Inflamm 2012; 2012:762840.
91. Danzl DF, Pozos RS, Auerbach PS, et al. Multicenter hypothermia survey. Ann Emerg Med 1987;16:1042–55.
92. Beilman GJ, Blondet JJ, Nelson TR, et al. Early hypothermia in severely injured trauma patients is a significant risk factor for multiple organ dysfunction syndrome but not mortality. Ann Surg 2009;249:845–50.
93. Waibel BH, Schlitzkus LL, Newell MA, et al. Impact of hypothermia (below 36 degrees C) in the rural trauma patient. J Am Coll Surg 2009;209:580–8.
94. ROSOMOFF HL. Protective effects of hypothermia against pathological processes of the nervous system. Ann N Y Acad Sci 1959;80:475–86.
95. Hypothermia after Cardiac Arrest Study Group. Mild therapeutic hypothermia to improve the neurologic outcome after cardiac arrest. N Engl J Med 2002;346: 549–56.
96. Bernard SA, Gray TW, Buist MD, et al. Treatment of comatose survivors of out-of-hospital cardiac arrest with induced hypothermia. N Engl J Med 2002;346:557–63.
97. Holzer M, Bernard SA, Hachimi-Idrissi S, et al. Hypothermia for neuroprotection after cardiac arrest: systematic review and individual patient data meta-analysis. Crit Care Med 2005;33:414–8.

98. Marion DW, Leonov Y, Ginsberg M, et al. Resuscitative hypothermia. Crit Care Med 1996;24:S81–9.
99. Nolan JP, Morley PT, Vanden Hoek TL, et al. Therapeutic hypothermia after cardiac arrest: an advisory statement by the advanced life support task force of the International Liaison Committee on Resuscitation. Circulation 2003;108: 118–21.
100. Merchant RM, Soar J, Skrifvars MB, et al. Therapeutic hypothermia utilization among physicians after resuscitation from cardiac arrest. Crit Care Med 2006; 34(7):1935–40.
101. Tisherman SA. Hypothermia and injury. Curr Opin Crit Care 2004;10:512–9.
102. Meyer DM, Horton JW. Effect of moderate hypothermia in the treatment of canine hemorrhagic shock. Ann Surg 1988;207:462–9.
103. Crippen D, Safar P, Porter L, et al. Improved survival of hemorrhagic shock with oxygen and hypothermia in rats. Resuscitation 1991;21:271–81.
104. Leonov Y, Safar P, Sterz F, et al. Extending the golden hour of hemorrhagic shock tolerance with oxygen plus hypothermia in awake rats. An exploratory study. Resuscitation 2002;52:193–202.
105. Prueckner S, Safar P, Kentner R, et al. Mild hypothermia increases survival from severe pressure-controlled hemorrhagic shock in rats. J Trauma 2001;50:253–62.
106. Wu X, Kochanek PM, Cochran K, et al. Mild hypothermia improves survival after prolonged, traumatic hemorrhagic shock in pigs. J Trauma 2005;59:291–9.
107. Mizushima Y, Wang P, Cioffi WG, et al. Should normothermia be restored and maintained during resuscitation after trauma and hemorrhage? J Trauma 2000;48:58–65.
108. Theusinger OM, Madjdpour C, Spahn DR. Resuscitation and transfusion management in trauma patients: emerging concepts. Curr Opin Crit Care 2012. [Epub ahead of print].
109. Schreiber MA. Coagulopathy in the trauma patient. Curr Opin Crit Care 2005;11: 590–7.
110. Patt A, McCroskey BL, Moore EE. Hypothermia-induced coagulopathies in trauma. Surg Clin North Am 1988;68:775–85.
111. Gubler KD, Gentilello LM, Hassantash SA, et al. The impact of hypothermia on dilutional coagulopathy. J Trauma 1994;36:847–51.
112. Rohrer MJ, Natale AM. Effect of hypothermia on the coagulation cascade. Crit Care Med 1992;20:1402–5.
113. Watts DD, Trask A, Soeken K, et al. Hypothermic coagulopathy in trauma: effect of varying levels of hypothermia on enzyme speed, platelet function, and fibrinolytic activity. J Trauma 1998;44:846–54.
114. Wolberg AS, Meng ZH, Monroe DM III, et al. A systematic evaluation of the effect of temperature on coagulation enzyme activity and platelet function. J Trauma 2004;56:1221–8.
115. Misgav M, Martinowitz U. Trauma-induced coagulopathy–mechanisms and state of the art treatment. Harefuah 2011;150:99–103, 207. [in Hebrew].
116. Lee KR, Chung SP, Park IC, et al. Effect of induced and spontaneous hypothermia on survival time of uncontrolled hemorrhagic shock rat model. Yonsei Med J 2002;43:511–7.
117. Resnick DK, Marion DW, Darby JM. The effect of hypothermia on the incidence of delayed traumatic intracerebral hemorrhage. Neurosurgery 1994;34:252–5.
118. Roberts I, Shakur H, Afolabi A, et al. The importance of early treatment with tranexamic acid in bleeding trauma patients: an exploratory analysis of the CRASH-2 randomised controlled trial. Lancet 2011;377:1096–101, 1101.

119. Roberts I, Shakur H, Ker K, et al. Antifibrinolytic drugs for acute traumatic injury. Cochrane Database Syst Rev 2011;(1):CD004896.
120. Sorensen B, Fries D. Emerging treatment strategies for trauma-induced coagulopathy. Br J Surg 2012;1(Suppl 99):40–50.
121. Perel P, Prieto-Merino D, Shakur H, et al. Predicting early death in patients with traumatic bleeding: development and validation of prognostic model. BMJ 2012;345:e5166.
122. Torossian A, Ruehlmann S, Middeke M, et al. Mild preseptic hypothermia is detrimental in rats. Crit Care Med 2004;32:1899–903.
123. Hashiguchi N, Shiozaki T, Ogura H, et al. Mild hypothermia reduces expression of heat shock protein 60 in leukocytes from severely head-injured patients. J Trauma 2003;55:1054–60.
124. Gregory JS, Flancbaum L, Townsend MC, et al. Incidence and timing of hypothermia in trauma patients undergoing operations. J Trauma 1991;31:795–8.
125. Little RA, Stoner HB. Body temperature after accidental injury. Br J Surg 1981;68:221–4.
126. Bernabei AF, Levison MA, Bender JS. The effects of hypothermia and injury severity on blood loss during trauma laparotomy. J Trauma 1992;33:835–9.
127. Jurkovich GJ, Greiser WB, Luterman A, et al. Hypothermia in trauma victims: an ominous predictor of survival. J Trauma 1987;27:1019–24.
128. Luna GK, Maier RV, Pavlin EG, et al. Incidence and effect of hypothermia in seriously injured patients. J Trauma 1987;27:1014–8.
129. Martin RS, Kilgo PD, Miller PR, et al. Injury-associated hypothermia: an analysis of the 2004 National Trauma Data Bank. Shock 2005;24:114–8.
130. Shafi S, Elliott AC, Gentilello L. Is hypothermia simply a marker of shock and injury severity or an independent risk factor for mortality in trauma patients? Analysis of a large national trauma registry. J Trauma 2005;59:1081–5.
131. Wang HE, Callaway CW, Peitzman AB, et al. Admission hypothermia and outcome after major trauma. Crit Care Med 2005;33:1296–301.
132. Gentilello LM, Jurkovich GJ, Stark MS, et al. Is hypothermia in the victim of major trauma protective or harmful? A randomized, prospective study. Ann Surg 1997;226:439–47.
133. Clifton GL, Miller ER, Choi SC, et al. Lack of effect of induction of hypothermia after acute brain injury. N Engl J Med 2001;344:556–63.
134. Shiozaki T, Hayakata T, Taneda M, et al. A multicenter prospective randomized controlled trial of the efficacy of mild hypothermia for severely head injured patients with low intracranial pressure. Mild Hypothermia Study Group in Japan. J Neurosurg 2001;94:50–4.
135. Henderson WR, Dhingra VK, Chittock DR, et al. Hypothermia in the management of traumatic brain injury. A systematic review and meta-analysis. Intensive Care Med 2003;29:1637–44.
136. McIntyre LA, Fergusson DA, Hebert PC, et al. Prolonged therapeutic hypothermia after traumatic brain injury in adults: a systematic review. JAMA 2003;289:2992–9.
137. Sydenham E, Roberts I, Alderson P. Hypothermia for traumatic head injury. Cochrane Database Syst Rev 2009;(2):CD001048.
138. Fox JL, Vu EN, Doyle-Waters M, et al. Prophylactic hypothermia for traumatic brain injury: a quantitative systematic review. CJEM 2010;12:355–64.
139. Polderman KH, Tjong Tjin JR, Peerdeman SM, et al. Effects of therapeutic hypothermia on intracranial pressure and outcome in patients with severe head injury. Intensive Care Med 2002;28:1563–73.

140. Jiang JY, Xu W, Li WP, et al. Effect of long-term mild hypothermia or short-term mild hypothermia on outcome of patients with severe traumatic brain injury. J Cereb Blood Flow Metab 2006;26:771–6.
141. Zhi D, Zhang S, Lin X. Study on therapeutic mechanism and clinical effect of mild hypothermia in patients with severe head injury. Surg Neurol 2003;59: 381–5.
142. Clifton GL, Valadka A, Zygun D, et al. Very early hypothermia induction in patients with severe brain injury (the National Acute Brain Injury Study: Hypothermia II): a randomised trial. Lancet Neurol 2011;10:131–9.

Nonsurgical Techniques to Control Massive Bleeding

Christian Zentai, MD[a,*], Oliver Grottke, MD, PhD, MPH[a], Donat R. Spahn, MD, FRCA[b], Rolf Rossaint, MD[a]

KEYWORDS

• Trauma • Shock • Traumatic hemorrhage • Embolization • Angiography • Hemostatic therapy • Coagulation factors

KEY POINTS

- Despite new therapeutic approaches to prevent and overcome trauma-associated coagulopathy, morbidity and mortality remain unacceptably high.
- Studies from recent years have shown that coagulation factors and factor concentrates may be useful for reducing the need for fresh frozen plasma, platelet, and red blood cell transfusions.
- It is necessary to identify the cause of the coagulation deficiency to tailor the therapy for terminating coagulopathy using coagulation factor concentrates to each patient's specific needs. Further research and randomized controlled trials are urgently needed to better understand and develop clear strategies to overcome coagulopathy.

C.Z. and O.G. equally contributed to this article.
Conflict of interest: Statement CZ declares no conflict of interest. RR received lecture and consulting fees as well as financial support of research projects from Novo Nordisk, CSL Behring and Bayer Healthcare. OG received lecture and financial support of research projects from CSL Behring, Bayer Healthcare, Nycomed, Biotest and Novo Nordisk. DRS's academic department is receiving grant support from the Swiss National Science Foundation, Berne, Switzerland (grant numbers: 33CM30_124117 and 406440-131268), the Swiss Society of Anesthesiology and Reanimation (SGAR), Berne, Switzerland (no grant numbers are attributed), the Swiss Foundation for Anesthesia Research, Zurich, Switzerland (no grant numbers are attributed), Bundesprogramm Chancengleichheit, Berne, Switzerland (no grant numbers are attributed), CSL Behring, Berne, Switzerland (no grant numbers are attributed), Vifor, Villars-sur-Glâne, Switzerland (no grant numbers are attributed). DRS was the chairman of the ABC Faculty and is a member of the ABC Trauma Faculty, which are both managed by Thomson Physicians World, Mannheim, Germany and sponsored by an unrestricted educational grant from Novo Nordisk A/S, Bagsvärd, Denmark and CSL Behring, Hattersheim am Main, Germany. In the past 5 years, DRS has received honoraria or travel support for consulting or lecturing from the following companies: Abbott, Baar, Switzerland, AstraZeneca, Zug, Switzerland, Bayer (Schweiz), Zürich, Switzerland, Baxter, Roma, Italy, B. Braun Melsungen, Melsungen, Germany, Boehringer Ingelheim (Schweiz), Basel, Switzerland, Bristol-Myers-Squibb, Rueil, Malmaison, France and Baar, Switzerland, CSL Behring, Hattersheim am Main, Germany and Bern, Switzerland, Curacyte, Munich, Germany, Ethicon Biosurgery, Sommerville, New Jersey, USA, Fresenius, Bad Homburg v.d.H., Germany, Galenica, Bern, Switzerland (including Vifor, Villars-sur-Glâne, Switzerland), GlaxoSmithKline, Hamburg, Germany, Janssen-Cilag, Baar, Switzerland, Janssen-Cilag EMEA, Beerse, Belgium, Merck Sharp & Dohme-Chibret, Opfikon-Glattbrugg, Switzerland, Novo Nordisk A/S, Bagsvärd, Denmark, Octapharma, Lachen, Switzerland, Organon, Pfäffikon/SZ, Switzerland, Oxygen Biotherapeutics, Costa Mesa, CA, Pentapharm (now tem Innovations), Munich, Germany, ratiopharm Arzneimittel Vertriebs, Vienna, Austria, Roche Pharma (Schweiz), Reinach, Switzerland, Schering- Plow International, Kenilworth, New Jersey, USA, Vifor Pharma Deutschland, Munich, Germany, Vifor Pharma Österreich, Vienna, Austria, Vifor (International), St. Gallen, Switzerland.
[a] Department of Anesthesiology, RWTH Aachen University Hospital, Pauwelsstraße 30, Aachen 52074, Germany; [b] Institute of Anesthesiology, University of Zurich, Ramistraße 100, Zurich CH-8091, Switzerland
* Corresponding author.
E-mail address: czentai@ukaachen.de

Anesthesiology Clin 31 (2013) 41–53
http://dx.doi.org/10.1016/j.anclin.2012.10.005 **anesthesiology.theclinics.com**
1932-2275/13/$ – see front matter

INTRODUCTION

Trauma is responsible for most deaths worldwide and is the leading cause of death before the age of 45 years in the United States.[1] Uncontrolled bleeding still poses a major challenge and is second in the list of early overall causes of trauma-related death,[2] accounting for almost half of all trauma deaths within the first 24 hours.[3]

In recent years, significant improvements in the nonsurgical and surgical treatment of trauma patients have been made. For example, damage control surgery is aimed at increasing the survival of severely injured patients and stopping life-threatening hemorrhage. The principles of damage control surgery incorporate the choice of the appropriate type and timing of surgical procedures. The repair of minor injuries is deferred because prolonged surgical treatment might initiate or exacerbate a preexisting coagulopathy. Coagulopathy occurs early after injury,[4] is associated with a 4-fold to 5-fold increased mortality,[5–7] and is present in approximately one-fourth to one-third of trauma patients at admission to a hospital.[5,6,8] Thus, the management of bleeding in the first hours after trauma is crucial to prevent death from hemorrhage. The combination of surgery, principles of damage control, external fixation, and angiographic embolization may sufficiently arrest bleeding from vascular damage in some cases of traumatic injury. Nonsurgical approaches are urgently required to successfully manage diffuse bleeding in the presence of coagulopathy or to prevent the fortification of coagulopathy. The overarching goals are to reverse the existing coagulopathy and to regain physiologic conditions to facilitate hemostasis, and these goals require more specific treatment in most cases. The directed use of coagulation factors and factor concentrates can support the correction of coagulopathy associated with massive blood loss in severely injured patients. Trauma-induced coagulopathy is complex and therefore requires a wide-ranging approach to therapy. However, the best treatment options and their timing are still under debate. Therefore, this article considers new developments in the contemporary, nonsurgical management of critical trauma bleeding.

TOURNIQUET AND PELVIC BINDER

Studies from military settings have shown that the use of tourniquets is highly effective for controlling life-threatening arterial bleeding from mangled extremities.[9–14] Overall, the studies show a low rate of complications after the use of tourniquets.[15] To reduce the potential side effects of tourniquets, such as limb ischemia and nerve paralysis, it is advised to keep the time of tourniquet application to a minimum.[16,17] Lacking published evidence, the role of the prehospital use of tourniquets remains unclear, although positive results have been reported for certain indications, such as severe trauma from firearms and industrial machinery as well as in cases of multiple casualties with limited resources.[18]

Several circumferential pelvic binders have been introduced in recent years. Their application is fast and simple and allows a temporary and quick pelvic closure. The stabilization of pelvic fractures in the emergency department with commercial compression devices or simple bed sheets in hemodynamically unstable patients is also advised according to the advanced trauma life support guidelines.[19] Although the prehospital application of a pelvic binder as initial treatment of a diagnosed or suspected unstable pelvis (for example, after high-energy trauma) might be advantageous, few studies have shown a benefit to clinically relevant end points.[20]

ANGIOGRAPHY AND EMBOLIZATION

In addition to surgery as the cornerstone of bleeding control, transcatheter angiographic embolization (TAE) is an established, minimally invasive technique used to control arterial bleeding from solid organ injury or pelvic fracture.[21–25]

This continuously evolving technique is used to arrest posttraumatic hemorrhage from solitary organs such as the spleen[26–28] and liver.[29–33] However, the main indication for the use of embolization is the control of bleeding resulting from pelvic fractures. This technique is regarded as part of the multidisciplinary treatment of severely injured patients, and success rates of more than 90%[25,34–37] have been reported. For instance, Fangio and colleagues[38] reported a radiologic success rate of 96% in a series of 25 patients with pelvic injuries. Using this technique, hemodynamic stabilization was achieved in 84% of patients. Hagiwara and colleagues[39] documented a successful outcome after TAE in 19 patients with blunt multiple trauma who showed only a transient response to fluid resuscitation.

Hemodynamically unstable patients with pelvic fractures should be considered for pelvic angiography/embolization if nonpelvic sources of bleeding have been excluded.[40]

The Technique and its Safety

The widespread use of multidetector computed tomography scanners within the initial diagnostic testing of trauma patients can provide early evidence for arterial contrast extravasation. This finding supports the identification of injuries that require embolization regardless of the hemodynamic status of the patient. To perform angiography, arterial access has to be gained first. An abdominal flush can then be used to assess abdominal sites. This procedure is followed by a pelvic flush and more selective evaluations in the internal and external iliac arteries.[41] Using angiography, the signs of vascular injuries in need of embolization include the extravasation of injected contrast, false aneurysm, vasospasm, and arteriovenous fistula.[42,43] The embolization of large vessels (main arteries and branches) is achieved using gelatin sponges or steel coils. Smaller vessels can be embolized with particles, gelatin sponges, or microcoils. Temporary agents such as a gelatin sponge suspension can also be used for multiple arterial injuries to allow subsequent recanalization.[42] After the initial treatment, angiography should then be repeated to ensure successful occlusion and exclude new sites of bleeding or ongoing bleeding fed by collateral pathways.

In general, pelvic embolization is associated with low morbidity.[24,25,44,45] However, serious complications have been reported, including necrosis of the distal colon and ureter, uterine and bladder necrosis, perineal wound sepsis,[46] ischemic damage to the gluteal muscle,[47] and paresis.[48] Risks should be considered if angiographic embolization is an option for the treatment of the patient, and the likelihood of nontarget embolization has to be minimized by assiduously performing the procedure and using (super-) selective techniques whenever feasible. The success of angiographic embolization highly depends on the experience with this technique. Furthermore, not all trauma centers can provide emergency angiographic diagnostic and treatment facilities that operate day and night.

Timing and Management

Delayed intervention (>3 hours) increases mortality from 14% to 75%.[34] Angiography and embolization should be conducted early after admission in hemodynamically unstable patients with ongoing or suspected bleeding.[41] However, the most beneficial sequence of angiographic embolization for controlling bleeding relative to surgical interventions is controversial.[49,50] For the early detection of the main source of hemorrhage, the best sequence is dependent on the individual patient. Whereas bleeding from veins, smaller arteries, and cancellous bone may be effectively controlled by external fixation, arterial bleeding may be successfully treated using surgery or angiographic embolization. Each of these therapeutic options is primarily concerned with a different site of bleeding. At best, the initial treatment should address the predominant source of bleeding and determine whether it is arterial or venous. In several studies, angiography detected arterial lesions in 44% to 76% of patients.[24,25,34,49–53] A retrospective case series of bleeding pelvic fractures identified positive angiographic findings in 73% of patients who remained hypotensive despite resuscitation.[49] The investigators concluded that an adequate response to resuscitation makes arterial bleeding unlikely. Furthermore, the investigators found arterial bleeding amenable to embolization in 7 of 16 patients (44%) who underwent external fixation before angiography. In these cases, treatment might have been delayed.[49] A retrospective multicenter study including 217 patients showed the need for TAE in 23 of 24 patients (96%) with severe injuries that could not be controlled by various surgical interventions.[50] The investigators concluded that nontherapeutic laparotomy should be avoided.

To determine the best sequence of management, several investigators have studied the underlying pattern of pelvic fractures according to the Young-Burgess classification to predict the potential requirement for acute embolization.[52,54,55] Eastridge and colleagues[52] retrospectively analyzed 86 patients with pelvic fractures (40 stable, 46 unstable) who presented in shock with an ongoing resuscitative requirement. Patients with unstable fractures undergoing laparotomy before angiography had a higher mortality (60% vs 25%). These findings suggest that angiography should be considered before laparotomy in patients with unstable fracture patterns.[52] In contrast, a study performed by Sarin and colleagues[54] including 283 patients with pelvic fracture and a systolic blood pressure 90 mm Hg or less at admission did not show a correlation between the fracture pattern, the order of embolization, external fixation, or laparotomy and the outcome. Accordingly, no correlation was found between specific fracture classes, outcome variables, and the need for early angiography.[55] A more recent prospective observational study identified the presence of sacroiliac joint disruption, female gender, and the duration of hypotension as reliable and simple risk factors to predict the need for therapeutic TAE.[56]

Typically, angiographic embolization is performed in a specialized angiography suite. The spatial distance between the emergency department, the angiography suite, and the operation theater requires the transport of a potentially hemodynamically unstable patient. To address this problem, an intra-aortic balloon occlusion procedure for hemodynamically unstable patients has been described.[57] Morozumi and colleagues[58] reported the use of mobile angiography and embolization in the emergency department to improve resuscitation intervals. C-arm digital subtraction angiography may also be used to perform emergency angiographic embolization in the operating theater.[45] This procedure enables the simultaneous surgical treatment of extrapelvic injuries if the institutional concepts are defined and logistical problems are solved.

Therefore, in most institutions, it is necessary to determine which treatment should be performed first. Nonetheless, it is generally agreed that the optimal resuscitation of these severely injured patients requires a multidisciplinary approach. Further clinical studies are needed to aid clinical decision making and refine the optimal timing of embolization relative to surgical bleeding control.

COAGULOPATHY AFTER TRAUMA

Life-threatening bleeding in polytraumatized patients is typically caused by a combination of traumatic injury and coagulopathy. Several mechanisms contributing to trauma-induced coagulopathy have been described (**Box 1**).[59] Immediately after trauma, shock and tissue hypoperfusion can cause metabolic changes affecting the initiation of coagulation.[60] Tissue hypoperfusion also leads to increased concentrations of activated protein C and thrombomodulin. The activation of this pathway overstimulates anticoagulation with a downregulation of thrombin generation.[4] Coagulopathy is further aggravated by hypothermia, anemia, low concentrations of calcium, acidosis, and the dilution and loss of coagulation factors.[61] To restore the coagulation system, fresh frozen plasma (FFP), cryoprecipitate, platelets, and coagulation factor concentrates are used. There are well-known drawbacks to the use of FFP,[62] including the induction of transfusion-related acute lung injury, transfusion-associated circulatory overload, and multiorgan failure.[63] In recent years, there has been a shift from empiric coagulation therapy toward an early targeted therapy using thromboelastometry and a more intense replacement of coagulation factors using recombinant and lyophilized coagulation factors. The application of recombinant and plasma-derived coagulation factor concentrates is argued by their immediate availability, decreased volume, rapid administration, and good viral safety.

BLOOD COMPONENT REPLACEMENT THERAPY

Antifibrinolytics

Antifibrinolytic agents include the serine protease inhibitor aprotinin, the synthetic lysine analogue e-aminocaproic acid and tranexamic acid.[64] The antifibrinolytic mechanism of the lysine analogues is mediated by competitive binding to the lysine binding site of the fibrin clot. Thereby, they block the binding of plasminogen to tissue plasminogen activator. This process hampers the conversion of plasminogen to plasmin and the subsequent plasmin-mediated fibrinolysis. In a large randomized study, the CRASH-2 (Clinical Randomisation of an Antifibrinolytic in Significant Haemorrhage 2) trial investigated the impact of tranexamic acid in 20,211 patients (admitted to 274 hospitals in 40 different countries) with major trauma who had or were at risk of severe hemorrhage.[65] Within 8 hours of injury, patients were treated with either tranexamic acid (1 g over 10 minutes followed by an additional 1 g over 8 hours) or with placebo. Overall, treatment with tranexamic acid decreased the rate of mortality and the risk of death as a result of hemorrhage. In addition, it was shown that early tranexamic acid treatment (within 1 hour) reduced the rate of death as a result of

Box 1
The factors contributing to trauma-induced coagulopathy are multifactorial and interrelated

- Loss and consumption of coagulation factors
- Shock-induced activation of the protein-C pathway
- Hyperfibrinolysis
- Dilution of coagulation factors
- Anemia and low platelet counts
- Metabolic changes (acidosis)
- Hypothermia
- Hypocalcemia

bleeding compared with its late application (1–3 hours).[66] A nested control study also showed that patients with traumatic brain injury showed a decrease in the mean intracranial size of hemorrhage.[67] Overall, treatment with tranexamic acid did not result in major adverse or thrombotic complications. Even before the results of these studies were published, the European guidelines for the management of bleeding recommended considering the use of tranexamic acid in bleeding trauma patients.[68] Based on the findings of the CRASH-2 trial, it is likely that the early administration of antifibrinolytic treatment using tranexamic acid will be recommended as a first-line treatment of established or suspected hyperfibrinolysis in patients presenting with major blood loss after trauma.

Fibrinogen

In normal plasma, fibrinogen is one of the most abundant coagulation factors with a concentration of 150 to 400 mg/dL. On dilution, fibrinogen is the first factor to reach critically low concentrations, as shown by Hiippala and colleagues.[69] Similarly, in severely injured patients with massive bleeding, fibrinogen typically reaches critical concentrations at an early stage. Next to the loss and consumption of fibrinogen after trauma, hyperfibrinolysis, hypothermia, and acidosis may further compromise the fibrinogen concentration.[70] Experimental data from animal studies and in vitro studies have shown that the application of exogenous fibrinogen increases clot firmness and reduces blood loss after blunt liver injury.[71–74] Several retrospective and prospective clinical studies performed in an array of clinical areas have shown that fibrinogen levels less than 150 to 200 mg/dL enhance the risk of perioperative and postoperative hemorrhage tendency.[75,76] In patients with postpartum hemorrhage, the fibrinogen level has also been shown to predict the severity of hemorrhage.[77] Evidence supporting the administration of fibrinogen to traumatized patients is derived from a retrospective study including 252 seriously injured soldiers and civilians who received a massive transfusion (defined as >10 units of red blood cells [RBC] in 24 hours).[78] The analysis of these data showed that the strategy of increasing the fibrinogen/RBC ratio was independently associated with improved survival to hospital discharge, primarily by decreasing death from hemorrhage. Despite the current evidence showing that the early use of fibrinogen concentrate exerts a protective effect against blood loss in severely bleeding patients, no prospective confirmatory data in traumatized patients are available. In addition, the critical threshold value is a matter of debate. Recent international recommendations suggest that the trigger of 100 mg/dL may be too low and that fibrinogen concentrations of 150 to 200 mg/dL may be appropriate.[68]

FFP, cryoprecipitate, and fibrinogen may be used to restore low concentrations of fibrinogen. However, large volumes of FFP are needed to efficiently resolve low levels of fibrinogen. Compared with FFP, the concentration of fibrinogen in fibrinogen concentrates is approximately 10-fold higher. As an alternative, cryoprecipitate containing factor VIII, fibrinogen, fibronectin, Von Willebrand factor, and factor XIII may be used.[79] A dose of approximately 10 single bags of cryoprecipitate derived from units of whole blood typically increases the plasma fibrinogen level by up to 60 to 100 mg/dL. However, because of the risk of blood-borne pathogen transmission, the use of cryoprecipitate for this indication should be considered with caution. Compared with FFP and cryoprecipitate, pasteurized fibrinogen is virus inactivated and has had a good overall safety profile.

Prothrombin Complex Concentrate

Prothrombin complex concentrates (PCCs) are concentrates of the vitamin K-dependent clotting factors (II, VII, IX, and X). Although PCCs with low amounts of factor VII are available (3-factor PCCs), PCCs containing higher concentrations of factor VII (4-factor PCCs) are more commonly used in Europe for the acute reversal of vitamin K antagonists. PCCs may also contain heparin, proteins C, S, and Z, and antithrombin, and the levels of these constituents differ markedly between PCCs.[80] The indications for the use of PCC are a fast reversal of oral anticoagulation with warfarin or a known deficiency of the vitamin K-dependent factors in potentially life-threatening bleeding.[81] The substitution should be supplemented by intravenous vitamin K to induce the endogenous synthesis of vitamin K-dependent factors. Because PCCs are highly efficacious thrombin generators, there is a growing interest in their use in trauma-related coagulopathy with multifactor deficiencies. Nevertheless, no prospective studies have investigated the use of PCC as a first-line monosubstance therapy for trauma-related coagulopathy. All evidence supporting the use of PCCs in trauma-related coagulopathy has been provided by observational and animal studies.[82–88] The results of these animal studies show that the application of PCC reduces blood loss, shortens bleeding time, and enhances thrombin generation. However, one animal study also showed that high concentrations of PCC increased the risk of thrombosis and disseminated intravascular coagulation.[83] This finding was attributed to an imbalance of procoagulatory and anticoagulatory proteins.

In addition to these experimental studies, three observational studies investigated the use of PCC as part of coagulation therapy in different surgical areas. Although the results also imply that PCC may effectively terminate severe bleeding, the evidence is limited by the retrospective design of the studies and the small number of patients.

For instance, a retrospective analysis investigated the efficacy of PCC in patients with severe bleeding not related to coumadin.[87] The data were mainly obtained from patients undergoing different surgical interventions, and PCC was administered at a median dose of 2000 IU. A coagulation analysis revealed a significant reduction in international normalized ratio after PCC infusion that was associated with bleeding termination in 36% of patients with surgical bleeding and in 96% of patients with signs of diffuse bleeding. However, 32% of patients received FFP before PCC was administered, and 29% of patients received FFP after PCC. Another observational trial investigated the effects of fibrinogen and PCC in trauma patients using a thromboelastometry-guided algorithm[88]; 77% of patients received fibrinogen followed by PCC infusion. PCC was administered at a median dose of 1800 IU to patients with prolonged clot initiation. This therapeutic approach significantly decreased mortality compared with that predicted by the trauma injury severity score. PCC may be useful for correcting trauma-induced coagulopathy, but given the lack of clinical safety data for PCCs for trauma-associated coagulopathy, clinical studies, particularly in patients with comorbidities, are needed to optimize dosing and ascertain the safety of PCCs for the treatment of severely injured patients.

Activated Recombinant Factor VII

The current understanding of hemostasis according to the cell-based model attributes a pivotal role of factor VII to coagulation. Eptacog alfa (activated recombinant factor VII [rFVIIa]) is structurally almost identical to endogenous FVIIa and is produced through recombination by baby hamster kidney cell lines. rFVIIa binds to thrombin-activated platelets in supraphysiologic doses, leading to the activation of factor X and prothrombin (thrombin burst).[89] Through enhanced thrombin generation, platelet activation and platelet adhesion are greatly increased.[90] Therapy with rFVIIa is licensed for the treatment of patients with hemophilia, inhibitory antibodies, and Glanzmann thrombasthenia.[91] rFVIIa has gained popularity as an adjunct for the treatment of coagulopathy in a wide array of clinical conditions with serious or life-threatening bleeding. The number of case reports and case series documenting the successful off-label use of rFVIIa as a last resort to terminate uncontrollable bleeding has steadily grown.[92] The results from a multicenter phase II randomized controlled trial (RCT), stratifying for severe blunt and penetrating trauma, showed a significant reduction in the primary end points (ie, RBC units transfused and the need for massive transfusion) in patients with blunt trauma who survived for more than 48 hours after rFVIIa treatment.[93] The need for massive transfusion was reduced by nearly 20%. Another multicenter phase III trial (CONTROL) was stopped after an analysis predicted the low likelihood of reaching a successful outcome in the primary end points (mortality and morbidity).[94] Because rFVIIa is a potent hemostatic agent, there is concern that its use may increase the risk for adverse events, particularly in patients with known risk factors for thromboembolic disease or a history of thrombosis. According to a report from the US Food and Drug Administration, 168 of 431 reports of approved and off-label uses of rFVIIa described 185 thromboembolic events between 1999 and 2004; 90% of the reports accounted for the off-label use of rFVIIa, and in part, these adverse events resulted in serious morbidity and mortality.[95] However, in 38% of these reports, a concomitant hemostatic medication was documented. A large and comprehensive study systematically analyzed data from 35 RCTs including 4468 subjects.[96] rFVIIa was administered to treat or prevent bleeding. The investigators found increased rates of arterial thromboembolic events among those who were treated with rFVIIa compared with placebo (5.5% vs 3.2%, respectively; $P = .003$), particularly in the elderly population. In contrast, Dutton and colleagues[97] did not find an association between the administration of rFVIIa to trauma patients for active hemorrhagic shock and thromboembolic events. However, the European Medicines Agency (EMEA) has advised that rFVIIa should not be administered outside the approved indications. Therefore, rFVIIa should be considered as a final rescue therapy attempt if first-line treatment with a combination of surgical approaches and best-practice use of blood products fails to control bleeding. To enhance rFVIIa efficacy, normothermia, hematocrit level greater than 24%, platelet count greater than 50,000/μL, pH 7.2 or greater, and fibrinogen 150 to 200 mg/dL or greater should be targeted.[68]

SUMMARY

Despite new therapeutic approaches to prevent and overcome trauma-associated coagulopathy, morbidity and mortality remain unacceptably high. However, the use of new nonsurgical techniques in addition to traditional surgical procedures may help rapidly stop hemorrhage and exsanguination. Studies from recent years have shown that coagulation factors and factor concentrates may be useful for reducing the need for FFP, platelet, and RBC transfusions. It is necessary to identify the cause of the coagulation deficiency to tailor the therapy for terminating coagulopathy using coagulation factor concentrates to each patient's specific needs. Further research and RCTs are urgently needed to better understand and develop clear strategies to overcome coagulopathy.

REFERENCES

1. Centers for Disease Control and Prevention, National Center for Injury Prevention and Control. Web-based Injury Statistics Query and Reporting System (WISQARS). 2007. Available at: http://www.cdc.gov/injury/wisqars. Accessed October 21, 2012.
2. Pfeifer R, Tarkin IS, Rocos B, et al. Patterns of mortality and causes of death in polytrauma patients–has anything changed? Injury 2009;40(9):907–11.

3. Kauvar DS, Lefering R, Wade CE. Impact of hemorrhage on trauma outcome: an overview of epidemiology, clinical presentations, and therapeutic considerations. J Trauma 2006;60(Suppl 6):S3–11.
4. Brohi K, Cohen MJ, Ganter MT, et al. Acute coagulopathy of trauma: hypoperfusion induces systemic anticoagulation and hyperfibrinolysis. J Trauma 2008; 64(5):1211–7 [discussion: 7].
5. Brohi K, Singh J, Heron M, et al. Acute traumatic coagulopathy. J Trauma 2003; 54(6):1127–30.
6. MacLeod JB, Lynn M, McKenney MG, et al. Early coagulopathy predicts mortality in trauma. J Trauma 2003;55(1):39–44.
7. Maegele M, Lefering R, Yucel N, et al. Early coagulopathy in multiple injury: an analysis from the German Trauma Registry on 8724 patients. Injury 2007;38(3):298–304.
8. Nystrup KB, Windelov NA, Thomsen AB, et al. Reduced clot strength upon admission, evaluated by thrombelastography (TEG), in trauma patients is independently associated with increased 30-day mortality. Scand J Trauma Resusc Emerg Med 2011;19(1):52.
9. Lakstein D, Blumenfeld A, Sokolov T, et al. Tourniquets for hemorrhage control on the battlefield: a 4-year accumulated experience. J Trauma 2003;54(Suppl 5): S221–5.
10. Beekley AC, Sebesta JA, Blackbourne LH, et al. Prehospital tourniquet use in Operation Iraqi Freedom: effect on hemorrhage control and outcomes. J Trauma 2008;64(Suppl 2):S28–37 [discussion: S37].
11. Brodie S, Hodgetts TJ, Ollerton J, et al. Tourniquet use in combat trauma: U.K. military experience. J Spec Oper Med 2009;9(1):74–7.
12. Kragh JF Jr, Littrel ML, Jones JA, et al. Battle casualty survival with emergency tourniquet use to stop limb bleeding. J Emerg Med 2011;41(6):590–7.
13. Kragh JF Jr, Walters TJ, Baer DG, et al. Survival with emergency tourniquet use to stop bleeding in major limb trauma. Ann Surg 2009;249(1):1–7.
14. Swan KG Jr, Wright DS, Barbagiovanni SS, et al. Tourniquets revisited. J Trauma 2009;66(3):672–5.
15. Kragh JF Jr, O'Neill ML, Walters TJ, et al. Minor morbidity with emergency tourniquet use to stop bleeding in severe limb trauma: research, history, and reconciling advocates and abolitionists. Mil Med 2011;176(7):817–23.
16. Clasper JC, Brown KV, Hill P. Limb complications following pre-hospital tourniquet use. J R Army Med Corps 2009;155(3):200–2.
17. Dayan L, Zinmann C, Stahl S, et al. Complications associated with prolonged tourniquet application on the battlefield. Mil Med 2008;173(1):63–6.
18. Lee C, Porter KM, Hodgetts TJ. Tourniquet use in the civilian prehospital setting. Emerg Med J 2007;24(8):584–7.
19. Kortbeek JB, Al Turki SA, Ali J, et al. Advanced trauma life support, 8th edition, the evidence for change. J Trauma 2008;64(6):1638–50.
20. National Association of Emergency Medical Technicians (US), Pre-Hospital Trauma Life Support Committee, American College of Surgeons, Committee on Trauma. PHTLS: prehospital trauma life support. 7th edition. St Louis (MO): Mosby Jems/Elsevier; 2011.
21. Bauer JR, Ray CE. Transcatheter arterial embolization in the trauma patient: a review. Semin Intervent Radiol 2004;21(1):11–22.
22. Panetta T, Sclafani SJ, Goldstein AS, et al. Percutaneous transcatheter embolization for massive bleeding from pelvic fractures. J Trauma 1985;25(11):1021–9.
23. Geeraerts T, Chhor V, Cheisson G, et al. Clinical review: initial management of blunt pelvic trauma patients with haemodynamic instability. Crit Care 2007;11(1):204.

24. Velmahos GC, Chahwan S, Falabella A, et al. Angiographic embolization for intraperitoneal and retroperitoneal injuries. World J Surg 2000;24(5):539–45.
25. Velmahos GC, Toutouzas KG, Vassiliu P, et al. A prospective study on the safety and efficacy of angiographic embolization for pelvic and visceral injuries. J Trauma 2002;53(2):303–8 [discussion: 8].
26. Hagiwara A, Yukioka T, Ohta S, et al. Nonsurgical management of patients with blunt splenic injury: efficacy of transcatheter arterial embolization. AJR Am J Roentgenol 1996;167(1):159–66.
27. Haan J, Scott J, Boyd-Kranis RL, et al. Admission angiography for blunt splenic injury: advantages and pitfalls. J Trauma 2001;51(6):1161–5.
28. Shanmuganathan K, Mirvis SE, Boyd-Kranis R, et al. Nonsurgical management of blunt splenic injury: use of CT criteria to select patients for splenic arteriography and potential endovascular therapy. Radiology 2000;217(1):75–82.
29. Greco L, Francioso G, Pratichizzo A, et al. Arterial embolization in the treatment of severe blunt hepatic trauma. Hepatogastroenterology 2003;50(51):746–9.
30. Kanakis MA, Thomas T, Martinakis VG, et al. Successful management of severe blunt hepatic trauma by angiographic embolization. Updates Surg 2011. Available at: http://link.springer.com/article/10.1007/s13304-011-0122-3/fulltext.html. Accessed November 10, 2011.
31. Letoublon C, Morra I, Chen Y, et al. Hepatic arterial embolization in the management of blunt hepatic trauma: indications and complications. J Trauma 2011; 70(5):1032–6 [discussion: 1036–7].
32. Monnin V, Sengel C, Thony F, et al. Place of arterial embolization in severe blunt hepatic trauma: a multidisciplinary approach. Cardiovasc Intervent Radiol 2008; 31(5):875–82.
33. Wang YC, Fu CY, Chen YF, et al. Role of arterial embolization on blunt hepatic trauma patients with type I contrast extravasation. Am J Emerg Med 2011; 29(9):1147–51.
34. Agolini SF, Shah K, Jaffe J, et al. Arterial embolization is a rapid and effective technique for controlling pelvic fracture hemorrhage. J Trauma 1997;43(3):395–9.
35. Wong YC, Wang LJ, Ng CJ, et al. Mortality after successful transcatheter arterial embolization in patients with unstable pelvic fractures: rate of blood transfusion as a predictive factor. J Trauma 2000;49(1):71–5.
36. Shapiro M, McDonald AA, Knight D, et al. The role of repeat angiography in the management of pelvic fractures. J Trauma 2005;58(2):227–31.
37. O'Neill PA, Riina J, Sclafani S, et al. Angiographic findings in pelvic fractures. Clin Orthop Relat Res 1996;329:60–7.
38. Fangio P, Asehnoune K, Edouard A, et al. Early embolization and vasopressor administration for management of life-threatening hemorrhage from pelvic fracture. J Trauma 2005;58(5):978–84 [discussion: 84].
39. Hagiwara A, Murata A, Matsuda T, et al. The usefulness of transcatheter arterial embolization for patients with blunt polytrauma showing transient response to fluid resuscitation. J Trauma 2004;57(2):271–6 [discussion: 276–7].
40. Cullinane DC, Schiller HJ, Zielinski MD, et al. Eastern Association for the Surgery of Trauma practice management guidelines for hemorrhage in pelvic fracture–update and systematic review. J Trauma 2011;71(6):1850–68.
41. Heetveld MJ, Harris I, Schlaphoff G, et al. Guidelines for the management of haemodynamically unstable pelvic fracture patients. ANZ J Surg 2004;74(7): 520–9.
42. Lopera JE. Embolization in trauma: principles and techniques. Semin Intervent Radiol 2010;27(1):14–28.

43. Tanizaki S, Maeda S, Hayashi H, et al. Early embolization without external fixation in pelvic trauma. Am J Emerg Med 2012;30(2):342–6.
44. Vassiliu P, Sava J, Toutouzas KG, et al. Is contrast as bad as we think? Renal function after angiographic embolization of injured patients. J Am Coll Surg 2002; 194(2):142–6.
45. Teo LT, Punamiya S, Chai CY, et al. Emergency angio-embolisation in the operating theatre for trauma patients using the C-Arm digital subtraction angiography. Injury 2012;43(9):1492–6.
46. Perez JV, Hughes TM, Bowers K. Angiographic embolisation in pelvic fracture. Injury 1998;29(3):187–91.
47. Yasumura K, Ikegami K, Kamohara T, et al. High incidence of ischemic necrosis of the gluteal muscle after transcatheter angiographic embolization for severe pelvic fracture. J Trauma 2005;58(5):985–90.
48. Hare WS, Holland CJ. Paresis following internal iliac artery embolization. Radiology 1983;146(1):47–51.
49. Miller PR, Moore PS, Mansell E, et al. External fixation or arteriogram in bleeding pelvic fracture: initial therapy guided by markers of arterial hemorrhage. J Trauma 2003;54(3):437–43.
50. Verbeek D, Sugrue M, Balogh Z, et al. Acute management of hemodynamically unstable pelvic trauma patients: time for a change? Multicenter review of recent practice. World J Surg 2008;32(8):1874–82.
51. Hamill J, Holden A, Paice R, et al. Pelvic fracture pattern predicts pelvic arterial haemorrhage. Aust N Z J Surg 2000;70(5):338–43.
52. Eastridge BJ, Starr A, Minei JP, et al. The importance of fracture pattern in guiding therapeutic decision-making in patients with hemorrhagic shock and pelvic ring disruptions. J Trauma 2002;53(3):446–50 [discussion: 450–1].
53. Biffl WL, Smith WR, Moore EE, et al. Evolution of a multidisciplinary clinical pathway for the management of unstable patients with pelvic fractures. Ann Surg 2001;233(6):843–50.
54. Sarin EL, Moore JB, Moore EE, et al. Pelvic fracture pattern does not always predict the need for urgent embolization. J Trauma 2005;58(5):973–7.
55. Starr AJ, Griffin DR, Reinert CM, et al. Pelvic ring disruptions: prediction of associated injuries, transfusion requirement, pelvic arteriography, complications, and mortality. J Orthop Trauma 2002;16(8):553–61.
56. Salim A, Teixeira PG, DuBose J, et al. Predictors of positive angiography in pelvic fractures: a prospective study. J Am Coll Surg 2008;207(5):656–62.
57. Martinelli T, Thony F, Declety P, et al. Intra-aortic balloon occlusion to salvage patients with life-threatening hemorrhagic shocks from pelvic fractures. J Trauma 2010;68(4):942–8.
58. Morozumi J, Homma H, Ohta S, et al. Impact of mobile angiography in the emergency department for controlling pelvic fracture hemorrhage with hemodynamic instability. J Trauma 2010;68(1):90–5.
59. Hess JR, Brohi K, Dutton RP, et al. The coagulopathy of trauma: a review of mechanisms. J Trauma 2008;65(4):748–54.
60. Lier H, Krep H, Schroeder S, et al. Preconditions of hemostasis in trauma: a review. The influence of acidosis, hypocalcemia, anemia, and hypothermia on functional hemostasis in trauma. J Trauma 2008;65(4):951–60.
61. Grottke O, Henzler D, Rossaint R. Use of blood and blood products in trauma. Best Pract Res Clin Anaesthesiol 2007;21(2):257–70.
62. Stanworth SJ, Hyde CJ, Murphy MF. Evidence for indications of fresh frozen plasma. Transfus Clin Biol 2007;14(6):551–6.

63. Sokolovic M, Pastores SM. Transfusion therapy and acute lung injury. Expert Rev Respir Med 2010;4(3):387–93.
64. Mannucci PM, Levi M. Prevention and treatment of major blood loss. N Engl J Med 2007;356(22):2301–11.
65. Shakur H, Roberts I, Bautista R, et al. Effects of tranexamic acid on death, vascular occlusive events, and blood transfusion in trauma patients with significant haemorrhage (CRASH-2): a randomised, placebo-controlled trial. Lancet 2010;376(9734):23–32.
66. Roberts I, Shakur H, Afolabi A, et al. The importance of early treatment with tranexamic acid in bleeding trauma patients: an exploratory analysis of the CRASH-2 randomised controlled trial. Lancet 2011;377(9771):1096–101, 1101.e1–2.
67. CRASH-2 Collaborators, Intracranial Bleeding Study. Effect of tranexamic acid in traumatic brain injury: a nested randomised, placebo controlled trial (CRASH-2 Intracranial Bleeding Study). BMJ 2011;343:d3795.
68. Rossaint R, Bouillon B, Cerny V, et al. Management of bleeding following major trauma: an updated European guideline. Crit Care 2010;14(2):R52.
69. Hiippala ST, Myllyla GJ, Vahtera EM. Hemostatic factors and replacement of major blood loss with plasma-poor red cell concentrates. Anesth Analg 1995; 81(2):360–5.
70. Fries D, Martini WZ. Role of fibrinogen in trauma-induced coagulopathy. Br J Anaesth 2010;105(2):116–21.
71. Fries D, Krismer A, Klingler A, et al. Effect of fibrinogen on reversal of dilutional coagulopathy: a porcine model. Br J Anaesth 2005;95(2):172–7.
72. Grottke O, Braunschweig T, Henzler D, et al. Effects of different fibrinogen concentrations on blood loss and coagulation parameters in a pig model of coagulopathy with blunt liver injury. Crit Care 2010;14(2):R62.
73. Fenger-Eriksen C, Anker-Moller E, Heslop J, et al. Thrombelastographic whole blood clot formation after ex vivo addition of plasma substitutes: improvements of the induced coagulopathy with fibrinogen concentrate. Br J Anaesth 2005; 94(3):324–9.
74. Fenger-Eriksen C, Tonnesen E, Ingerslev J, et al. Mechanisms of hydroxyethyl starch-induced dilutional coagulopathy. J Thromb Haemost 2009;7(7):1099–105.
75. Gerlach R, Tolle F, Raabe A, et al. Increased risk for postoperative hemorrhage after intracranial surgery in patients with decreased factor XIII activity: implications of a prospective study. Stroke 2002;33(6):1618–23.
76. Blome M, Isgro F, Kiessling AH, et al. Relationship between factor XIII activity, fibrinogen, haemostasis screening tests and postoperative bleeding in cardiopulmonary bypass surgery. Thromb Haemost 2005;93(6):1101–7.
77. Charbit B, Mandelbrot L, Samain E, et al. The decrease of fibrinogen is an early predictor of the severity of postpartum hemorrhage. J Thromb Haemost 2007; 5(2):266–73.
78. Stinger HK, Spinella PC, Perkins JG, et al. The ratio of fibrinogen to red cells transfused affects survival in casualties receiving massive transfusions at an army combat support hospital. J Trauma 2008;64(Suppl 2):S79–85 [discussion: S85].
79. Callum JL, Karkouti K, Lin Y. Cryoprecipitate: the current state of knowledge. Transfus Med Rev 2009;23(3):177–88.
80. Kalina U, Bickhard H, Schulte S. Biochemical comparison of seven commercially available prothrombin complex concentrates. Int J Clin Pract 2008;62(10):1614–22.
81. Colomina MJ, Diez Lobo A, Garutti I, et al. Perioperative use of prothrombin complex concentrates. Minerva Anestesiol 2012;78(3):358–68.

82. Honickel M, Rieg A, Rossaint R, et al. Prothrombin complex concentrate reduces blood loss and enhances thrombin generation in a pig model with blunt liver injury under severe hypothermia. Thromb Haemost 2011;106(4):724–33.
83. Grottke O, Braunschweig T, Spronk HM, et al. Increasing concentrations of prothrombin complex concentrate induce disseminated intravascular coagulation in a pig model of coagulopathy with blunt liver injury. Blood 2011;118(7):1943–51.
84. Dickneite G, Pragst I. Prothrombin complex concentrate vs fresh frozen plasma for reversal of dilutional coagulopathy in a porcine trauma model. Br J Anaesth 2009;102(3):345–54.
85. Dickneite G, Doerr B, Kaspereit F. Characterization of the coagulation deficit in porcine dilutional coagulopathy and substitution with a prothrombin complex concentrate. Anesth Analg 2008;106(4):1070–7 [table of contents].
86. Bruce D, Nokes TJ. Prothrombin complex concentrate (Beriplex P/N) in severe bleeding: experience in a large tertiary hospital. Crit Care 2008;12(4):R105.
87. Schick KS, Fertmann JM, Jauch KW, et al. Prothrombin complex concentrate in surgical patients: retrospective evaluation of vitamin K antagonist reversal and treatment of severe bleeding. Crit Care 2009;13(6):R191.
88. Schochl H, Nienaber U, Hofer G, et al. Goal-directed coagulation management of major trauma patients using thromboelastometry (ROTEM)-guided administration of fibrinogen concentrate and prothrombin complex concentrate. Crit Care 2010; 14(2):R55.
89. Monroe DM, Hoffman M, Oliver JA, et al. Platelet activity of high-dose factor VIIa is independent of tissue factor. Br J Haematol 1997;99(3):542–7.
90. Lisman T, Adelmeijer J, Cauwenberghs S, et al. Recombinant factor VIIa enhances platelet adhesion and activation under flow conditions at normal and reduced platelet count. J Thromb Haemost 2005;3(4):742–51.
91. Grottke O, Henzler D, Rossaint R. Activated recombinant factor VII (rFVIIa). Best Pract Res Clin Anaesthesiol 2010;24(1):95–106.
92. Lin Y, Stanworth S, Birchall J, et al. Use of recombinant factor VIIa for the prevention and treatment of bleeding in patients without hemophilia: a systematic review and meta-analysis. CMAJ 2011;183(1):E9–19.
93. Boffard KD, Riou B, Warren B, et al. Recombinant factor VIIa as adjunctive therapy for bleeding control in severely injured trauma patients: two parallel randomized, placebo-controlled, double-blind clinical trials. J Trauma 2005; 59(1):8–15 [discussion:15–8].
94. Hauser CJ, Boffard K, Dutton R, et al. Results of the CONTROL trial: efficacy and safety of recombinant activated Factor VII in the management of refractory traumatic hemorrhage. J Trauma 2010;69(3):489–500.
95. O'Connell KA, Wood JJ, Wise RP, et al. Thromboembolic adverse events after use of recombinant human coagulation factor VIIa. JAMA 2006;295(3):293–8.
96. Levi M, Levy JH, Andersen HF, et al. Safety of recombinant activated factor VII in randomized clinical trials. N Engl J Med 2010;363(19):1791–800.
97. Dutton RP, Parr M, Tortella BJ, et al. Recombinant activated factor VII safety in trauma patients: results from the CONTROL trial. J Trauma 2011;71(1):12–9.

Point of Care Devices for Assessing Bleeding and Coagulation in the Trauma Patient

Oliver M. Theusinger, MD[a,*], Jerrold H. Levy, MD, FAHA, FCCM[b]

KEYWORDS

- Thromboelastometry • Blood coagulation • Hemostasis • ROTEM • Trauma
- Point of care devices

KEY POINTS

- Routine coagulation tests in the laboratory only reflect the initiation phase of hemostasis and cannot be used to monitor coagulopathy.
- Viscoelastic devices (such as thromboelastography or rotation thromboelastometry) measure clot formation and dissolution in whole blood and thus should be used to monitor trauma patients.
- Hypocoagulable results in viscoelastic devices predict the need for massive transfusion and correlate with increased rate of mortality; hence, therapy aiming at restoring clot strength is recommendable.
- Actual available devices to measure hemoglobin noninvasively have problems regarding the accuracy and thus are not really to be used in trauma patients.

INTRODUCTION

On admission to the hospital, about 40% of trauma patients will present with trauma-induced coagulopathy, with an increased risk of bleeding and an associated several-fold increase in rates of morbidity and mortality.[1–4] Rates of mortality in patients with trauma-induced coagulopathy is up to 4 times higher than in patients not presenting this state. Some studies even claim that 20% of deaths in trauma could be preventable because most deaths are linked to uncontrolled bleeding.[5,6] For this reason, as management of trauma-induced coagulopathy differs from center to center, the crucial goal remains to prevent, identify, and correct this type of coagulopathy by early aggressive treatment to increase chances of survival. Therefore the need of point-of-care (POC) devices to monitor coagulation in these cases seems obvious.

[a] Institute of Anesthesiology, University Zurich, University Hospital Zurich, Zurich CH-8091, Switzerland; [b] Emory University School of Medicine, Atlanta, GA, USA
* Corresponding author.
E-mail address: oliver.theusinger@usz.ch

Anesthesiology Clin 31 (2013) 55–65
http://dx.doi.org/10.1016/j.anclin.2012.10.006 **anesthesiology.theclinics.com**

Classical laboratory tests such as activated partial thromboplastin time or prothrombin time are plasma-based coagulation tests that can take from 30 minutes up to 90 minutes before getting the results. Recent reviews have shown that the plasma-based tests are inappropriate for monitoring trauma-induced coagulopathy or guiding goal-directed transfusions, therefore, supporting the use of POC devices. The purpose of this review is to give a brief overview on actually available POC devices to be used in trauma patients, to assess bleeding, platelet function, and coagulation in the trauma patient as well as to inform how to put the results into the context of goal-directed transfusions.

POINT OF CARE DEVICE FOR NONINVASIVE HEMOGLOBIN CONCENTRATION MEASUREMENTS

For standard monitoring, pulse oximetry is used to calculate the O_2 hemoglobin fraction by 2 wavelengths, 660 nm and 940 nm.[7,8] The pulse oximeter uses a correction factor that was calculated from measurements in healthy volunteers.[9] It would be of interest to use these properties to measure the hemoglobin concentration continuously and noninvasively. So far, the development of such devices has encountered some problems, which include the consistency of tissues through which light has to go through, size of fingers, resulting in inappropriate finger position, establishment of references measurements in healthy volunteers, and so on.

In 2002, Astrim (Sysmex, Kobe, Japan) was the first device to be launched to try to measure total hemoglobin concentration in a noninvasive way. This device uses 3 wavelengths, 660 nm, 805 nm, and 880 nm. A study performed by Saigo and colleagues[10–12] in healthy volunteers and patients with hematological diseases showed several problems in the precision of measurements and discovered, as mentioned earlier, problems caused by the finger position and temperature. This device is no longer used to measure hemoglobin concentration. The next attempt was made 3 years later by Noiri and colleagues,[8] using 4 wavelengths, 660 nm, 805 nm, 940 nm, and 1300 nm, to compare laboratory levels of hemoglobin to noninvasive measurements in patients and volunteers showing a better sensitivity (84%) and specificity (85%) but still not acceptable levels for clinical use. The next step was made in 2006 by Suzaki and colleagues by increasing the number of wavelengths to 7, ranging from 600 nm to 1300 nm.[12] This increase made it possible to measure the saturation of hemoglobin in oxygen, reduced hemoglobin, carbon monoxide hemoglobin, methemoglobin, and water with fairly good results.[12–14] A pulse oximeter using 2 wavelengths, allowing measurement under motion and low perfusion (Masimo, Irvine, CA, USA),[13,14] was further developed, culminating in the current Rainbow device (Masimo), which measures, using up to 12 wavelengths, oxygen saturation, pulse rate, and perfusion index, in addition to total hemoglobin, total arterial oxygen content, plethysmographic variability index, carboxyhemoglobin, methemoglobin, and acoustic respiration rate.[15]

Different studies have shown thus far that, although changing and improving the sensors, reliable results can be recorded only in healthy volunteers. In patients confounding problems such as hemodilution, lower body temperature, use of catecholamines, low blood pressure, and low hemoglobin lead to clinically unacceptable results.[14–21] The idea of measuring hemoglobin noninvasively was to reduce the number of blood-gas analysis or laboratory measurements, to save the patient's red blood cell count, and to reduce the number of red blood cell transfusions, but because no clinically satisfying results can be achieved, these ideas had to be dismissed. A possible trend measurement of hemoglobin could be a clinical advantage even if accuracy regarding these devices is not given.

PLATELET MONITORING

As patients are increasingly treated with antiplatelet drugs (ie, for ischemic cardiovascular disease), platelet function monitoring has become increasingly important in trauma. Platelet counts are useful information in the treatment of traumatic bleeding and, if available by POC testing, critical time can be gained compared with the laboratory testing. Indications are not evidence based in part due to the lack of readily available platelet function testing. Recommendations for platelet transfusion are $\leq$50,000/μl if the patient is bleeding without traumatic brain injury and $\leq$100,000/μl in cases of traumatic brain injury.[22–25] In the laboratory, platelet aggregation is measured by light transmission aggregometry to evaluate bleeding disorders or to assess the effect of antiplatelet drugs.[26,27] Platelet function testing is time consuming and may not be accurate with dilutional coagulopathy, thus not useful in acute traumatic bleeding. Three POC devices are available to monitor platelet function: (1) the PFA-100 (Siemens Healthcare Diagnostics Inc, Deerfield, IL, USA); (2) Multiplate (Dynabyte, Munich, Germany) (**Fig. 1**); and (3) Ultegra rapid platelet function analyzer (Accumetrics, San Diego, CA, USA).

In the PFA-100, the occlusion time of a micropore membrane by platelets after activation with adenosine diphosphate or collagen epinephrine is measured. This time, called closure time, will be prolonged in patients using an antiplatelet drug or having a platelet dysfunction.[28,29] This information may be useful for transfusing platelets in trauma patients.

The second device, Multiplate (see **Fig. 1**), works with a cup containing 4 electric filaments, measuring in hirudin whole blood time-dependent changes of the electrical impedance between 2 filaments. Platelets can be stimulated by different tests, including arachidonic acid, adenosine diphosphate, collagen, and thrombin receptor–activating peptide. The results of the platelet aggregometry are displayed as the area under the curve by plotting electrical impedance versus time. The Multiplate allows the detection of the action of aspirin, glycoprotein IIb-IIIa inhibitors, and thienopyridines and offers, compared with the PFA-100, 5 measurements simultaneously.[30,31]

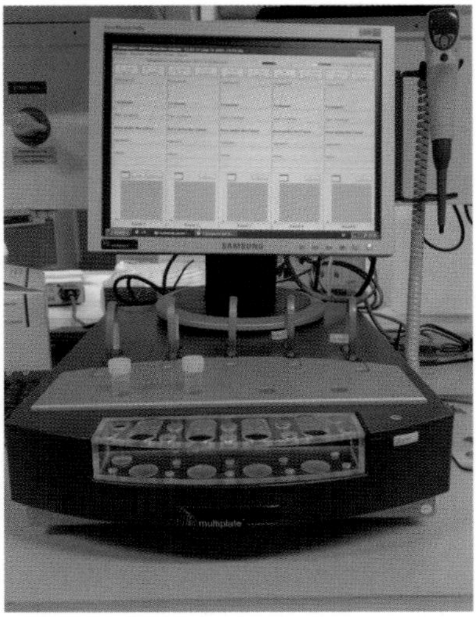

Fig. 1. Showing 1 Multiplate (Dynabyte, Munich, Germany) in the University Hospital in Zürich, Switzerland.

ROTATION THROMBELASTOMETRY, THROMBELASTOGRAPHY, AND COAGULATION/PLATELET FUNCTION ANALYZER

Thrombelastography, first described by Hartert in 1948, is a method to assess coagulation in a single whole blood sample.[32] Different terms to be found in the literature for this initial technique are thrombelastograph, thrombelastography, and thromboelastography (TEG). Since 1996, the term TEG is registered by the Hemoscope Corporation in Niles, IL and thus describes only the test method by Hemoscope, which presents 2 channels. Rotation thromboelastometry (ROTEM) (**Fig. 2**) is a modified device with 4 channels, which was first introduced in the year 2000 by Pentapharm GmbH, now TEM International GmbH (Munich, Germany).[33] Between the 2 devices, some differences must be mentioned: first, the way they function, and second, the terminology (**Table 1**).

TEG uses a stationary cup containing the blood sample, which oscillates with an angle of 4.45°. The pin, in which motion is measured, is suspended in the blood sample by a torsion wire. The movement of the pin is converted by a mechanical-electrical transducer into an electric signal that is then displayed in a curve. The firmness of the clot limits the movement. One problem in TEG compared with ROTEM, where no resting of the citrated sample for at least 30 minutes is required, is that results and measurements are delayed.[34]

In ROTEM, the signal of the pin that is suspended in the whole blood sample is transmitted via an optical detector system and not a torsion wire. In ROTEM, the pin moves 4.75° and not the cup,[35] leading to a shock resistance. In addition, the instrument is equipped with an automatic pipette, making it much more user-friendly. A typical ROTEM trace is displayed in **Fig. 3**.[35]

Both devices graphically represent changes in viscoelasticity and show all phases of the clot formation, including lysis, hyperfibrinolysis, and hypercoagulable states. The terminology of both devices is different as well as the available tests and their reference values (see **Table 1**).[36–38] One of the most important details these devices provide in trauma is whether hyperfibrinolysis is present, allowing rapid treatment.

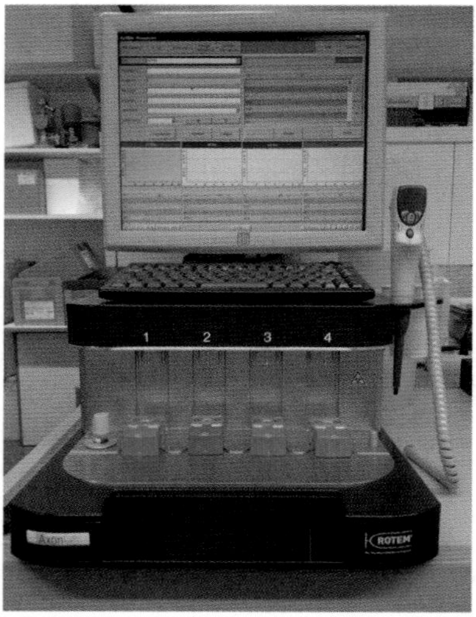

Fig. 2. Showing 1 ROTEM (TEM International GmbH, Munich, Germany) in the University Hospital in Zürich, Switzerland.

Table 1
Showing differences in terms between ROTEM and TEG

Parameter	ROTEM	TEG
Clot time period to 2 mm amplitude	Clotting time (CT)	Reaction time (R)
Clot kinetics period from 2 to 20 mm amplitude	Clot formation time (CFT)	Kinetics (K)
α-angle	Slope of tangent at 2 mm amplitude (α)	Slope between R and K (α)
Maximum clot strength	Maximum clot firmness (MCF)	Maximum amplitude (MA)
Clot elasticity	Maximum clot elasticity (MCE)	G
Lysis at certain points of time	Amplitude reduction after 30 or 60 min after MCF (CL30, CL60)	Amplitude reduction after 30 or 60 min after MA (Ly30, Ly60)
Clot lysis	Maximum lysis (ML)	Estimated percent lysis (EPL)

ROTEM tests that should be performed in trauma are the extrinsic system activated by tissue factor as well as the intrinsic system (INTEM) activated by the contact activator. Functionality and levels of fibrinogen can be tested by a fibrinogen specific essay (FIBTEM), a test in which the platelets are inhibited by cytochalasin D.[35,39] The results have been proven to correlate well with levels of fibrinogen measured in the laboratory. One weakness of the laboratory-measured levels of fibrinogen, typically the optical method of Clauss, is that hemodilution with colloids interferes with this method, causing falsely higher levels of fibrinogen with Claus testing.[40]

The Sonoclot Coagulation and Platelet Function Analyzer (Sienco Inc, Arvada, CO, USA) has existed since 1975.[41] The measurements of this POC device are also based on changes in viscoelasticity of whole blood or plasma and are performed in a disposable plastic probe mounted on a transducer head. The sample to be analyzed is added to a cuvette containing different coagulation activators/inhibitors. The mixing process is automated and samples are oscillated vertically, measuring changes in impedance because of the developing clot.

Compared with the TEG and ROTEM, the Sonoclot Analyzer not only provides quantitative results on hemostasis in a graph but also qualitative results, including

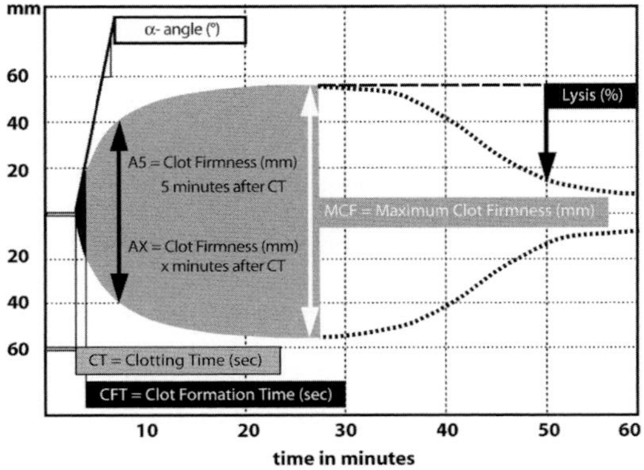

Fig. 3. Typical ROTEM curve modified, with authorization of TEM International GmbH, Munich, Germany. Terms are explained in **Table 1**.

the activated clotting time (ACT), platelet function, and the rate of clot formation.[42–44] Platelet function, derived from the timing and quality of the clot retraction, is an additional piece of useful information. The maximum possible clot strength represents a platelet function of 5, whereas no clot would represent a platelet function of 0.[45] The results of the Sonoclot Analyzer are influenced by gender, age, and platelet count. Results are poorly reproducible but still have a precision that is very close to thrombelastography.[46–49]

MONITORING ANTICOAGULATION IN TRAUMA

Many patients receive chronic anticoagulation therapy and therefore additional testing should be considered. The ACT measurement should be considered when treating trauma patients, in addition to the earlier mentioned platelet inhibitor monitoring. Devices measuring the ACT are used to guide heparin therapy. They can be modified with heparinase to assess coagulation in the absence of the anticoagulatory effects of heparin. ROTEM and TEG have heparinase-modified tests that allow clearing heparin/low molecular weight heparin effects. In ROTEM, the combination of INTEM and HEPTEM (test with heparinase) makes it easy to point out the influence of heparin.[50] Recently, the use of direct thrombin inhibitors, including the new oral agent dabigatran (Pradaxa), is increasing and monitoring with viscoelastic devices using ecarin clotting time specifically can assess hemostasis in these patients.[51,52]

CRITIQUES OF POINT OF CARE MONITORING

Because of the difficulty of standardizing POC tests, concerns have been raised regarding their use as bedside tests. Further confusing the issue are the different additives in the collection tubes (hirudin, citrate, or serum). The influence of gender and age, as reported by Theusinger and colleagues,[35] on ROTEM is a critical consideration. Possible additional effects of the activators used in ROTEM could also alter the results. Standardization for POC devices is essential and includes quality controls and maintenance, as recommended by the manufacturer. However, moving these POC devices into the central laboratory to be operated by laboratory technicians does not seem to be an adequate solution because of the transportation time, delays in processing the sample, and transferring real-time data or even online data to the bedside.

WHAT IS DONE WITH THE RESULTS OF THESE DEVICES—WHY ARE THEY CONSIDERED STATE OF THE ART?

Initial coagulopathy in the traumatized patient is not due to hypothermia, metabolic acidosis, dilutional or consumptive coagulopathy, but rather a phenomenon named "acute traumatic coagulopathy."[53,54] Up to 60% of Emergency Department patients following major trauma present this type of coagulopathy and early detection by POC devices is needed for effective diagnosis and treatment. For example, hyperfibrinolysis increases the rate of mortality, rate of morbidity, and transfusion requirements but can be treated easily if detected early (eg, by rotation thrombelastometry or thrombelastography).[55–58] Tissue hypoperfusion in the first half hour after trauma increases tissue plasminogen activator and thrombomodulin.[59,60] Thrombomodulin by activating protein C and protein S to an inhibition of factor Va and VIIa as well as to an inhibition of plasminogen activator inhibitor-1 results in an imbalance of tissue plasminogen activator and plasminogen activator inhibitor-1, leading to hyperfribinolysis.[1,59–62] Because of the complexity of bleeding management in trauma, algorithms with POC devices integrated in them are needed for a logical, standardized, and clear pathway/algorithm.[25]

Treatment with blood products, red blood cells, fresh frozen plasma, and platelets is known to be associated with an increased length of stay, infections, multiorgan failure, rate of mortality, rate of morbidity, infections, sepsis, transfusion-related acute lung injury, and transfusion overload.[63] Thus appropriate use is critical, considering the risks and benefits of those products. POC devices reduce blood product use and are ideal for goal-directed transfusion therapy with factor concentrates. The problem is that in the United States and several other countries outside of Europe coagulation factor concentrates are not available or cannot be substituted selectively as this use would be off-label. Fibrinogen administration has been shown to improve survival in several clinical studies in trauma patients with hemorrhage and dilutional coagulopathy.[64–66] As demonstrated by others, hyperfibrinolysis can be stopped by tranexamic acid[55]; its benefit has been shown in the CRASH-2 trail in which more than 20,000 patients were included, examining the effect of placebo compared with tranexamic acid on transfusion needs, bleeding, and rate of mortality.[67,68] Factor XIII, which stabilizes the clot, has been recently proven to have an influence on hyperfibrinolysis. Furthermore, trauma and massive bleeding may lead to an acquired factor XIII deficiency, thus suggesting an early substituting of factor XIII and thereby improving clot firmness, reducing bleeding, and minimizing the use of blood products.[69–72]

The use of prothrombin complex concentrates (PCC), which provide a source of factor II, VII, IX, and X in 4-factor PCC in Europe and only II, IX, and X in 3-factor PCC in the United States, is also ideally monitored by TEG or ROTEM.[73] The role of PCCs in controlling trauma-related bleeding is being elucidated because this indication is currently off-label. Because of potential thrombotic complications, the use has to be evaluated carefully. Current studies showed that the use of PCCs in trauma patients reduces allogeneic transfusions, improves survival, and reduces bleeding.[74] Goal-directed algorithms have been proven to reduce the use of blood products and to lead to a better outcome in nonsurgical trauma bleeding. The university hospital of Zurich, Switzerland, has recently published their second version of a goal-directed transfusion algorithm, including patient's history, clinical presentation, coagulation laboratory tests, and bedside viscoelastic coagulation tests.[25] Using POC devices for bleeding and coagulation management in trauma will increase costs in the beginning because of the administration of specific coagulation factors and running those tests, but in the long term, will be a cost-saving measure.[57,75]

SUMMARY

Viscoelastic POC devices and platelet function analyzers are ideal for the management of bleeding in trauma patients, especially for guiding goal-directed transfusions.

Viscoelastic POC devices and platelet function analyzers provide, within a very short time (ie, ROTEM and Multiplate within 10 minutes) useful information in massive hemorrhage and the assessment of hypocoagulable states and hypercoagulable states, and allow and monitor goal-directed transfusions using predefined algorithms.[25] Compared to time-consuming laboratory measurements, which measure coagulation in plasma only, these POC devices represent the entire clotting process as they work with whole blood. The fact that these tests are made under static conditions in vitro, the interpretation of the results must be made carefully and must be correlated to clinical conditions. Devices for noninvasive hemoglobin measurements have improved, but may not be reliable in trauma patients. In the future it would be desirable if certain POC devices could be regrouped, making it easier for the users or even acquiring full automated devices for reducing possible handling mistakes, to make the handling of the blood sample easier.

REFERENCES

1. Brohi K, Cohen MJ, Davenport RA. Acute coagulopathy of trauma: mechanism, identification and effect. Curr Opin Crit Care 2007;13:680–5.
2. Ganter MT, Brohi K, Cohen MJ, et al. Role of the alternative pathway in the early complement activation following major trauma. Shock 2007;28:29–34.
3. Johansson PI, Ostrowski SR, Secher NH. Management of major blood loss: an update. Acta Anaesthesiol Scand 2010;54:1039–49.
4. Cothren CC, Moore EE, Hedegaard HB, et al. Epidemiology of urban trauma deaths: a comprehensive reassessment 10 years later. World J Surg 2007;31:1507–11.
5. Esposito TJ, Sanddal TL, Reynolds SA, et al. Effect of a voluntary trauma system on preventable death and inappropriate care in a rural state. J Trauma 2003;54: 663–9 [discussion: 669–70].
6. Holcomb JB, McMullin NR, Pearse L, et al. Causes of death in U.S. Special operations forces in the global war on terrorism: 2001-2004. Ann Surg 2007;245:986–91.
7. Mannheimer PD. The light-tissue interaction of pulse oximetry. Anesth Analg 2007;105:S10–7.
8. Noiri E, Kobayashi N, Takamura Y, et al. Pulse total-hemoglobinometer provides accurate noninvasive monitoring. Crit Care Med 2005;33:2831–5.
9. Bland JM, Altman DG. Comparing methods of measurement: why plotting difference against standard method is misleading. Lancet 1995;346:1085–7.
10. Saigo K, Imoto S, Hashimoto M, et al. Noninvasive monitoring of hemoglobin. The effects of WBC counts on measurement. Am J Clin Pathol 2004;121:51–5.
11. Kanashima H, Yamane T, Takubo T, et al. Evaluation of noninvasive hemoglobin monitoring for hematological disorders. J Clin Lab Anal 2005;19:1–5.
12. Suzaki H, Kobayashi N, Nagaoka T, et al. Noninvasive measurement of total hemoglobin and hemoglobin derivatives using multiwavelength pulse spectrophotometry -In vitro study with a mock circulatory system. Conf Proc IEEE Eng Med Biol Soc 2006;1:799–802.
13. Causey MW, Miller S, Foster A, et al. Validation of noninvasive hemoglobin measurements using the Masimo Radical-7 SpHb Station. Am J Surg 2011; 201:592–8.
14. Goldman JM, Petterson MT, Kopotic RJ, et al. Masimo signal extraction pulse oximetry. J Clin Monit Comput 2000;16:475–83.
15. Macknet MR, Allard M, Applegate RL 2nd, et al. The accuracy of noninvasive and continuous total hemoglobin measurement by pulse CO-Oximetry in human subjects undergoing hemodilution. Anesth Analg 2010;111:1424–6.
16. Shamir MY, Kaplan L, Marans RS, et al. Urine flow is a novel hemodynamic monitoring tool for the detection of hypovolemia. Anesth Analg 2011;112:593–6.
17. Miller RD, Ward TA, Shiboski SC, et al. A comparison of three methods of hemoglobin monitoring in patients undergoing spine surgery. Anesth Analg 2011;112: 858–63.
18. Lamhaut L, Apriotesei R, Combes X, et al. Comparison of the accuracy of noninvasive hemoglobin monitoring by spectrophotometry (SpHb) and HemoCue(R) with automated laboratory hemoglobin measurement. Anesthesiology 2011; 115:548–54.
19. Frasca D, Dahyot-Fizelier C, Catherine K, et al. Accuracy of a continuous noninvasive hemoglobin monitor in intensive care unit patients. Crit Care Med 2011;39:2277–82.

20. Berkow L, Rotolo S, Mirski E. Continuous noninvasive hemoglobin monitoring during complex spine surgery. Anesth Analg 2011;113:1396–402.
21. Gayat E, Bodin A, Sportiello C, et al. Performance evaluation of a noninvasive hemoglobin monitoring device. Ann Emerg Med 2011;57:330–3.
22. British Committee for Standards in Haematology, Blood Transfusion Task Force. Guidelines for the use of platelet transfusions. Br J Haematol 2003;122:10–23.
23. Rebulla P. Revisitation of the clinical indications for the transfusion of platelet concentrates. Rev Clin Exp Hematol 2001;5:288–310 [discussion 311–2].
24. Rebulla P. Platelet transfusion trigger in difficult patients. Transfus Clin Biol 2001; 8:249–54.
25. Theusinger OM, Madjdpour C, Spahn DR. Resuscitation and transfusion management in trauma patients: emerging concepts. Curr Opin Crit Care 2012;18:661–70.
26. Cattaneo M, Hayward CP, Moffat KA, et al. Results of a worldwide survey on the assessment of platelet function by light transmission aggregometry: a report from the platelet physiology subcommittee of the SSC of the ISTH. J Thromb Haemost 2009;7:1029.
27. Cattaneo M. Light transmission aggregometry and ATP release for the diagnostic assessment of platelet function. Semin Thromb Hemost 2009;35:158–67.
28. Homoncik M, Jilma B, Hergovich N, et al. Monitoring of aspirin (ASA) pharmacodynamics with the platelet function analyzer PFA-100. Thromb Haemost 2000;83: 316–21.
29. Koessler J, Kobsar AL, Rajkovic MS, et al. The new INNOVANCE(R) PFA P2Y cartridge is sensitive to the detection of the P2Y(1)(2) receptor inhibition. Platelets 2011;22:19–25.
30. Jambor C, Weber CF, Gerhardt K, et al. Whole blood multiple electrode aggregometry is a reliable point-of-care test of aspirin-induced platelet dysfunction. Anesth Analg 2009;109:25–31.
31. Sibbing D, Schulz S, Braun S, et al. Antiplatelet effects of clopidogrel and bleeding in patients undergoing coronary stent placement. J Thromb Haemost 2010;8:250–6.
32. Hartert H. Blutgerinnungsstudie mit der Thrombelastographie, einem neuen Untersuchungsverfahren. Klin Wochenschr 1948;26:577–83.
33. Luddington RJ. Thrombelastography/thromboelastometry. Clin Lab Haematol 2005;27:81–90.
34. Camenzind V, Bombeli T, Seifert B, et al. Citrate storage affects Thrombelastograph analysis. Anesthesiology 2000;92:1242–9.
35. Theusinger OM, Nurnberg J, Asmis LM, et al. Rotation thromboelastometry (ROTEM) stability and reproducibility over time. Eur J Cardiothorac Surg 2010; 37:677–83.
36. Mallett SV, Cox DJ. Thrombelastography. Br J Anaesth 1992;69:307–13.
37. Di Benedetto P, Baciarello M, Cabetti L, et al. Present and future perspectives in clinical practice. Minerva Anestesiol 2003;69:501–9, 9–15.
38. Nielsen VG. A comparison of the Thrombelastograph and the ROTEM. Blood Coagul Fibrinolysis 2007;18:247–52.
39. Kettner SC, Panzer OP, Kozek SA, et al. Use of abciximab-modified thrombelastography in patients undergoing cardiac surgery. Anesth Analg 1999;89:580–4.
40. Hiippala ST. Dextran and hydroxyethyl starch interfere with fibrinogen assays. Blood Coagul Fibrinolysis 1995;6:743–6.
41. von Kaulla KN, Ostendorf P, von Kaulla E. The impedance machine: a new bedside coagulation recording device. J Med 1975;6:73–88.

42. Dalbert S, Ganter MT, Furrer L, et al. Effects of heparin, haemodilution and aprotinin on kaolin-based activated clotting time: in vitro comparison of two different point of care devices. Acta Anaesthesiol Scand 2006;50:461–8.
43. Ganter MT, Dalbert S, Graves K, et al. Monitoring activated clotting time for combined heparin and aprotinin application: an in vitro evaluation of a new aprotinin-insensitive test using SONOCLOT. Anesth Analg 2005;101:308–14 [table of contents].
44. Ganter MT, Hofer CK. Coagulation monitoring: current techniques and clinical use of viscoelastic point-of-care coagulation devices. Anesth Analg 2008;106: 1366–75.
45. Tucci MA, Ganter MT, Hamiel CR, et al. Platelet function monitoring with the Sonoclot analyzer after in vitro tirofiban and heparin administration. J Thorac Cardiovasc Surg 2006;131:1314–22.
46. Horlocker TT, Schroeder DR. Effect of age, gender, and platelet count on Sonoclot coagulation analysis in patients undergoing orthopedic operations. Mayo Clin Proc 1997;72:214–9.
47. McKenzie ME, Gurbel PA, Levine DJ, et al. Clinical utility of available methods for determining platelet function. Cardiology 1999;92:240–7.
48. Ekback G, Carlsson O, Schott U. Sonoclot coagulation analysis: a study of test variability. J Cardiothorac Vasc Anesth 1999;13:393–7.
49. Forestier F, Belisle S, Contant C, et al. Reproducibility and interchangeability of the Thromboelastograph, Sonoclot and Hemochron activated coagulation time in cardiac surgery. Can J Anaesth 2001;48:902–10 [in French].
50. Coppell JA, Thalheimer U, Zambruni A, et al. The effects of unfractionated heparin, low molecular weight heparin and danaparoid on the thromboelastogram (TEG): an in-vitro comparison of standard and heparinase-modified TEGs with conventional coagulation assays. Blood Coagul Fibrinolysis 2006;17:97–104.
51. Carroll RC, Chavez JJ, Simmons JW, et al. Measurement of patients' bivalirudin plasma levels by a thrombelastograph ecarin clotting time assay: a comparison to a standard activated clotting time. Anesth Analg 2006;102:1316–9.
52. Nielsen VG, Steenwyk BL, Gurley WQ, et al. Argatroban, bivalirudin, and lepirudin do not decrease clot propagation and strength as effectively as heparin-activated antithrombin in vitro. J Heart Lung Transplant 2006;25:653–63.
53. Lier H, Krep H, Schroeder S, et al. Preconditions of hemostasis in trauma: a review. The influence of acidosis, hypocalcemia, anemia, and hypothermia on functional hemostasis in trauma. J Trauma 2008;65:951–60.
54. Mitra B, Cameron PA, Mori A, et al. Acute coagulopathy and early deaths post major trauma. Injury 2012;43:22–5.
55. Theusinger OM, Wanner GA, Emmert MY, et al. Hyperfibrinolysis diagnosed by rotational thromboelastometry (ROTEM) is associated with higher mortality in patients with severe trauma. Anesth Analg 2011;113:1003–12.
56. Kashuk JL, Moore EE, Sawyer M, et al. Primary fibrinolysis is integral in the pathogenesis of the acute coagulopathy of trauma. Ann Surg 2010;252:434–42 [discussion: 443–4].
57. Schochl H, Nienaber U, Hofer G, et al. Goal-directed coagulation management of major trauma patients using thromboelastometry (ROTEM)-guided administration of fibrinogen concentrate and prothrombin complex concentrate. Crit Care 2010; 14:R55.
58. Schochl H, Frietsch T, Pavelka M, et al. Hyperfibrinolysis after major trauma: differential diagnosis of lysis patterns and prognostic value of thrombelastometry. J Trauma 2009;67:125–31.

59. Theusinger OM, Spahn DR, Ganter MT. Transfusion in trauma: why and how should we change our current practice? Curr Opin Anaesthesiol 2009;22: 305–12.
60. Brohi K, Cohen MJ, Ganter MT, et al. Acute coagulopathy of trauma: hypoperfusion induces systemic anticoagulation and hyperfibrinolysis. J Trauma 2008;64: 1211–7 [discussion: 1217].
61. Brohi K, Singh J, Heron M, et al. Acute traumatic coagulopathy. J Trauma 2003; 54:1127–30.
62. Hayakawa M, Sawamura A, Gando S, et al. Disseminated intravascular coagulation at an early phase of trauma is associated with consumption coagulopathy and excessive fibrinolysis both by plasmin and neutrophil elastase. Surgery 2011;149:221–30.
63. Lelubre C, Piagnerelli M, Vincent JL. Association between duration of storage of transfused red blood cells and morbidity and mortality in adult patients: myth or reality? Transfusion 2009;49:1384–94.
64. Haas T, Fries D, Velik-Salchner C, et al. The in vitro effects of fibrinogen concentrate, factor XIII and fresh frozen plasma on impaired clot formation after 60% dilution. Anesth Analg 2008;106:1360–5 [table of contents].
65. Haas T, Fries D, Velik-Salchner C, et al. Fibrinogen in craniosynostosis surgery. Anesth Analg 2008;106:725–31 [table of contents].
66. Haas T, Fries D, Holz C, et al. Less impairment of hemostasis and reduced blood loss in pigs after resuscitation from hemorrhagic shock using the small-volume concept with hypertonic saline/hydroxyethyl starch as compared to administration of 4% gelatin or 6% hydroxyethyl starch solution. Anesth Analg 2008;106: 1078–86 [table of contents].
67. Shakur H, Roberts I, Bautista R, et al. Effects of tranexamic acid on death, vascular occlusive events, and blood transfusion in trauma patients with significant haemorrhage (CRASH-2): a randomised, placebo-controlled trial. Lancet 2010;376:23–32.
68. Ker K, Kiriya J, Perel P, et al. Avoidable mortality from giving tranexamic acid to bleeding trauma patients: an estimation based on WHO mortality data, a systematic literature review and data from the CRASH-2 trial. BMC Emerg Med 2012;12:3.
69. Dirkmann D, Gorlinger K, Gisbertz C, et al. Factor XIII and tranexamic acid but not recombinant factor VIIa attenuate tissue plasminogen activator-induced hyperfibrinolysis in human whole blood. Anesth Analg 2012;114:1182–8.
70. Theusinger OM. The inhibiting effect of factor XIII on hyperfibrinolysis. Anesth Analg 2012;114:1149–50.
71. Egbring R, Kroniger A, Seitz R. Factor XIII deficiency: pathogenic mechanisms and clinical significance. Semin Thromb Hemost 1996;22:419–25.
72. Nielsen VG, Gurley WQ Jr, Burch TM. The impact of factor XIII on coagulation kinetics and clot strength determined by thrombelastography. Anesth Analg 2004;99:120–3.
73. Honickel M, Rieg A, Rossaint R, et al. Prothrombin complex concentrate reduces blood loss and enhances thrombin generation in a pig model with blunt liver injury under severe hypothermia. Thromb Haemost 2011;106:724–33.
74. Patanwala AE, Acquisto NM, Erstad BL. Prothrombin complex concentrate for critical bleeding. Ann Pharmacother 2011;45:990–9.
75. Schochl H, Forster L, Woidke R, et al. Use of rotation thromboelastometry (ROTEM) to achieve successful treatment of polytrauma with fibrinogen concentrate and prothrombin complex concentrate. Anaesthesia 2010;65:199–203.

Advances in the Management of the Critically Injured Patient in the Operating Room

Kristen Carey Rock, MD*, Magdalena Bakowitz, MD, MPH, Maureen McCunn, MD, MIPP, FCCM

KEYWORDS

• Trauma • Critical care • Invasive monitoring • APRV
• Abdominal compartment syndrome

KEY POINTS

- The pathophysiology of trauma as a longitudinal illness continues to be elucidated. After initial injury, secondary injury occurs through a complex cascade of acute inflammatory reactants, cytokines, and immunomodulators that can lead to multi-organ system failure and death.
- Optimizing fluid management and aggressively treating coagulopathy may prevent up to 20% of deaths from traumatic hemorrhage.
- A new generation of invasive monitoring, including brain tissue oxygenation monitoring and echocardiography, are important new guides to clinical decision-making for critically ill trauma patients.

INTRODUCTION

Trauma remains the leading cause of death among people aged 1 to 44 years and is one of the top 10 causes for all other age groups in the United States. It is also a leading cause of morbidity and mortality worldwide.[1] Through advances in trauma care during the "golden hour," more patients survive and are transferred to the ICU and often return to the operating room (OR) for additional procedures (**Fig. 1**). Operative management of these patients after initial stabilization continues to be a challenge for the anesthesiologist. This article provides an evidence-based update of anesthetic considerations for the critically ill trauma patient after initial presentation, including management of intracranial pressure (ICP), cardiac monitoring, management of the

---

Disclosures: The authors report no financial disclosures.
Department of Anesthesiology and Critical Care, University of Pennsylvania, 6 Dulles, 3400 Spruce Street, Philadelphia, PA 19104, USA
* Corresponding author.
E-mail address: Kristen.carey@uphs.upenn.edu

Anesthesiology Clin 31 (2013) 67–83
http://dx.doi.org/10.1016/j.anclin.2012.11.001 **anesthesiology.theclinics.com**

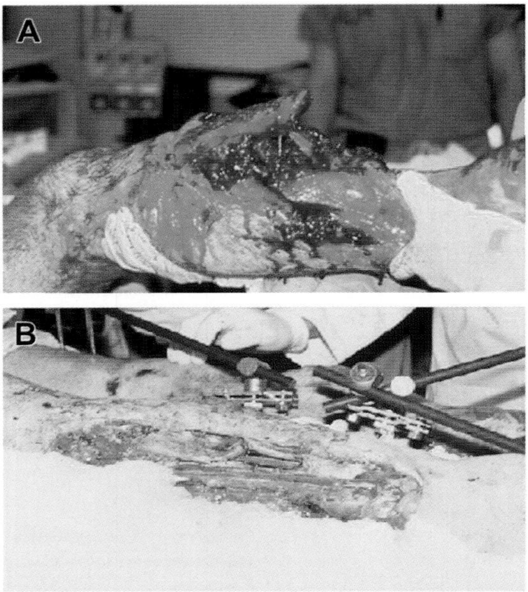

Fig. 1. A severe extremity injury with fracture (especially long bones) can lead to pulmonary-cardiac dysfunction from fat-marrow emboli. Unexplained hypotension in the OR should lead the anesthesiologist to look under all drapes for nonoperative sources of blood loss. (*A*) Acute injury with severe bony, soft tissue and neurovascular compromise. (*B*) Patient on return to the OR for one of multiple washouts and debridements.

damage control abdomen, fluid and hemodynamic management, and control of coagulopathies.

HEAD AND SPINE INJURY

Patients with severe traumatic brain injury (TBI) have three times the mortality compared with patients with other types of traumatic injury.[2] The secondary injuries resulting from the initial insult, including edema, uncontrolled inflammatory cascades, release of excitatory neurotransmitters, tissue hypoxia, and ischemia, are responsible for much of the morbidity of TBI and thus are targets for anesthetic modulation.[3]

Pharmacologic management of TBI is a mainstay of the anesthesiologist's role in the OR. Management of elevated intracranial pressure (ICP) intraoperatively may be accomplished with mannitol or hypertonic saline. There seems to be no difference in long-term morbidity and mortality between the two drugs at 6 months, although hypertonic saline may potentiate small short-term improvements in cerebral blood flow and cerebral perfusion pressure.[4,5] Meyer and colleagues[3] recently performed a meta-analysis of many common drugs used in intraoperative management of TBI, including propofol, barbiturates, opioids, benzodiazepines, and corticosteroids. Corticosteroids were the only drug which increased mortality. The others had acute benefit in reductions in ICP and sedation but no appreciable long-term benefit.

Prevention of secondary brain injury is a primary goal after TBI. The generally accepted goals to achieve optimal cerebral perfusion and oxygenation are systolic blood pressure greater than 90 mm Hg and Pa_{O_2} greater than 60 (SpO_2 >90%).

ICP may be monitored through the use of a ventricular catheter and should be maintained at less than 20 mm Hg. A variety of monitoring devices have been developed to measure cerebral perfusion pressure and cerebral oxygenation, including polarographic cerebral oxygen (Licox [Integra life sciences, Plainsboro NJ]) monitors, jugular venous oxygen saturation, positron emission tomography, near-infrared spectroscopy, and brain tissue oxygenation monitoring ($PbtO_2$).[6] Although controversy exists in the neurosurgery literature on how best to use Licox catheters, the assumption is that a $PbtO_2$ less than 20 mm Hg signifies brain tissue hypoxia, which then may be corrected by increasing the fraction of inspired oxygen, blood transfusion, inotropic support, or sedation if increased ICP results in decreased cerebral blood flow.[6,7] Research is ongoing, but $PbtO_2$ monitoring and treatment to optimize $PbtO_2$ has been shown to improve Glasgow outcome scores and mortality.[6–10]

A retrospective review of 209 consecutive patients with isolated TBI demonstrated the high incidence of subsequent organ failure—89% developed dysfunction of at least one nonneurologic organ system.[11] A recently described syndrome called Takotsubo cardiomyopathy may lead to severe myocardial dysfunction in the brain-injured patient. The reasons for development are likely multifactorial, including interplay between the neuroendocrine system and the injured brain. A catecholamine surge occurs after TBI that may manifest as subendocardial ischemia and lead to biventricular heart failure, even in young, previously healthy patients. This cycle may be exacerbated during OR procedures if vasoactive agents are administered.

Beta blockade has been suggested to be protective in human studies in subjects with brain injuries. Retrospective database reviews indicated improved neurologic outcome and reduced morbidity and mortality in patients receiving peri-insult beta blockade.[12–14] Beta blockade in head injuries was initially thought to be deleterious insofar as it may decrease mean arterial pressure (MAP). However, because catecholamine surge is greater in head injury, beta blockers may be protective in reducing cerebral oxygen consumption, MAP, and ICP, all of which may mitigate progression of secondary brain injury.[15] However, intraoperative initiation of beta blockers has not been investigated nor have there been any randomized controlled trials (RCTs) or prospective trials with beta blockers in TBI. The data for beta blockers are promising, but studies are small and have design flaws.[16]

Similar to TBI, spinal cord injury has a primary and secondary injury pattern. The effects of secondary ischemia, inflammation, excitotoxicity, and apoptosis peak between 4 and 6 days after the initial injury.[17] Augmentation of blood pressure to a MAP of 85 to 90 mm Hg for the first 7 days after injury continues to be the guidelines suggested by the American Association of Neurologic Surgeons.[18] Depending on the level of spinal cord injury, inotropes, chronotropes (cervical injuries), and peripheral vasoconstrictors (thoracic and lumbar injuries) should be used in addition to fluids to counter the interruption of sympathetic innervations of the heart and vasodilation resulting from spinal cord injury.[17] Euvolemia is the goal with fluid management. High-dose steroids remain controversial in this population. Although the latest Cochrane review suggests that high-dose methylprednisolone succinate (30 mg/kg intravenously) given within 8 hours of injury followed by a continuous infusion for 48 hours may enhance neurologic recovery,[19] much of the contemporary literature suggests that steroids are of no benefit.[20,21] The National Acute Spinal Cord Injury Study (NASCIS) trials during the 1990s did not show a difference in neurologic outcome at 1 year, but did show a greater incidence of pulmonary complications, sepsis, and gastrointestinal bleeding in the steroid group.[20] A recent survey of surgeons found that 76% of surgeons were no longer prescribing methylprednisolone, although a minority of surgeons continued the practice, citing litigation concerns.[22] Finally, the anesthesiologist should be comfortable with the increased use of multimodal intraoperative monitoring, including electromyography sensory-evoked potentials and motor-evoked potentials, and familiar with how to design an anesthetic to optimize these monitoring modalities. However, evidence is currently weak that these monitors prevent the worsening of a previous insult.[23]

CARDIOVASCULAR MONITORING AND TRANSESOPHAGEAL ECHOCARDIOGRAPHY

Anesthesiologist assessment of critically ill patients' intravascular volume status is crucial to providing conditions for adequate tissue perfusion. Controversy continues regarding which monitors beyond American Society of Anesthesiologists (ASA) standards should be used to guide therapy. Central venous pressure (CVP) and its trends are no longer considered to be the gold standard to guide volume responsiveness and fluid management.[24] Although the use of pulmonary artery catheters has declined over the past decade, the use of central venous oxygen saturation measurements as surrogates for oxygen extraction by the tissues continues.[25,26] Minimally invasive methods that measure cardiac output, including pulse contour techniques, esophageal Doppler, partial carbon dioxide rebreathing, and transthoracic bioimpedance, lack sufficient precision and accuracy compared with the established reference standard of the thermodilution method to replace the latter.[27] A systematic review and meta-analysis concluded that passive leg raising induced changes in cardiac output that predicted fluid responsiveness better than arterial pulse pressure.[26] Furthermore, inferior vena cava diameter and collapsibility on transthoracic echocardiography has shown to be a predictor of volume responsiveness.[28] A recent systematic review suggests that the institution of hemodynamic protocols affects outcome to a greater degree than the choice of monitor.[29] Practice is changing in that anesthesiologists are less likely to believe transduced pressure values than a dynamic two- or three-dimensional view of the heart and of the great vessels during the cardiac and respiratory cycle.

Hemodynamic instability, despite what is thought to be adequate fluid resuscitation perioperatively, or a mechanism of injury suggestive of cardiac injury, should prompt an investigation of possible cardiovascular causes. By the time trauma victims reach the ICU or the OR, they frequently have undergone a (transthoracic) Focused Cardiac Ultrasound (FOCUS) as part of the Focused Assessment with Sonography in Trauma (FAST) in the emergency room, followed by a full-body CT scan.[29] The American Society of Echocardiography lists "severe deceleration injury or chest trauma when valve injury, pericardial effusion, or cardiac injury are possible or suspected" as appropriate use criteria for transthoracic echocardiography (TTE) in trauma patients, but "routine evaluation in the setting of mild chest trauma with no electrocardiographic changes or biomarker elevation" as an inappropriate indication.[30]

Transesophageal echocardiography (TEE) solves many of the limitations of TTE, including suboptimal imaging due to pneumothoraces, chest tubes, dressings, surgical drapes, chronic obstructive pulmonary disease, or obesity. TEE in 389 trauma subjects at the University of Maryland lead to a reported change in management in over 30% of patients.[31] Of note, 50% of trauma patients with pulmonary artery catheters received TEE nonetheless for unknown volume status.[31] There are several findings on TEE that will alter therapy and thus prognosis of patients in critical condition. Acute systolic anterior motion of the anterior mitral leaflet that exacerbates dynamic left ventricular outflow obstruction can easily be alleviated by intravascular volume administration and ventricular filling (**Fig. 2**). Mildly impaired ventricular

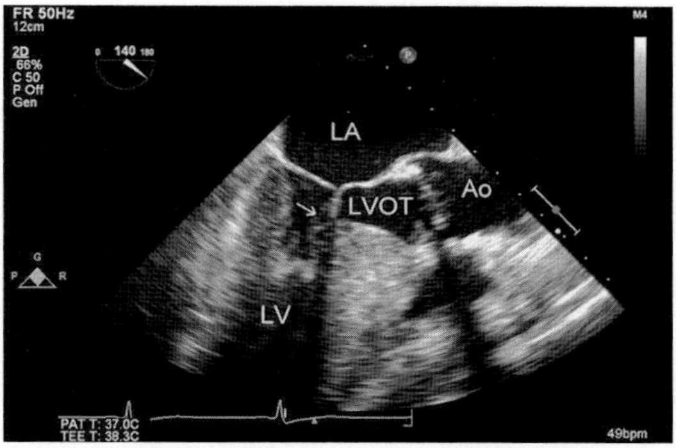

Fig. 2. Midesophageal left ventricular outflow view. The arrow points at the left anterior mitral valve leaflet obstructing left ventricular outflow during systole (systolic anterior motion). Ao, aorta; LA, left atrium; LV, left ventricle; LVOT, left ventricular outflow tract.

function resulting from blunt myocardial injury or Takotsubo cardiomyopathy is managed differently than acute right heart failure in the septic patient. The latter is usually addressed with titration of inotropes and afterload reduction. Diagnoses of ventricular rupture or tamponade can be made within minutes and requires immediate surgical intervention.

Frequently, the consultant in anesthesia encounters competing priorities. For example, emergent surgery is classically indicated in right ventricular rupture after blunt chest wall trauma from a motor vehicle accident. Surgery may have to be delayed due to concomitant injuries (ie, traumatic brain or solid organ injuries) because of a concern of anticoagulation that precludes cardiopulmonary bypass (although centers with heparinized circuits may avoid the need for systemic heparinization). In these situations, TEE can provide reassuring monitoring of the status of the cardiac injury (**Figs. 3** and **4**). If function of the ruptured ventricle deteriorates, timing of surgery can be revisited (Benjamin Kohl, MD, personal communication, 2012).

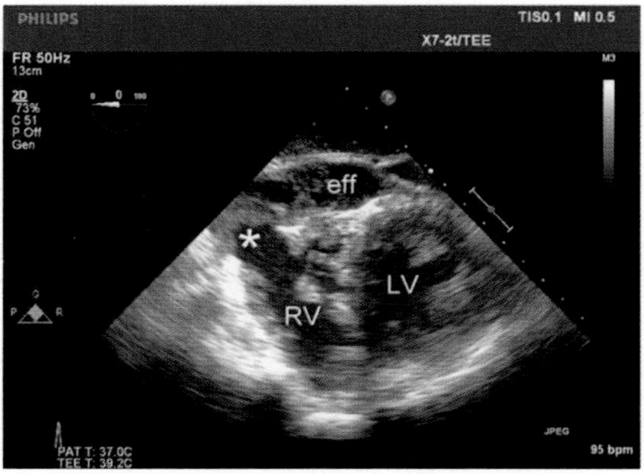

Fig. 3. Transgastric midpapillary short-axis view. The asterisk denotes right ventricular rupture site. eff, posterior effusion with thrombus; LV, left ventricle; RV, right ventricle.

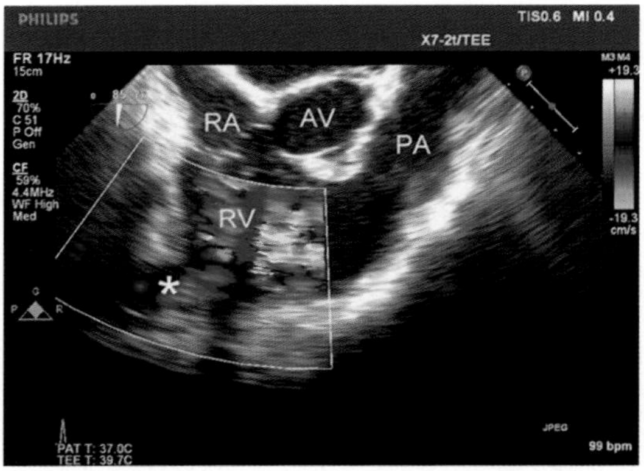

Fig. 4. Midesophageal right ventricular inflow-outflow with color flow Doppler. The asterisk denotes right ventricular rupture site. AV, aortic valve; PA, pulmonary artery; RA, right atrium; RV, right ventricle.

THE DAMAGE CONTROL ABDOMEN AND ABDOMINAL COMPARTMENT SYNDROME

The damage control abdomen is a strategy used in trauma to address life-threatening hemorrhage and fecal contamination during an initial exploratory laparotomy. The abdominal fascia is left open and a return to the OR is planned after the patient is stabilized for repair of injuries that are not life-threatening. Damage control resuscitation (DCR) decreases the amount of time the unstable patient spends in the OR and allows for correction of coagulopathy, hypothermia, and acidosis—the triad of death-in the ICU. As surgeons have gained experience in taking care of patients using DCR, the early complications of enterocutaneous fistulas, evaporative losses, loss of domain, and incisional hernias have improved.[32] Temporary abdominal closure devices (ie, wound vacuum-assisted closures) are in large part responsible for this improvement in protecting the viscera from infection and removal of proinflammatory fluids (**Figs. 5** and **6**).[32,33]

DCR has been shown to reduce the number of cases of intra-abdominal hypertension (IAH) and abdominal compartment syndrome (ACS).[34] IAH is defined using a graded scale of intra-abdominal pressures between 12 to 15 mm Hg for Grade I IAH, to greater than 25 mm Hg for grade IV IAH. Abdominal pressures should be measured with serial bladder pressures at end-expiration in the supine position with the transducer at the level of the midaxillary line. ACS is defined as elevated intra-abdominal pressures greater than 20 mm Hg with signs of end-organ dysfunction.[35] Trauma patients are among the highest risk for developing either primary ACS (with an abdominal pathological condition as the inciting factor) or secondary ACS (shock).[36] Recent studies estimate that up to three-fourths of trauma patients may develop IAH, leading to renal dysfunction, gut ischemia, and bacterial translocation. Anesthesiologists can increase the risk of developing ACS with large-volume crystalloid resuscitations.[36] Intraoperative signs of developing ACS include hypothermia, acidosis (base deficit greater than 14 mmol/L), hemoglobin less than 8 gm/dL and oliguria.[36,37] All of these signs are relatively nonspecific, so a high index of suspicion must be maintained.

Decompressive laparotomy is not a cure for ACS. ACS can recur with an open abdomen, particularly with injudicious fluid administration. If a patient is taken to the

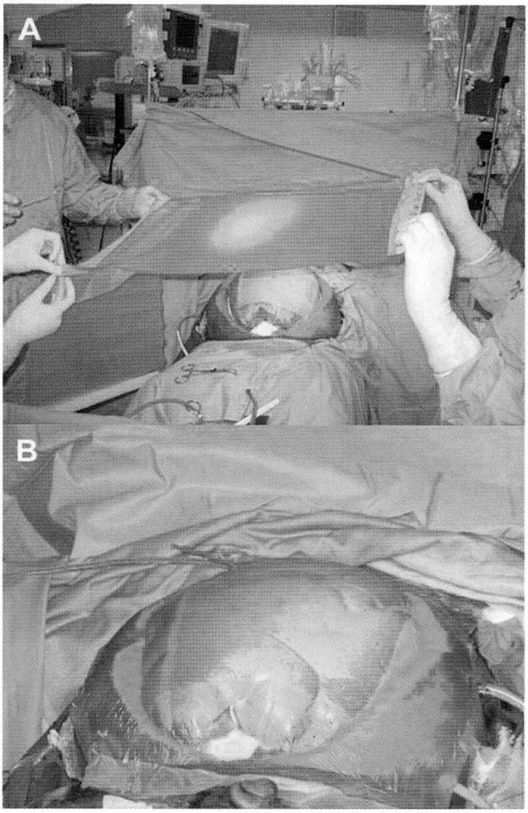

Fig. 5. (*A, B*) Temporary abdominal closure after DCR with towels and sterile dressing.

OR with ACS for abdominal decompression, the anesthesiologist should be aware of "reperfusion syndrome," a period of hypotension as ischemic tissues release a milieu of acid and cytokines.[34]

DCR and ACS can present considerable challenges for mechanical ventilation in the form of increased work of breathing, alteration of chest wall mechanics, and interference with gas exchange.[38] Animal models have shown double the incidence of pulmonary edema, high-grade atelectasis, and increased lung neutrophil activation with abdominal pressures greater than 16 mm Hg.[38] Controlled mechanical ventilation is likely preferable to Pressure support ventilation (PSV) with ACS.[38] The old understanding of ventilation strategies for patients with IAH and ACS was to add Positive end-expiratory pressure (PEEP) to ventilation to overcome the transpulmonary pressure at end-expiration. PEEP was thought to combat the increase in abdominal pressure that the expanding diaphragm was working against, thus improving oxygenation. However, in porcine studies PEEP worsened IAH by increasing abdominal venous and capillary pressures and compromising thoracic duct drainage.[39] Animal studies are currently inconclusive as to whether prone positioning may be protective.[39] Aggressive diuresis following DCR can improve oxygenation and ventilation, and it allows for early closure of the abdominal fascia (**Fig. 7**).

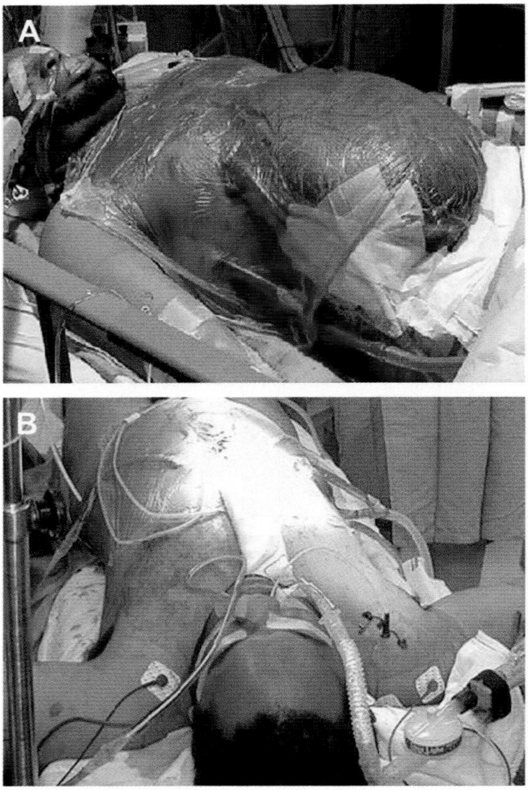

Fig. 6. Abdominal closure with wound vacuum-assisted closure (V A C, KCI, San Antonio, TX) system. (*A*) Postinjury day 2 at completion of resuscitation. (*B*) Same patient on postinjury day 4 after diuresis on return to or for abdominal closure.

HEMODYNAMIC AND FLUID MANAGEMENT

Hemorrhage is responsible for up to 40% of trauma deaths and coagulopathies are attributed to an additional percentage of deaths in the first few days postinjury.[40,41] Optimization of fluid management and prevention and treatment of coagulopathy are posited as possibly preventing up to 10% to 20% of trauma deaths by exsanguination.[41,42]

Over the past 10 to 15 years, the accepted view on trauma resuscitation has been to limit crystalloid in lieu of a near even balance of packed cells, Fresh frozen plasma (FFP), and platelets.[42–44] Large-volume crystalloid resuscitation contributes to hemodilution, coagulopathy, and IAH. The Saline versus Albumin Fluid Evaluation (SAFE) trial demonstrated no difference in outcomes with colloid versus crystalloid administration.[45] Hetastarch, dextran, and gelatin are well documented as causing fibrinogen dysfunction and deficiency.[41,46] Despite several studies, there is no defined optimal hemoglobin goal for trauma patients. The ASA recommends transfusion to maintain hemoglobin level greater than 6 g/dL. Higher thresholds to transfuse may be appropriate if ongoing blood loss is anticipated, there are signs of end-organ ischemia, hypovolemia, or patient risk factors for developing ischemia such as coronary disease, low cardiopulmonary reserve or high oxygen consumption, eg, sepsis.[47] A recent large

RCT as part of the FOCUS trial showed no difference between a liberal transfusion (hemoglobin >10) and restrictive transfusion strategy (symptoms of anemia or at physician discretion for a hemoglobin level of less than 8 g/dL) in terms of morbidity and mortality, particularly in patients with cardiovascular risk factors.[48]

Although translated from the sepsis literature, a generally accepted MAP goal for chronically ill trauma patients is greater than 65 mg Hg and Central venous pressure (CVP) of 8 mm Hg (12 mm Hg if mechanically ventilated), notwithstanding preexisting comorbidities.[49] Guides to adequate resuscitation should extend beyond vital sign stability to markers of adequate tissue perfusion, such as serum lactate, pH, and mixed venous oxygen saturation.[43] There is debate as to whether permissive hypotension confers a survival advantage by minimizing dilutional coagulopathy and reducing blood loss by maintaining lower MAPs. A 2003 Cochrane review of RCTs examining immediate versus delayed fluid resuscitation found insufficient evidence to support either strategy[50] although more recent animal data are supportive of lower MAP goals for trauma.[41] There are a few prospective controlled trials in humans that suggested faster control of hemorrhage and reduced morbidity with lower blood pressure goals.[43] Morrison and colleagues[51] recently published a RCT of 90 trauma subjects randomized to MAP of 50 versus MAP of 65. The lower MAP cohort had a reduction in transfusion requirements, postoperative coagulopathy, and a mortality benefit.

Even after seemingly adequate initial resuscitation at the time of injury, trauma patients often remain hypotensive and hemodynamic management remains difficult. Initially described as systemic inflammatory immune response (SIRS), critically ill patients with prolonged ICU stays develop what is increasingly known as persistent inflammation, immunosuppression, and catabolism syndrome (PICS). Simplistically, PICS is characterized by persistent imbalance of proinflammatory and antiinflammatory cytokines, macrophage and T-cell dysfunction, endothelial cell damage all of which lead to multiorgan system dysfunction (MODS).[52] There is some suggestion that the degree of vasodilatation and the severity of the initial SIRS response correlate with the extent of later PICS and MODS.[53]

Although continued volume resuscitation remains important, appropriate treatment of a trauma patient who has developed PICS syndrome would include pressors to combat the vasodilatation associated with this inflammatory response. The patient should be adequately resuscitated before initiating vasoactive agents because premature use of pressors of any kind has been associated with up to an 80% increase in mortality, unless cardiovascular collapse is imminent.[54,55] At this time, there is no definitive evidence for the superiority of one vasopressor over another in chronically ill trauma patients. The Surviving Sepsis guidelines suggest norepinephrine or dopamine as first-line vasopressors. Epinephrine or vasopressin is suggested as second-line agents or adjuvants.[49]

Norepinephrine, a potent alpha and beta-1 agonist that has less effect on beta-2 receptors, has been proposed as the agent of choice. Studies suggest that norepinephrine constricts the somatic circulation and redistributes blood volume to the viscera.[56] Norepinephrine improves MAP, cardiac output and stroke volume index, global end-diastolic volume index, and ventriculoarterial coupling.[57,58] Rat models have also suggested a reduction in lactate levels connoting improvement in tissue oxygenation in septic shock, contrary to a widely held belief that systemic vasoconstriction has the opposite effect.[59]

Epinephrine is a more potent beta-2 agonist than norepinephrine and also improves MAP, cardiac output and stroke volume, and ventriculoarterial coupling.[57] Because beta-2 receptors lead to vasodilatation in the somatic circulation, this agent is less effective than norepinephrine in translocating blood away from muscle and skin and

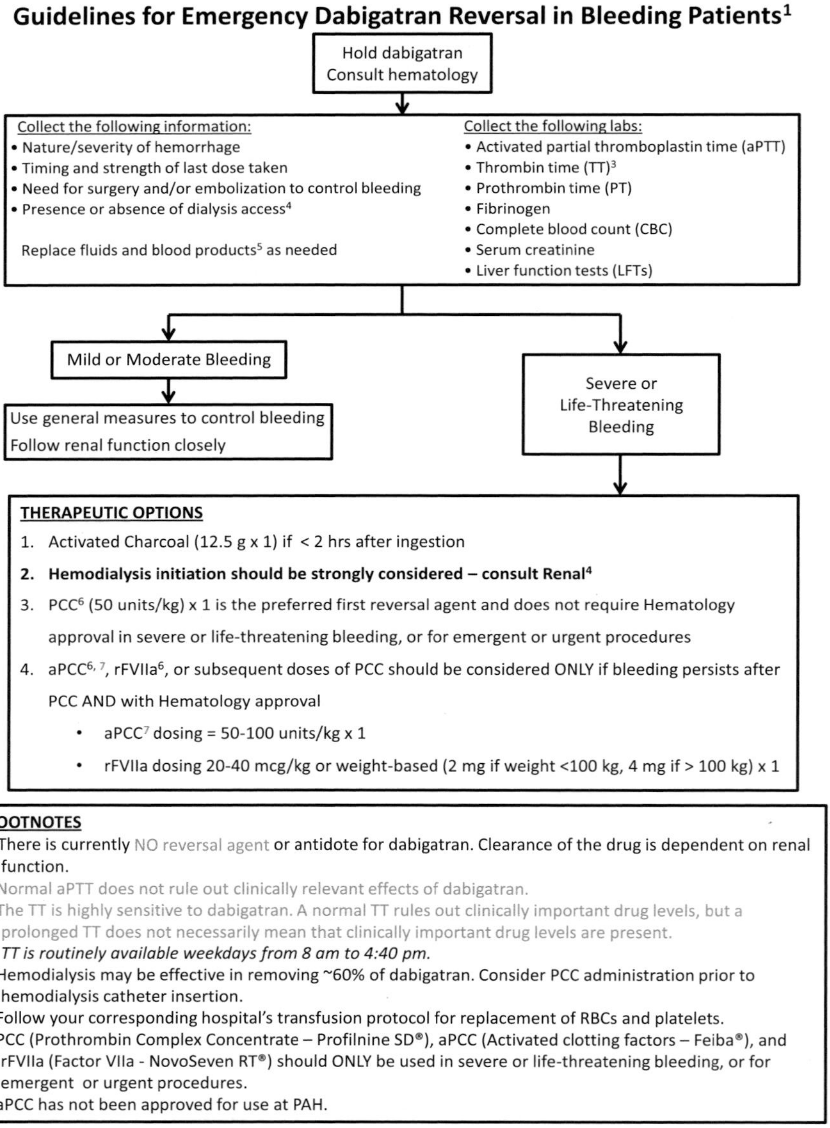
Guidelines for Emergency Dabigatran Reversal in Bleeding Patients1
Hold dabigatran
Consult hematology
Collect the following information:
• Nature/severity of hemorrhage
• Timing and strength of last dose taken
• Need for surgery and/or embolization to control bleeding
• Presence or absence of dialysis access4
Replace fluids and blood products5 as needed
Collect the following labs:
• Activated partial thromboplastin time (aPTT)
• Thrombin time (TT)3
• Prothrombin time (PT)
• Fibrinogen
• Complete blood count (CBC)
• Serum creatinine
• Liver function tests (LFTs)
Mild or Moderate Bleeding
Use general measures to control bleeding
Follow renal function closely
Severe or Life-Threatening Bleeding
THERAPEUTIC OPTIONS
1. Activated Charcoal (12.5 g x 1) if < 2 hrs after ingestion
2. Hemodialysis initiation should be strongly considered – consult Renal4
3. PCC6 (50 units/kg) x 1 is the preferred first reversal agent and does not require Hematology approval in severe or life-threatening bleeding, or for emergent or urgent procedures
4. aPCC6, 7, rFVIIa6, or subsequent doses of PCC should be considered ONLY if bleeding persists after PCC AND with Hematology approval
• aPCC7 dosing = 50-100 units/kg x 1
• rFVIIa dosing 20-40 mcg/kg or weight-based (2 mg if weight <100 kg, 4 mg if > 100 kg) x 1
FOOTNOTES
1 There is currently NO reversal agent or antidote for dabigatran. Clearance of the drug is dependent on renal function.
2 Normal aPTT does not rule out clinically relevant effects of dabigatran.
3 The TT is highly sensitive to dabigatran. A normal TT rules out clinically important drug levels, but a prolonged TT does not necessarily mean that clinically important drug levels are present.
TT is routinely available weekdays from 8 am to 4:40 pm.
4 Hemodialysis may be effective in removing ~60% of dabigatran. Consider PCC administration prior to hemodialysis catheter insertion.
5 Follow your corresponding hospital's transfusion protocol for replacement of RBCs and platelets.
6 PCC (Prothrombin Complex Concentrate – Profilnine SD®), aPCC (Activated clotting factors – Feiba®), and rFVIIa (Factor VIIa - NovoSeven RT®) should ONLY be used in severe or life-threatening bleeding, or for emergent or urgent procedures.
7 aPCC has not been approved for use at PAH.

Fig. 7. Hospital of the University of Pennsylvania guidelines for emergency dabigatran reversal in bleeding patients.

toward the viscera, and there is concern that epinephrine-induced tachycardia and a demonstrated increase in myocardial oxygen consumption may be deleterious.[49,57]

Recent studies indicate that dopamine, long a mainstay in trauma management, may be deleterious.[60,61] The highly nonspecific nature of this agent (it can stimulate a host of dopamine receptors as well as alpha, beta-1, and beta-2 receptors) makes it difficult to use. In a recent multicenter RCT of dopamine versus norepinephrine in patients with shock, there was no difference in mortality at 28 days. However, patients

Guidelines for Emergency Dabigatran Reversal in Peri-Procedural Patients[1]

Hold dabigatran
Consult hematology

↓

Collect the following:
- Urgency of procedure[7]
- Timing and strength of last dose taken
- Obtain activated partial thromboplastin time (aPTT)[2], thrombin time (TT)[3], CBC, creatinine, and LFTs
- Presence or absence of dialysis access[4]

↓

- Discuss above parameters with Hematology to decide on timing of procedure and therapeutic interventions
- See Therapeutic Options Box for therapeutic choices

↓

THERAPEUTIC OPTIONS

1. Activated Charcoal (12.5 g x 1) if < 2 hrs after ingestion
2. **Hemodialysis initiation should be strongly considered – consult Renal[4]**
3. PCC[6] (50 units/kg) x 1 is the preferred first reversal agent and does not require Hematology approval in severe or life-threatening bleeding, or for emergent or urgent procedures
4. aPCC[6,7], rFVIIa[6], or subsequent doses of PCC should be considered ONLY if bleeding persists after PCC AND with Hematology approval
   - aPCC[7] dosing = 50-100 units/kg x 1
   - rFVIIa dosing 20-40 mcg/kg or weight-based (2 mg if weight <100 kg, 4 mg if > 100 kg) x 1

FOOTNOTES

[1] There is currently NO reversal agent or antidote for dabigatran. Clearance of the drug is dependent on renal function.
[2] Normal aPTT does not rule out clinically relevant effects of dabigatran.
[3] The TT is highly sensitive to dabigatran. A normal TT rules out clinically important drug levels, but a prolonged TT does not necessarily mean that clinically important drug levels are present.
TT is routinely available weekdays from 8 am to 4:40 pm.
[4] Hemodialysis may be effective in removing ~60% of dabigatran. Consider PCC administration prior to hemodialysis catheter insertion.
[5] Follow your corresponding hospital's transfusion Protocol for replacement of RBCs and platelets.
[6] PCC (Prothrombin Complex Concentrate – Profilnine SD®), aPCC (Activated clotting factors – Feiba®), and rFVIIa (Factor VIIa - NovoSeven RT®) should ONLY be used in severe or life-threatening bleeding, or for emergent or urgent procedures.
[7] aPCC has not been approved for use at PAH.
**This is a draft of guidelines that have not yet received final approval at the University of Pennsylvania

[7] Guide to dabigatran cessation before elective procedures:

Renal Function (CrCl, mL/min)	Half-life (hours)	Timing of discontinuation after last dose of dabigatran before procedure	
		High Risk of Bleeding	Standard Risk of Bleeding
> 80	~13	2 – 4 days	24 hours
> 50 to ≤ 80	~15	2 – 4 days	24 hours
> 30 to ≤ 50	~18	4 days	at least 48 hours
≤ 30	~27	> 5 days	2 – 5 days

Fig. 7. (*continued*)

treated with dopamine had a higher incidence of adverse events, including arrhythmias.[61] In subset analysis, there was an increase in mortality in those patients with cardiogenic shock treated with dopamine.[61] Dopamine has not been shown to be beneficial for renal or mesenteric protection in traditional renal-protective doses and should not be used for this purpose.[49,60]

In sepsis or chronic critical illness, endogenous arginine vasopressin levels have shown to be inappropriately low,[62,63] causing profound vasodilatation and dysregulation of renal fluid balance. In vasodilatory shock, low doses (0.01–0.04 U/min) of vasopressin increased the mean MAP through a V_1-mediated baroreceptor effect, stimulated renal resorption of water by way of an aquaporin-2 effect, yet also increased urine output.[62,64] Vasopressin also reduced norepinephrine requirements when used as an adjuvant.[62] Vasopressin comes with the caveats of possible decrease in cardiac output, decreased heart rate, arrhythmias, and myocardial, mesenteric, and digital ischemia, particularly when used in doses greater than 0.04 U/min.

As a pure alpha 1 agonist, phenylephrine will increase MAP through vasoconstriction, yet will also increase afterload, reduce venous compliance, and reduce renal blood flow.[65] It cannot be recommended as a first-line agent.

Beta blockers are gaining increasing attention in trauma patients, particularly because many elderly trauma patients are prescribed them preadmission. Beta blockers are thought to mitigate hypermetabolism, tachycardia, and increased oxygen demand.[15] Friese and colleagues[66] suggested that beta blockade may modulate catecholamine levels that then produce an immunomodulatory response, specifically IL-6. In a retrospective cohort study by Arbabi and colleagues,[15] those trauma subjects on beta blockers during their ICU stay had a statistically significant reduction in mortality compared with subjects who did not receive a beta blocker. Beta blockade was only initiated after hemodynamic stability and volume resuscitation were achieved in both studies. Data are far from conclusive, however. A retrospective cohort study by Neideen and colleagues[67] included geriatric patients on admission beta blockers and suggested an increase in mortality. More prospective research must be done to characterize if and when beta blockers are appropriate for trauma patients.

COAGULATION

The presence of a coagulopathy on presentation portends an increased morbidity and mortality. In one study, patients with a coagulopathy on presentation had fourfold increase in mortality.[40] The nature of the coagulopathy manifested by trauma patients is still being defined but is physiologically distinct from the disseminated intravascular coagulation (DIC) of sepsis or other described coagulopathies, earning it the name acute coagulopathy of trauma shock (ACoTS) or trauma-induced coagulopathy. ACoTS is defined as a partial thromboplastin time (PTT) greater than 35 seconds and/or International Normalized Ratio (INR) greater than 1.2 and is thought to be related to the activation of thrombin and protein C, and inhibition of factors V and VII, which eventually leads to decreased fibrinogen use and increased fibrinolysis.[68] However, unlike DIC, there is a relative sparing of platelets and fibrinogen, and the microvascular thrombosis associated with DIC is not present in ACoTS.[68] These mechanisms occur independently of the coagulopathy resulting from hemodilution, academia, hypothermia, and loss of coagulation factors through hemorrhage.[69]

Although trauma patients often present with an incomplete history, efforts should be made to obtain a history on use of anticoagulants or antiplatelet therapy before a return to the OR. Particularly in older patients, there is an increasing use of the low-molecular-weight heparins (LMWHs) or newer direct thrombin inhibitors such as dabigatran and oral factor Xa inhibitors, rivaroxaban, and apixaban. Dabigatran has a half-life of 11 to 14 hours; rivaroxaban and apixaban have half-lives of 5.7 to 9.2 and 8 to 15 hours, respectively, with few clinically relevant drug interactions.[70] The anesthesiologist should also be mindful that prothrombin time (PT) and PTT will not reflect the activity of factor Xa or direct thrombin inhibitors, and that administration of plasma will not correct bleeding caused by these agents. Factor Xa levels can be measured, but these often take longer to return than is clinically relevant for a patient in an OR. Dabigatran will prolong the PTT but will not do so in a dose-dependent fashion.[70]

Administration of vitamin K and FFP for warfarin and protamine for heparin have been the mainstays for anticoagulant reversal. There are currently few options for the reversal LMWH and direct thrombin and oral factor Xa inhibitors. Evidence-based guidelines for the reversal of the newer anticoagulants are not yet available, yet research with a variety of alternative therapies is ongoing. Although protamine will not completely reverse LMWH, the American College of Chest Physicians recommends 1 mg protamine for every 1 mg enoxaparin in the first 8 hours after administration and 0.5 mg of protamine after that time.[71,72] Recombinant activated factor VII (rFVIIa) has been shown to normalize PTT, PT, and INR when administered to patients with warfarin and fondaparinux-induced coagulopathies. However, it has not been shown to reduce surgical bleeding in these situations.[70,73] rFVIIa may show some promise in reversal of factor Xa inhibitors, but this has only been shown in animal models.[74] Prothrombin complex concentrates (PCCs) have been available since the 1970s, and their use has been validated in prospective RCTs as having a statistically significant advantage over FFP in reducing INR, correcting clinically significant bleeding, and reducing the incidence of volume overload.[75] However, dosing is more complex and there is a higher risk of thrombotic complications.[75] In an RCT of healthy volunteers receiving rivaroxaban or dabigatran, PCCs were successful in significantly reducing bleeding for patients receiving rivaroxaban but not dabigatran.[76]

The anesthesiologist should be mindful that the antiplatelet agents aspirin, clopidogrel, and ticlopidine bind irreversibly to the COX-1 enzyme and P2Y ADP receptors, respectively. Thus, these drugs can cause platelet dysfunction despite normal platelet counts for days after cessation of therapy. One dose of platelets is thought to reverse the effects of salicylates.[77] Desmopressin has not been well studied, but is likely effective, as well.[77] Clopidogrel and ticlopidine have active metabolites with long half-lives, so their antiplatelet function may extend much further than the salicylates. Therefore, platelet transfusion may be beneficial up to 5 days after cessation of therapy, although there are no good studies to support this recommendation.[77]

SUMMARY

Care of trauma patients in the OR and the ICU continues to improve though better understanding of optimal timing of OR interventions, improved monitoring for patients with head injury and hemodynamic compromise, optimization of volume status, and use of appropriate vasoactive agents. Continued investigation of the pathophysiology of trauma patients as they progress to the chronic phase of illness will continue to advance interventions in the field in the ICU and in the OR.

REFERENCES

1. Centers for Disease Control and Prevention, National Center for Injury Prevention and Control. Web-based injury statistics query and reporting system (WISQARS). Available at: http://www.cdc.gov/Injury/wisqars/pdf/10LCD-age-grp-US-2009-a.pdf. 2009. Accessed July 15, 2012.
2. Lefering R, Paffrath T, Linker R, et al. Deutsche gesellschaft fur unfallchirurgie/german society for trauma surgery. Head injury and outcome—what influence do concomitant injuries have? J Trauma 2008;65(5):1036–43 [discussion: 1043–4].
3. Meyer MJ, Megyesi J, Meythaler J, et al. Acute management of acquired brain injury part II: an evidence-based review of pharmacological interventions. Brain Inj 2010;24(5):706–21.

4. Cottenceau V, Masson F, Mahamid E, et al. Comparison of effects of equiosmolar doses of mannitol and hypertonic saline on cerebral blood flow and metabolism in traumatic brain injury. J Neurotrauma 2011;28(10):2003–12.
5. Sakellaridis N, Pavlou E, Karatzas S, et al. Comparison of mannitol and hypertonic saline in the treatment of severe brain injuries. J Neurosurg 2011;114(2):545–8.
6. McCarthy MC, Moncrief H, Sands JM, et al. Neurologic outcomes with cerebral oxygen monitoring in traumatic brain injury. Surgery 2009;146(4):585–91.
7. Bohman LE, Heuer GG, Macyszyn L, et al. Medical management of compromised brain oxygen in patients with severe traumatic brain injury. Neurocrit Care 2011; 14(3):361–9.
8. Stiefel MF, Spiotta A, Gracias VH, et al. Reduced mortality rate in patients with severe traumatic brain injury treated with brain tissue oxygen monitoring. J Neurosurg 2005;103(5):805–11.
9. Martini RP, Deem S, Yanez ND, et al. Management guided by brain tissue oxygen monitoring and outcome following severe traumatic brain injury. J Neurosurg 2009;111(4):644–9.
10. Narotam PK, Morrison JF, Nathoo N. Brain tissue oxygen monitoring in traumatic brain injury and major trauma: outcome analysis of a brain tissue oxygen-directed therapy. J Neurosurg 2009;111(4):672–82.
11. Zygun DA, Kortbeek JB, Fick GH, et al. Non-neurologic organ dysfunction in severe traumatic brain injury. Crit Care Med 2005;33(3):654–60.
12. Bukur M, Lustenberger T, Cotton B, et al. Beta-blocker exposure in the absence of significant head injuries is associated with reduced mortality in critically ill patients. Am J Surg 2012;204(5):697–703.
13. Cotton BA, Snodgrass KB, Fleming SB, et al. Beta-blocker exposure is associated with improved survival after severe traumatic brain injury. J Trauma 2007; 62(1):26–33.
14. Schroeppel TJ, Fischer PE, Zarzaur BL, et al. Beta-adrenergic blockade and traumatic brain injury: protective? J Trauma 2010;69(4):776–80.
15. Arbabi S, Campion EM, Hemmila MR, et al. Beta-blocker use is associated with improved outcomes in adult trauma patients. J Trauma 2007;62(1):56–61 [discussion: 61–2].
16. Ker K, Perel P, Blackhall K. Beta-2 receptor antagonists for traumatic brain injury: a systematic review of controlled trials in animal models. CNS Neurosci Ther 2009;15(1):52–64.
17. Dooney N, Dagal A. Anesthetic considerations in acute spinal cord trauma. Int J Crit Illn Inj Sci 2011;1(1):36–43.
18. Blood pressure management after acute spinal cord injury. Neurosurgery 2002; 50(Suppl 3):S58–62.
19. Bracken MB. Steroids for acute spinal cord injury. Cochrane Database Syst Rev 2012;(1):CD001046.
20. Liu JC, Patel A, Vaccaro AR, et al. Methylprednisolone after traumatic spinal cord injury: yes or no? PM R 2009;1(7):669–73.
21. Felleiter P, Muller N, Schumann F, et al. Changes in the use of the methylprednisolone protocol for traumatic spinal cord injury in Switzerland. Spine (Phila Pa 1976) 2012;37(11):953–6.
22. Hurlbert RJ, Hamilton MG. Methylprednisolone for acute spinal cord injury: 5-year practice reversal. Can J Neurol Sci 2008;35(1):41–5.
23. Fehlings MG, Brodke DS, Norvell DC, et al. The evidence for intraoperative neurophysiological monitoring in spine surgery: does it make a difference? Spine (Phila Pa 1976) 2010;35(Suppl 9):S37–46.

24. Marik PE, Baram M, Vahid B. Does central venous pressure predict fluid responsiveness? A systematic review of the literature and the tale of seven mares. Chest 2008;134(1):172–8.
25. Walley KR. Use of central venous oxygen saturation to guide therapy. Am J Respir Crit Care Med 2011;184(5):514–20.
26. Koo KK, Sun JC, Zhou Q, et al. Pulmonary artery catheters: evolving rates and reasons for use. Crit Care Med 2011;39(7):1613–8.
27. Peyton PJ, Chong SW. Minimally invasive measurement of cardiac output during surgery and critical care: a meta-analysis of accuracy and precision. Anesthesiology 2010;113(5):1220–35.
28. Cavallaro F, Sandroni C, Marano C, et al. Diagnostic accuracy of passive leg raising for prediction of fluid responsiveness in adults: systematic review and meta-analysis of clinical studies. Intensive Care Med 2010;36(9):1475–83.
29. Gurgel ST, do Nascimento P Jr. Maintaining tissue perfusion in high-risk surgical patients: a systematic review of randomized clinical trials. Anesth Analg 2011; 112(6):1384–91.
30. American College of Cardiology Foundation Appropriate Use Criteria Task Force, American Society of Echocardiography, American Heart Association, et al. ACCF/ASE/AHA/ASNC/HFSA/HRS/SCAI/SCCM/SCCT/SCMR 2011 appropriate use criteria for echocardiography. A report of the American College of Cardiology Foundation Appropriate Use Criteria Task Force, American Society of Echocardiography, American Heart Association, American Society of Nuclear Cardiology, Heart Failure Society of America, Heart Rhythm Society, Society for Cardiovascular Angiography and Interventions, Society of Critical Care Medicine, Society of Cardiovascular Computed Tomography, Society for Cardiovascular Magnetic Resonance American College of Chest Physicians. J Am Soc Echocardiogr 2011; 24(3):229–67.
31. Boss M, Conti B, Hyder M, et al. Echocardiography in trauma: a five year experience at the R. Adams Cowley Shock Trauma Center. 105th Annual Meeting of the American Sociological Association in Atlanta GA. 2010.
32. Cheatham ML, Safcsak K. Intra-abdominal hypertension and abdominal compartment syndrome: the journey forward. Am Surg 2011;77(Suppl 1):S1–5.
33. De Waele JJ, Leppaniemi AK. Temporary abdominal closure techniques. Am Surg 2011;77(Suppl 1):S46–50.
34. Anand RJ, Ivatury RR. Surgical management of intra-abdominal hypertension and abdominal compartment syndrome. Am Surg 2011;77(Suppl 1):S42–5.
35. Malbrain ML, Cheatham ML. Definitions and pathophysiological implications of intra-abdominal hypertension and abdominal compartment syndrome. Am Surg 2011;77(Suppl 1):S6–11.
36. Balogh ZJ, Leppaniemi A. Patient populations at risk for intra-abdominal hypertension and abdominal compartment syndrome. Am Surg 2011;77(Suppl 1):S12–6.
37. Balogh ZJ, Martin A, van Wessem KP, et al. Mission to eliminate postinjury abdominal compartment syndrome. Arch Surg 2011;146(8):938–43.
38. Pelosi P, Luecke T, Rocco PR. Chest wall mechanics and abdominal pressure during general anaesthesia in normal and obese individuals and in acute lung injury. Curr Opin Crit Care 2011;17(1):72–9.
39. Hedenstierna G, Larsson A. Influence of abdominal pressure on respiratory and abdominal organ function. Curr Opin Crit Care 2012;18(1):80–5.
40. Johansson PI, Sorensen AM, Perner A, et al. Disseminated intravascular coagulation or acute coagulopathy of trauma shock early after trauma? An observational study. Crit Care 2011;15(6):R272.

41. Curry N, Davis PW. What's new in resuscitation strategies for the patient with multiple trauma? Injury 2012;43(7):1021–8.
42. Spinella PC, Holcomb JB. Resuscitation and transfusion principles for traumatic hemorrhagic shock. Blood Rev 2009;23(6):231–40.
43. Dutton RP. Current concepts in hemorrhagic shock. Anesthesiol Clin 2007;25(1): 23–34, viii.
44. Dutton RP. Resuscitative strategies to maintain homeostasis during damage control surgery. Br J Surg 2012;99(Suppl 1):21–8.
45. Finfer S, Bellomo R, Boyce N, et al. A comparison of albumin and saline for fluid resuscitation in the intensive care unit. N Engl J Med 2004;350(22):2247–56.
46. Sorensen B, Tang M, Larsen OH, et al. The role of fibrinogen: a new paradigm in the treatment of coagulopathic bleeding. Thromb Res 2011;128(Suppl 1): S13–6.
47. American Society of Anesthesiologists Task Force on Perioperative Blood Transfusion and Adjuvant Therapies. Practice guidelines for perioperative blood transfusion and adjuvant therapies: an updated report by the American Society of Anesthesiologists Task Force on Perioperative Blood Transfusion and Adjuvant Therapies. Anesthesiology 2006;105(1):198–208.
48. Carson JL, Terrin ML, Noveck H, et al. Liberal or restrictive transfusion in high-risk patients after hip surgery. N Engl J Med 2011;365(26):2453–62.
49. Dellinger RP, Levy MM, Carlet JM, et al. Surviving sepsis campaign: international guidelines for management of severe sepsis and septic shock: 2008. Crit Care Med 2008;36(1):296–327.
50. Kwan I, Bunn F, Roberts I, WHO Pre-Hospital Trauma Care Steering Committee. Timing and volume of fluid administration for patients with bleeding. Cochrane Database Syst Rev 2003;(3):CD002245.
51. Morrison CA, Carrick MM, Norman MA, et al. Hypotensive resuscitation strategy reduces transfusion requirements and severe postoperative coagulopathy in trauma patients with hemorrhagic shock: preliminary results of a randomized controlled trial. J Trauma 2011;70(3):652–63.
52. Gentile LF, Cuenca AG, Efron PA, et al. Persistent inflammation and immunosuppression: a common syndrome and new horizon for surgical intensive care. J Trauma Acute Care Surg 2012;72(6):1491–501.
53. Keel M, Trentz O. Pathophysiology of polytrauma. Injury 2005;36(6):691–709.
54. Plurad DS, Talving P, Lam L, et al. Early vasopressor use in critical injury is associated with mortality independent from volume status. J Trauma 2011;71(3): 565–70 [discussion: 570–2].
55. Sperry JL, Minei JP, Frankel HL, et al. Early use of vasopressors after injury: caution before constriction. J Trauma 2008;64(1):9–14.
56. Hannemann L, Reinhart K, Grenzer O, et al. Comparison of dopamine to dobutamine and norepinephrine for oxygen delivery and uptake in septic shock. Crit Care Med 1995;23(12):1962–70.
57. Ducrocq N, Kimmoun A, Furmaniuk A, et al. Comparison of equipressor doses of norepinephrine, epinephrine, and phenylephrine on septic myocardial dysfunction. Anesthesiology 2012;116(5):1083–91.
58. Hamzaoui O, Georger JF, Monnet X, et al. Early administration of norepinephrine increases cardiac preload and cardiac output in septic patients with life-threatening hypotension. Crit Care 2010;14(4):R142.
59. Sennoun N, Montemont C, Gibot S, et al. Comparative effects of early versus delayed use of norepinephrine in resuscitated endotoxic shock. Crit Care Med 2007;35(7):1736–40.

60. Segal JM, Phang PT, Walley KR. Low-dose dopamine hastens onset of gut ischemia in a porcine model of hemorrhagic shock. J Appl Physiol 1992;73(3): 1159–64.
61. De Backer D, Biston P, Devriendt J, et al. Comparison of dopamine and norepinephrine in the treatment of shock. N Engl J Med 2010;362(9):779–89.
62. Russell JA. Vasopressin in vasodilatory and septic shock. Curr Opin Crit Care 2007;13(4):383–91.
63. Landry DW, Levin HR, Gallant EM, et al. Vasopressin deficiency contributes to the vasodilation of septic shock. Circulation 1997;95(5):1122–5.
64. den Ouden DT, Meinders AE. Vasopressin: physiology and clinical use in patients with vasodilatory shock: a review. Neth J Med 2005;63(1):4–13.
65. Thiele RH, Nemergut EC, Lynch C 3rd. The clinical implications of isolated alpha(1) adrenergic stimulation. Anesth Analg 2011;113(2):297–304.
66. Friese RS, Barber R, McBride D, et al. Could beta blockade improve outcome after injury by modulating inflammatory profiles? J Trauma 2008;64(4):1061–8.
67. Neideen T, Lam M, Brasel KJ. Preinjury beta blockers are associated with increased mortality in geriatric trauma patients. J Trauma 2008;65(5):1016–20.
68. Hess JR, Brohi K, Dutton RP, et al. The coagulopathy of trauma: a review of mechanisms. J Trauma 2008;65(4):748–54.
69. Rourke C, Curry N, Khan S, et al. Fibrinogen levels during trauma hemorrhage, response to replacement therapy and association with patient outcomes. J Thromb Haemost 2012;10(7):1342–51.
70. Bauer KA. Reversal of antithrombotic agents. Am J Hematol 2012;87(Suppl 1): S119–26.
71. Hirsh J, Bauer KA, Donati MB, et al. Parenteral anticoagulants: American College of Chest Physicians evidence-based clinical practice guidelines (8th edition). Chest 2008;133(Suppl 6):141S–59S.
72. van Veen JJ, Maclean RM, Hampton KK, et al. Protamine reversal of low molecular weight heparin: clinically effective? Blood Coagul Fibrinolysis 2011;22(7): 565–70.
73. Skolnick BE, Mathews DR, Khutoryansky NM, et al. Exploratory study on the reversal of warfarin with rFVIIa in healthy subjects. Blood 2010;116(5):693–701.
74. Godier A, Miclot A, Le Bonniec B, et al. Evaluation of prothrombin complex concentrate and recombinant activated factor VII to reverse rivaroxaban in a rabbit model. Anesthesiology 2012;116(1):94–102.
75. Leissinger CA, Blatt PM, Hoots WK, et al. Role of prothrombin complex concentrates in reversing warfarin anticoagulation: a review of the literature. Am J Hematol 2008;83(2):137–43.
76. Eerenberg ES, Kamphuisen PW, Sijpkens MK, et al. Reversal of rivaroxaban and dabigatran by prothrombin complex concentrate: a randomized, placebo-controlled, crossover study in healthy subjects. Circulation 2011;124(14):1573–9.
77. Campbell PG, Sen A, Yadla S, et al. Emergency reversal of antiplatelet agents in patients presenting with an intracranial hemorrhage: a clinical review. World Neurosurg 2010;74(2–3):279–85.

Resuscitation in a Multiple Casualty Event

Roman Dudaryk, MD[a,b], Ernesto A. Pretto Jr, MD, MPH[c,*]

KEYWORDS

- Disaster • Multiple casualty event • Mass casualty event • Resuscitation
- Disaster medicine • Life-supporting first aid • Bystander response
- Advanced life support

KEY POINTS

- Increasingly, man-made disasters, such as wars, terrorism, and technologic disasters, are the cause of multiple casualty events.
- Resuscitation in a multiple casualty event consists of the life support chain spanning basic life support, in the form of bystander-administered life-supporting first aid, and advanced life support by professional rescuers in the field, to prolonged life support and definitive care by medical and surgical teams in hospitals.
- Bystander first aid continues to be the weakest link in the life support chain in everyday emergencies and multiple casualty events because of a lack of education and training programs for the public.
- Advances in triage methodology have improved the allocation of limited resources in these events.
- Common mechanisms of cardiac arrest among victims of a multiple casualty event are hypovolemia, traumatic brain injury, and airway obstruction.
- Portable ultrasound has revolutionized diagnostic traumatology.

No commercial interests to report.

[a] Division of Trauma Anesthesia, Department of Anesthesiology, Perioperative Medicine and Pain Management, Ryder Trauma Center, Jackson Memorial Hospital, University of Miami Miller School of Medicine, 1800 North West 10th Avenue T237, Miami, FL 33136, USA; [b] Division of Critical Care Medicine, Department of Anesthesiology, Perioperative Medicine and Pain Management, Ryder Trauma Center, Jackson Memorial Hospital, University of Miami Miller School of Medicine, 1800 North West 10th Avenue T237, Miami, FL 33136, USA; [c] Division of Transplant and Vascular Anesthesia, Department of Anesthesiology, Perioperative Medicine and Pain Management, Jackson Memorial Hospital, University of Miami Miller School of Medicine, 1800 North West 10th Avenue T237, Miami, FL 33136, USA

* Corresponding author.

E-mail address: eapretto@med.miami.edu

Anesthesiology Clin 31 (2013) 85–106

http://dx.doi.org/10.1016/j.anclin.2012.11.002 **anesthesiology.theclinics.com**

1932-2275/13/$ – see front matter

INTRODUCTION

A review of disasters resulting in mass or multiple casualty events in the first decade of the new millennium is striking in terms of the human and economic damage sustained, which leads to the following conclusions: (1) no geographic region of the globe or human society, developed or undeveloped, is invulnerable to the adverse health consequences of large-scale natural or man-made disasters; (2) no two events have the same outcome; (3) the recent trend is toward entirely preventable man-made disasters, such as wars (Iraq and Afghanistan), terrorism (9/11), and technologic disasters (Fukushima nuclear power plant), also known as "acts of man"; (4) natural disasters, such as hurricanes (Katrina 2005) and major earthquakes or tsunamis (Indonesia 2006, Haiti 2010, Japan 2011), continue to result in preventable morbidity and mortality and long-term disability; and (5) human societies have been unable to implement the sort of medical disaster response needed to significantly reduce morbidity and mortality in these events.

Depending on the number of casualties and local medical resources available a multiple casualty event may result in a medical disaster requiring mobilization of local, regional, or international resources to meet the needs of the affected population, who comprise the spectrum of injured and uninjured survivors. A major premise of this article is that anesthesiologists, who are experts in resuscitation and crisis management, are well suited to be at the forefront of multiple casualty planning, preparedness, and emergency response worldwide. This article provides a review of resuscitation in multiple casualty events, first considering the language of disaster.

DISASTER TERMINOLOGY

"Risk" is the probability of the occurrence of a disaster or its consequences. It is the product of the probability of the event multiplied by the seriousness or severity of the event, and thus focuses on the after-effects of disasters.

"Hazard" is a forceful natural or man-made event with the potential to adversely affect human life and property or the environment. Natural hazards are a normal consequence of the internal and external forces that are constantly transforming the earth (ie, earthquakes, hurricanes, tornadoes, volcanoes, and so forth). However, man-made hazards arise from deliberate human actions or inactions (war, terrorism, humanitarian emergencies, weapons of mass destruction, and so forth) that are usually predictable and entirely preventable. They may also arise from the unforeseen or unexpected consequences of human development and technology (ie, nuclear or industrial accidents).

"Disaster" is the result of the adverse interaction between a man-made or natural hazard and the environment, resulting in widespread human or structural damage that exceeds human capacity to respond in a timely and adequate manner. Health or medical disaster refers to the extent of human injury, illness, or death caused by a disaster and the damage sustained by medical facilities; consequently, the needs of surviving injured or ill and of uninjured survivors determine the resources required to provide necessary emergency support functions.

"Emergency support (societal) functions" entail the timely restoration of basic human needs in the form of food and potable water supply, sanitation, transportation, shelter, and emergency health and medical services to the affected population to prevent secondary illness, injury, or death.

There exist a qualitative and a quantitative difference between everyday trauma and emergency medical response for the multicasualty incident and disaster response for the multiple or mass casualty event. Because of these differences planning and preparedness for medical response to a multicasualty incident does not always translate into effective disaster planning and preparedness. Moreover, the ideal multiple casualty management response must aim for a seamless and timely escalation of local, regional, and national or international resources to meet the needs of casualties.

"Disaster planning and preparedness" is integral to the development and implementation of disaster prevention, preparedness, and mitigation programs, and is more effective when based on hazard and vulnerability risk analyses, and lessons learned through experience and comprehensive evaluations of disaster exercises, simulations, and actual events. During the past decades, much knowledge has been gained in the fields of comparing and measuring risk, but at the same time more doubt has arisen about the value of this quantification of risk. The perception of risk, or the subjective aspects of safety and risk, should also be taken into account. In terms of the human and economic costs, the severity, impact, and outcome of a disaster is highly dependent on the predisaster socioeconomic level of the community and its prior investment in quality infrastructure (buildings, highways, sewage systems, communication systems, trauma and emergency medical services, and so forth) and planning and prevention programs. Therefore, socioeconomic development is an important risk factor that must be incorporated into disaster planning and preparedness (eg, Haiti 2010).

"Disaster medicine" refers to the emergency health and medical response to surviving victims of disaster. However, there is also a distinction between civilian and military disaster medical response. Military medical teams, unlike civilian counterparts, train and work together. Chain of command is well established and understood by all members. Conventional wars are planned events and military casualties are usually healthy young men, not civilians of all ages with multiple comorbidities. Armed conflicts and complex humanitarian emergencies that arise from civil strife, however (ie, Syria 2012), can directly impact civilian populations. In contrast, peacetime civilian-military collaboration is essential to the logistics of planning, preparedness, and response to major disasters. Disaster medicine encompasses resuscitation medicine.

"Resuscitation medicine" may be defined as the science, technology, and practice of efforts to reverse acute terminal states and clinical death. The primary aim of disaster medicine is to prevent or mitigate morbidity, mortality, and long-term disability among the victims of disaster by immediately restoring emergency medical and public health services when these have been overwhelmed or interrupted. As in the other acute care medical specialties founded on the principles and practice of resuscitation medicine, anesthesiologists have played a pioneering role in the development of disaster medicine. Peter Safar was one of the first individuals to focus attention on lifesaving efforts in disaster.[1,2]

"Disaster reanimatology," a term coined by Safar, is the study of modern techniques of resuscitation as applied to the critically injured or ill victims of disaster. Safar advanced disaster medicine by viewing it from the perspective of resuscitation. He did so as cofounder of the World Association for Disaster and Emergency Medicine in 1976 and initiator of its official journal (*Prehospital and Disaster Medicine*), the first scientific publication exclusively devoted to disaster medicine, and of the Disaster Reanimatology Study Group, dedicated to the study of resuscitation in disaster. As Safar highlighted and as has been confirmed in several reports, the area of greatest life-saving potential remains the delivery of emergency medical care to the critically ill slowly dying victim of disaster. Furthermore, institutional planning for medical response to major disasters continues to neglect the resuscitation component by failing to incorporate basic emergency medical education and training programs aimed at the masses.[3]

CIRCUMSTANCES, CAUSES, AND MECHANISMS OF DEATH IN A MULTIPLE CASUALTY EVENT

The multidisciplinary Disaster Reanimatology Study Group was established in 1988 at the University of Pittsburgh. Over a period of 10 years this group performed post-disaster surveys of survivors (eyewitnesses) after earthquakes in Armenia (1988),[2,4] Costa Rica (1991),[5,6] and Turkey (1992).[7] Study design included qualitative survey methodology comprised of structured interviews of survivors who witnessed deaths in the out-of-hospital or prehospital setting (using a questionnaire or verbal autopsy instrument) and medical records reviews. The research team also reviewed thousands of nonstandard autopsy reports performed by medical examiners and other physicians after the Great Hanshin-Awaji earthquake in Japan (1995).[8] These studies determined circumstances, causes, mechanisms, and timing of prehospital deaths. Based on the findings of this series of survey studies, two distinct groups of earthquake deaths emerged: instant and protracted.[8] Instant death was defined as one occurring at the scene of injury immediately or within minutes of earthquake impact. Protracted death was defined as either a witnessed death or a death wherein autopsy report indicated no evidence of lethal traumatic injury.

Furthermore, instant deaths in major earthquakes were caused primarily by crush injury of vital anatomic areas (head, chest, or abdomen) and were considered not preventable when informed judgment of a panel of medical experts indicated that these victims would not have survived even if immediate emergency medical care to treat injuries had been provided. These could only be reduced with pre-earthquake engineering planning and mitigation (ie, antiseismic design and construction).

In contrast, approximately one-third of deaths were found to have occurred in a protracted manner (over a period of hours to days) in most events surveyed. This finding was also based on either a witnessed death (verbal autopsy instrument) whose eyewitness was interviewed by the research team, or an autopsy report indicating nonlethal injuries (superficial injuries or traumatic crush injury of extremities or of nonvital areas). The circumstances of these deaths most likely corresponded to two scenarios: lightly injured victim who was trapped or pinned under heavy rubble but was not readily accessible to rescuers using hand-held hydraulic tools and who later died of slow bleeding or environmental factors (dust inhalation, asphyxia, or hypothermia) within the first 24 to 48 hours after earthquake impact and before arrival of heavy rescue; or critically injured casualties who (according to eyewitnesses) were readily accessible and extricated from under light rubble by friends or relatives using bare hands or improvised tools but later died while awaiting emergency medical care or in transit to medical facilities, within hours or days of earthquake impact. These deaths were considered preventable if the informed judgment of a panel of medical experts concluded that, if immediate emergency medical care in the form of advanced life support (ALS) could have been rendered, these lives could potentially have been saved. Although lacking scientific rigor, these studies provided better than anecdotal evidence of a significant life-saving potential in earthquake disasters if more rapid emergency medical response is provided in the first few hours after impact.[5]

Crippen[9] elaborated on these findings and described four major classes of victims of multiple casualty events. Class 1 victims correspond to instant deaths and classes 2 to 4 correspond to potentially salvageable victims who, if left unaided, result in protracted deaths (**Table 1**).

Class 1 victims do not benefit from resuscitative efforts. Class 2 victims may be salvageable with immediate application of advanced resuscitative techniques

Table 1
Description of four major classes of victims in multiple casualty events (earthquake)

Class 1	Victims died immediately or within minutes after event
Class 2	Victims sustained serious traumatic injuries, are trapped, or require difficult, time-consuming manipulations to be extracted from the rubble and then need advanced life support
Class 3	Victims potentially salvageable if rendered immediate, simple first aid, such as hemostatic measures, stabilizing fractures, or maintaining the airway until further care is available
Class 4	Victims with minimal injuries that are trapped in protected coves where they have some protection from further trauma until rescued

Data from Crippen D. The World Trade Center attack. Similarities to the 1988 earthquake in Armenia: time to teach the public life-supporting first aid? Crit Care 2001;5(6):312–4.

requiring availability of specialists, usually physicians and technology (equipment for mechanical ventilation, massive transfusion, procedures of advanced trauma life support protocol). Generally, this can be done at trauma centers in civilian settings or mobile hospital units in military settings. At the present time no trauma or emergency medical services system in the world has the capacity to deliver adequate resources within a few minutes to a large population of critically injured casualties. Indeed, resuscitative effort geared toward class 2 victims hinders rescue of more salvageable victims and may be detrimental to overall success of the response.

Class 3 represents the group with the highest rescue potential. Life-supporting first aid (LSFA) applied by trained uninjured survivors can have the most profound impact. The set of simple maneuvers described later not only saves lives but also ensures good functional outcome preventing secondary injuries to brain, spinal cord, bones structures, and peripheral nerves.

Survival of class 4 victims depends not on medical personnel but mainly on search and rescue teams, sniff dogs, and work by structural engineers.

MAJOR COMPONENTS OF RESUSCITATION

Resuscitation in a multiple casualty event consists of the life-support chain that spans basic life support (BLS) in the field to definitive medical-surgical treatment with or without prolonged life support and intensive care in hospitals. Resuscitation is divided into three highly interdependent components: (1) BLS or LSFA, administered by uninjured bystanders or first responders; (2) ALS, administered by trained emergency medical personnel; and (3) prolonged life support (definitive and intensive care), administered by medical specialists functioning within the context of a well-organized emergency medical and trauma care system.

BLS is the entity with which most first responders in the United States are familiar. Basic trauma life support is an offshoot that adds emphasis on cerebral resuscitation and control of hemorrhage. LSFA, introduced and promulgated by Safar and Bircher[1] in the 1990s, is a relatively new term with a dual intent. As the name implies LSFA consists of potentially life-saving skills or maneuvers that can be applied in any emergency by anyone, anywhere, and with minimal to no equipment. LSFA focuses on the following techniques or procedures: (1) activating the emergency care system; (2) safe extrication of the trapped victim (rescue pull); (3) positioning for shock; (4) establishment and maintenance of the patent airway; (5) temperature control; (6) control of external hemorrhage; and (7) if applicable, cardiopulmonary resuscitation (CPR).

ALS usually delivered within 1 hour of injury (the golden hour) during everyday emergency and trauma care (scoop and run) is delayed for several hours or days and shifted almost entirely to the prehospital setting during multiple casualty events (stay and play or resuscitate while transporting). The objective of multiple casualty care in sudden-impact civilian disasters is different than in the nondisaster situation and is aimed at prolonging the window of opportunity for the delivery of resuscitative life support to the most salvageable (by triage) severely injured casualties, within 24 hours (golden 24 hours) of injury.

Prolonged life support consists of prompt definitive medical or surgical treatment of life-threatening injuries (ie, resuscitative or damage control surgery), also within 24 hours of injury, followed by intensive care over a period of days or weeks, and if necessary, rehabilitation over months to years.

Resuscitology (or reanimatology) is the science of resuscitation. When applied to the victims of multiple casualty events it encompasses the life support chain, which starts at the scene of injury with basic or LSFA response by trained bystanders and more advanced care provided by personnel of the emergency medical services system and is followed immediately by definitive medical-surgical treatment or prolonged life support and critical care (intensive care) medicine, as needed, in hospitals. There is a caveat: strict separation of these life-supporting steps into cardiac versus trauma life support is not advisable because the pathophysiologic derangements to be treated and the techniques to be realized are similar. Nevertheless, closed chest compression as a current cornerstone of the LSFA/BLS/advanced cardiac life support (ACLS) algorithms has major limitations in the setting of a multiple casualty event. At this time bystander (civilian) response remains the weakest link in the life support chain during everyday emergencies and especially in multiple casualty events. This is caused by lack of a concerted effort on the part of health authorities to mass educate and train the public in LSFA.

OPTIMAL TIMING OF RESUSCITATION

Time is the crucial risk factor for emergency medical response in multiple casualty events.

Prehospital Response (0–6 Hours)

Life-supporting first aid (LSFA)

LSFA must be provided at the scene within minutes of injury and can be mastered by any individual older than 12 years of age.[10] Before proceeding with rescue efforts hazards have to be assessed. The rescue potential of disaster is a function of the number of lives saved (deaths prevented), which in turn is highly dependent on the timing and quality of the intervention. However, lay rescuers must be taught that rescue efforts may pose a significant danger to them and should only be attempted if trained. LSFA consists of the key maneuvers discussed next.

External hemorrhage control

The control of external arterial or venous hemorrhage should be promptly done by direct compression to underlying tissue or elevation of the extremity. Widely described maneuvers for compression control of bleeding from major vessels requires some knowledge of anatomy and may be less effective in a crisis situation.

Tourniquets should be used only as a last resort and only in cases of extreme trauma to the extremities in which major vessels have been injured. Even in traumatic amputations severed vessels may retract and stop bleeding. When the tourniquet is in place over extended periods, nerves, blood vessels, and the entire extremity may be permanently damaged. When applied too loosely the tourniquet can increase bleeding by impeding venous drainage. To summarize, only trained medical personnel should apply tourniquets and its value for LSFA is limited.[11]

Airway control

Airway obstruction should be promptly recognized at the scene. Unconscious victims likely may have traumatic brain injury (TBI) of various degrees. Simple maneuvers, such as head tilt/chin lift/jaw thrust (the triple-airway maneuver) **Fig. 1**, can reverse airway obstruction and restore spontaneous ventilation and oxygenation. The triple-airway maneuver relieves soft tissue obstruction of the posterior hypopharynx. In the setting of suspected cervical spine injury, however, jaw thrust without head tilt should be used to avoid further spinal cord damage. Victims of a fall from a height are likely to have the highest percentage of cervical spine injury. In this case the two-handed jaw thrust should be initially attempted because it has been shown to be more successful.[12] There is growing evidence that chest compression is the most important component of CPR. However, this may not apply to the unconscious victims of a mass casualty event. Most of these casualties are unconscious because of TBI or profound hypotension, and not because of dysrhythmic cardiac events. Hypoventilation, hypercarbia, and hypoxia are well established and likely the most important determinants of morbidity, mortality, and functional status after TBI. Therefore, a patent airway and adequate ventilation become dominant factors for successful resuscitation of the victim.

Positioning and extrication of casualties (rescue pull)

A seriously injured person should not be moved by anyone not trained in field rescue, unless it is essential to avoid aggravating injuries or to protect the victim from further injury or death. If the injured person is conscious the victim should be placed in the horizontal and supine (face up) position with legs elevated. This may have a slight autotransfusion effect and counteracts postural hypotension. This effect is transient and increases cardiac output and blood pressure but lasts less than 10 minutes.[13] The head-down position is not recommended. Although it may increase blood pressure, cardiac output and tissue perfusion remain the same.[14] Normal body temperature should be maintained thereby avoiding overheating and hypothermia. Lightweight thermal blankets are used for this purpose. If the shocked victim is unconscious and breathing adequately the victim should be placed in the supported supine position or moved with head/neck/chest aligned into the stable side position, even when conscious, because vomiting and aspiration are possible. If the victim needs to be moved to safety, the rescue pull (ie, extrication without equipment) should be applied. During a rescue pull the injured limbs are displaced as little as possible and the head, neck, and chest immobilized in the aligned position, preferably with the assistance of helpers providing simultaneous airway management (head tilt, open mouth, and jaw

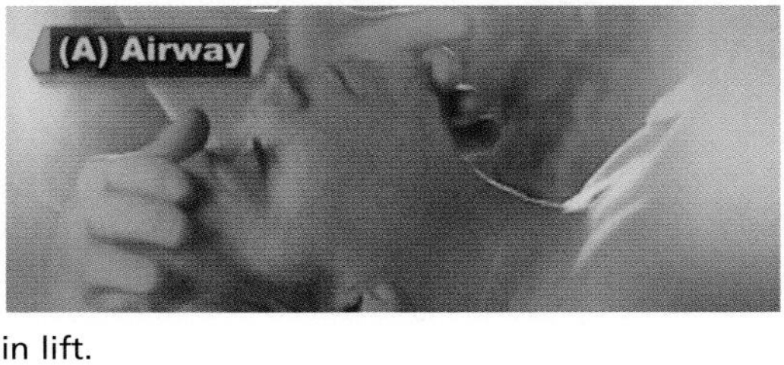

Fig. 1. Head tilt, chin lift.

thrust) in the unconscious victim. Ambulance personnel, whenever possible, should extricate with the help of a short backboard applied before gently moving the patient onto a longer backboard, using established methods of prehospital trauma care.

External cardiac resuscitation (CPR)
Classical CPR with chest compressions and defibrillation delivered to critically injured casualties in a multiple casualty event in the prehospital setting usually yields disappointing results in terms of survival and neurologic outcome.[15] External CPR alone in an exsanguinating victim is futile.[16] One should remember that the ACLS algorithm was designed mainly for the victim of cardiac arrest secondary to primary cardiac cause. Predominant mechanisms of cardiac arrest in victims of a multiple casualty event are hypovolemia, TBI, and airway obstruction. Therefore, depending on the scale of the event and the immediate availability of post-CPR resources, such as mechanical ventilation or immediate transport to tertiary care center, ACLS should be used only in selected cases.

ALS (0–12 Hours)

Airway management
In the comatose and unresponsive patient endotracheal intubation is the definitive step in airway management and remains the gold standard. A Glasgow Coma Scale (GCS) less than eight is a well-established indication for endotracheal intubation (**Fig. 2**) according to TBI guidelines.[17] The availability of mechanical ventilation must be determined in advance. Adequate mask ventilation is as important a skill to master as is direct laryngoscopy and endotracheal intubation. This has particular importance in the setting of TBI when even brief episodes of hypoxia and hypercarbia have deleterious potential. Recently, various supraglottic airway devices have been adopted by

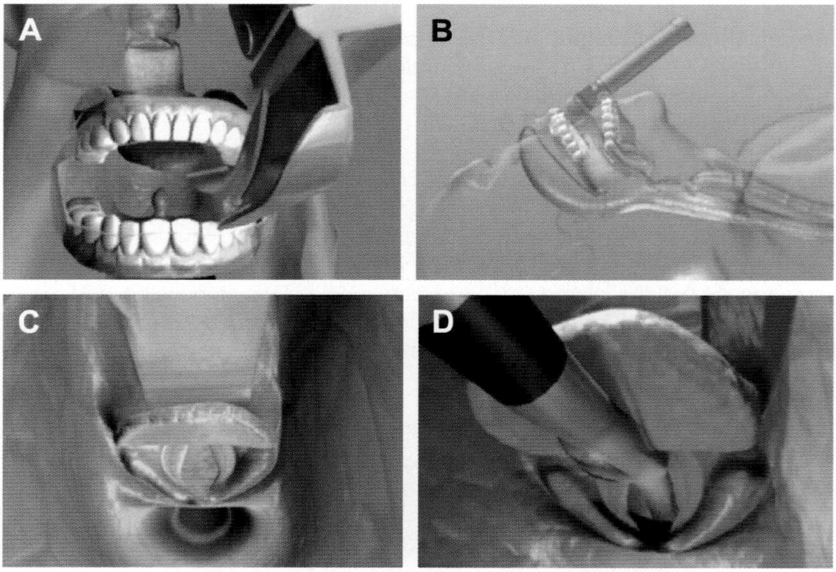

Fig. 2. Endotracheal intubation. (*A*) Curved blade inserted in the right corner of the mouth and tongue swept aside. (*B, C*) Tip of the blade placed into the valecula and vocal cords are visualized. (*D*) Endotracheal tube placed under direct vision into the trachea.

emergency medical services systems in the United States. These include different types of Laryngeal mask airway (LMA)s, the King airway, and so forth. Emergency medical care providers who are less experienced in endotracheal intubation usually use these devices. It is also used as a back-up airway rescue technique when endotracheal intubation fails.[18] If there is a need for prolonged mechanical ventilation these devices should be exchanged for an endotracheal tube, because they do not reliably protect from aspiration. The surgical airway, cricothyroidotomy, remains the option of last resort when all other measures of airway management fail. Again, timing of this life-saving intervention is crucial. It should be attempted before profound bradycardia develops, which is usually an indication of severe hypoxemia and impending cardiac arrest.[19] Any airway device placement should be confirmed by capnometry or capnography, because other methods of confirmation are not sufficiently reliable.[20]

Ventilation and oxygenation

During the last decade two ventilation concepts have changed significantly. First, the danger of dynamic hyperinflation or auto-peep has been recognized. In hypovolemic patients positive pressure ventilation (PPV) with inadequate expiratory time leading to incomplete deflation of the lung and step-wise increase in end-expiratory intrathoracic pressure may cause cardiovascular collapse. This is more common with aggressive bag-valve-mask ventilation of hemodynamically unstable patients.[21] Cardiac output is lower in hypovolemic patients. CO_2 transport is impaired with increase in dead space. Alveolar ventilation should be maintained at adequate level to avoid CO_2 accumulation and exacerbation of acidosis by adding respiratory component. If CPR is attempted providers should deliver a breath every 6 to 8 seconds, for 8 to 10 breaths per minute,[20] which allows enough time for exhalation. Second, there is increased incidence of oxygen toxicity with extended administration of high-inspired oxygen concentration. Fraction of inspired oxygen should be adjusted to maintain saturation above 90%, but not 100% in the postresuscitation period.[22,23] This approach is consistent with the latest evidence and recommendations regarding oxygen toxicity and concurrently it helps preserve oxygen supply for the victims in need.

Tube thoracostomy

Emergency tube thoracostomy is discussed in this section because tension pneumothorax may lead to immediate cardiopulmonary collapse and death with initiation of PPV. High clinical suspicion is the key for rapid diagnosis and life-saving treatment. Intervention should never be delayed for radiographic confirmation. Bedside ultrasound (US) is rapidly gaining popularity because methods to assess air or fluid in the pleural cavity with sensitivity of 90% and specificity of 98% are routinely obtained.[24] US units have become more portable and rugged, allowing use in extreme environments. As expertise and ease of US use grows within the medical community it is feasible that it will be used as a point-of-care or triage tool, including thoracic trauma, even in the setting of multiple casualty events.[25] Needle decompression in the second intercostal space with a 14-gague intravenous catheter should be done promptly, if development of tension pneumothorax is suspected. Tube thoracostomy is a definitive treatment (**Fig. 3**).

Volume resuscitation

The approach to fluid resuscitation has changed significantly with the development and implementation of the concept of damage control resuscitation. Damage control resuscitation is a strategy combining the techniques of permissive hypotension, hemostatic resuscitation, and damage control surgery, and has been widely adopted as the preferred method of resuscitation in patients with hemorrhagic shock. The main

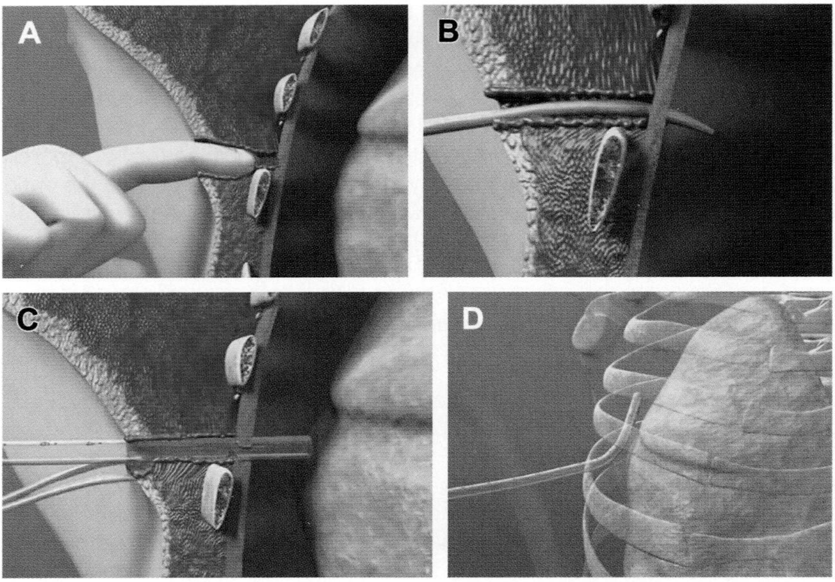

Fig. 3. Tube thoracostomy. (*A*) Incision is made at fifth intercostal space (nipple level) over superior aspect of the rib to avoid neurovascular bundle. (*B*) Bluntly dissect with Kelly clamp/finger angled superiorly remaining on superior border of the rib. (*C*) Grasp the end of the chest tube with the Kelly clamp and insert alongside index finger guiding away from lung parenchyma. (*D*) Direct anteroapical for pneumothorax and posterobasilar for fluid.

goal of damage control resuscitation is to prevent development of the "lethal triad" of trauma: (1) coagulopathy, (2) acidosis, and (3) hypothermia.[26,27] In the early prehospital and hospital phase of resuscitation of the hemorrhaging victim permissive hypotension should be allowed, with systolic blood pressure (SBP) goals of 80 to 90 mm Hg to minimize bleeding by damaged vessels. Aggressive crystalloid and colloid resuscitation in this phase has been linked to coagulopathy and worse outcome compared with restrictive fluid strategy. There are sufficient animal data to support this concept in blunt and penetrating injury. Human data exist to support its use in the setting of penetrating trauma.[28] This method should not be used in someone who is suffering from TBI. In this group SBP of 100 mm Hg should be targeted.

Transfusion practice in the setting of trauma and massive hemorrhage has changed dramatically during the last decade. Early transfusion of fresh frozen plasma (FFP) and platelets has been advocated to prevent development of trauma-induced coagulopathy. Optimal ratio of these blood products in relationship to packed red blood cells (PRBC) continues to be debated. Most evidence advocating "hemostatic protocols" comes from military experience with penetrating trauma in young men. A major concern with these studies, however, is the so called "survival bias," wherein patients who survive long enough to receive higher volumes of FFP result in high PRBC/FFP ratios.[29] Although the number of retrospective studies advocating high ratios of PRBC/FFP/platelet transfusion is impressive, the American Association of Blood Banks neither supports nor recommends this practice. In multiple casualty events blood product availability is limited. In this case, whole blood may be a better alternative to blood component therapy. Infrastructure and resources to ensure blood donation should be developed before such an event.[30] Massive transfusion frequently leads to hypocalcemia caused by chelation of calcium by citrate contained in PRBC and FFP. Correction of ionized calcium is a simple measure to avoid this problem. The amount of FFP transfused and the degree of metabolic acidosis were identified as major predictors of hypocalcemia. Sodium bicarbonate use is controversial in lactic acidosis and hypovolemic shock. It may lead to exacerbation of intracellular acidosis and hypercarbia if minute ventilation is not adequate. Although it may briefly correct metabolic acidosis there is no benefit in terms of survival. If it is used bicarbonate should be given for pH of less than 7 to 7.1.[31]

Tranexamic acid should be given to anyone requiring massive transfusion. Its value is increased in the setting of limited resources, when hemostatic transfusion protocols cannot be maintained, such as in multiple casualty events. If used, tranexamic acid should be initiated within 3 hours of the injury. Its use past this window has been associated with increased mortality.[32] However, in multiple casualty events with limited resources massive transfusion is not justifiable, and the use of blood and blood component products is very limited and highly dependent on the estimated number of critically injured casualties.

Vasoactive drugs

Catecholamines, such as epinephrine and norepinephrine, have limited use in the setting of hypovolemic shock. They may lead to worsening of metabolic acidosis, increase in lactate production, induce cardiac dysrhythmias, and increase myocardial oxygen consumption. Vasopressin is a potent vasoconstrictor and has been shown to improve outcomes in animal models of hypovolemic shock.[33] It is the most potent vasoconstrictor and has sparing effects on the cerebral, renal, and coronary microcirculations. Unlike cathecolamines vasopressin efficacy is not affected by acidosis, which is almost always observed in the setting of hypervolemia.[34] Some authors suggested low-dose vasopressin infusion as part of a resuscitation algorithm.[35] There is an ongoing European trial assessing administration of vasopressin versus normal saline in the prehospital phase during everyday trauma.[36] However, lack of evidence, logistical difficulties of setting-up infusion delivery systems, and monitoring hemodynamics, requiring experienced providers, significantly limit the use of vasoactive infusions in the field, and at this point they cannot be recommended for use in the prehospital phase of multiple casualty events.

Acute pain management

Adequate and safe pain relief in the prehospital phase during a multiple casualty event cannot be overemphasized. Definitive medical care addressing appropriate pain control can be delayed significantly. In addition to the alleviation of suffering adequate pain relief facilitates fracture immobilization and reduction, safe transport of the patient, and extraction of entrapped victims. Opioids, usually morphine sulfate, have been used extensively in the prehospital trauma setting for a long time. It has significant disadvantages, such as delayed onset of action, difficulty with titration, and hypotension with higher doses, especially in the patient who is hypovolemic. Ketamine has been successfully used for more effective pain relief, fracture immobilization, and to facilitate prolonged extrication of trapped or pinned victims by emergency personnel. It can be given as intramuscular injection. It does not depress ventilation and almost never leads to airway compromise requiring airway management. Several studies have confirmed the efficiency and safety of ketamine use in the prehospital setting. Median dose in one of the studies was 45 mg.[37] Ketamine has also been shown to be effective in combination with regional anesthesia.[38]

Hospital Phase: Prolonged Life Support (0–24 hours)

Triage

The main purpose of triage is the optimal use of available resources when the scale of human damage exceeds the capabilities of the emergency medical care delivery system, ensuring that the maximum lifesaving benefit is delivered to the largest number of salvageable victims with the minimal amount of resources. As the scale of the multiple casualty event increases more or sometimes all triage decisions are made in the field. There are two major triage models. One is based on short evacuation times and prompt access to definitive care, such as in a mass shooting or transport accident. Another is based on a multiple casualty event with significant damage to infrastructure, delay of outside assistance, and unknown arrival time of definitive care, such as in an earthquake or tsunami. The simple triage and rapid treatment (START) (**Fig. 4**) system has been rapidly adopted across the United States since the late 1980s. It has been shown to have acceptable levels of undertriage with 100% sensitivity and 90%

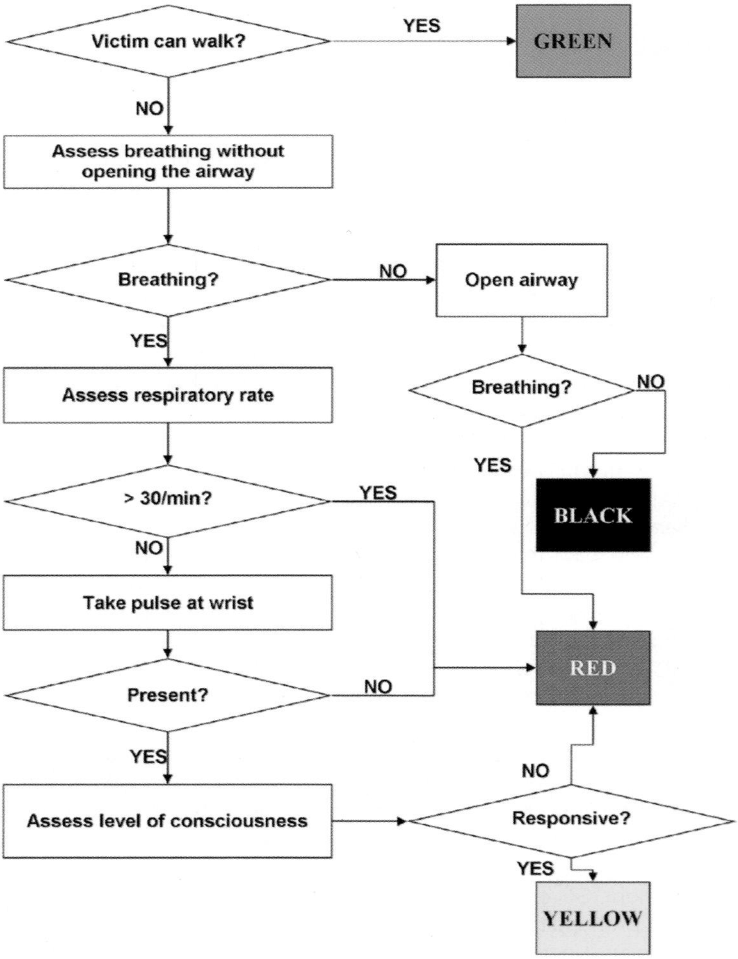

Fig. 4. START system algorithm.

specificity for the "red" life-threatening injury group. Amount of overtriaged patients was significant, reaching 44.6% in one study.[39] The START algorithm can be combined with secondary triage level (secondary assessment of victim endpoint). The latter method directs resources to the patient based on age, preexisting comorbidities, extent of injuries, and available trauma statistics to guide triage decisions, but a full description of this triage method is beyond the scope of this article.[40]

Cerebral resuscitation

Patients with suspected TBI should be immediately evaluated for appropriateness of hemodynamic and intracranial pressure (ICP) management. This is essential to prevent secondary brain injury, which may aggravate initial cerebral injury. Victims with GCS of eight or less should have elective endotracheal intubation. The nasal route should be avoided because of the possibility of basilar skull fractures. SBP less than 90 mm Hg, oxygen saturation less than 90 mm Hg, and Po_2 less than 60 should be avoided and corrected immediately if noticed. Patients with GCS of nine or less and high probability of intracranial hemorrhage should have an ICP monitor placed. Cerebral perfusion pressure should be maintained at 50 mm Hg or higher. If elevated ICP is diagnosed, it can be treated in several ways. Elevation of the head of the bed to improve venous outflow should be instituted. Normocarbia should be maintained. Hyperventilation may lead to profound cerebral vasoconstriction and worsening of brain perfusion and should be avoided. Hyperosmolar therapy with mannitol or hypertonic saline has been used extensively in this group of patients. Mannitol can be used as a temporizing measure to decrease ICP while awaiting completion of imaging studies or as an ongoing therapy for increases in ICP. Refractory ICP elevation may necessitate placement of a ventriculostomy (**Fig. 5**) and monitoring of serum

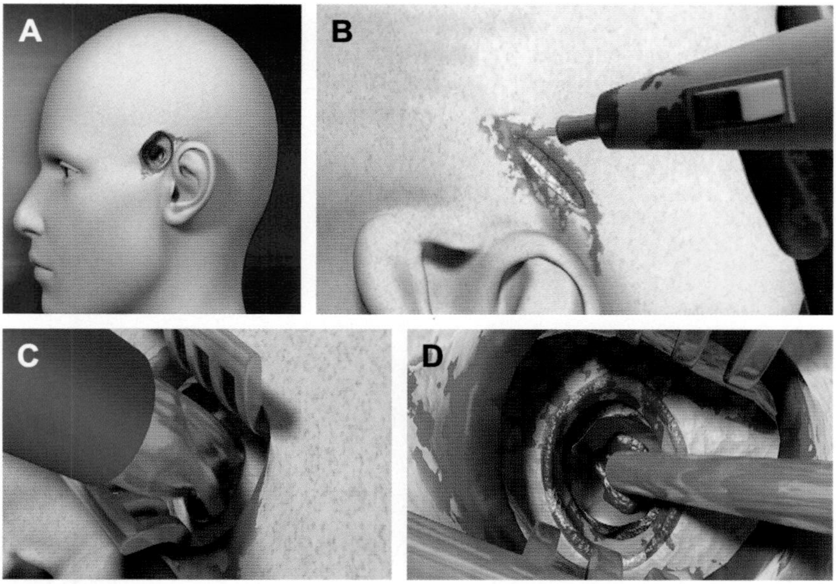

Fig. 5. Ventriculostomy. (*A*) Anterior insertion point: midpupilary line, 3 cm lateral to the sagittal suture and 2 cm anterior to the coronal suture. (*B*) Make 1-cm incision with the scalpel and extend down to the bone. (*C*) Hold the twist drill perpendicular to the skull and make a bur hole. (*D*) Advance the ventriculostomy catheter perpendicular to the brain surface toward median cantus of ipsilateral eye.

osmolality. Hypertonic saline has not been shown to be superior to mannitol for ICP reduction. One group of patients that may benefit from administration of hypertonic saline is those with moderate to severe TBI with coexisting hypovolemic shock.[17] The TBI resuscitation algorithm is shown in **Fig. 6**.

Focused assessment with sonography in trauma

Focused assessment with sonography in trauma (FAST) has revolutionized diagnostic traumatology. With the bedside US machine the diagnosis of hemoperitoneum can be made rapidly and reliably. Significant improvement in technology and availability of hand-held portable US machines can drastically improve the care of victims, even in the prehospital or field hospital setting. Recently, FAST examination has been modified to extended FAST, which includes evaluation of the chest for hemothorax and pneumothorax, and evaluation for pericardial effusion.[41] There is recent evidence of success with the FAST examination to screen earthquake victims in the field for intra-abdominal injuries, with sensitivity and specificity approaching that of a CT examination (**Fig. 7**).[42]

Resuscitative surgery

A description of resuscitative craniotomy, thoracotomy, and laparotomy procedures as forms of damage control surgery is beyond the scope of this article. These interventions are usually performed by trauma surgeons on patients with life-threatening head, chest, or abdominal injuries under emergency conditions. The reader is referred to other publications for a detailed treatise of these topics.[43–47]

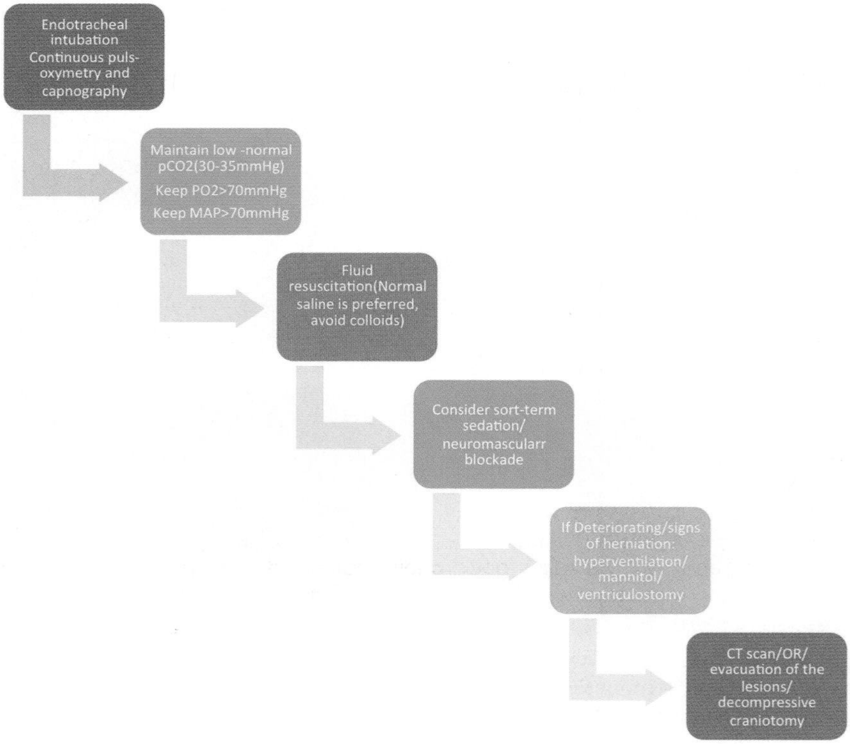

Fig. 6. TBI resuscitation algorithm.

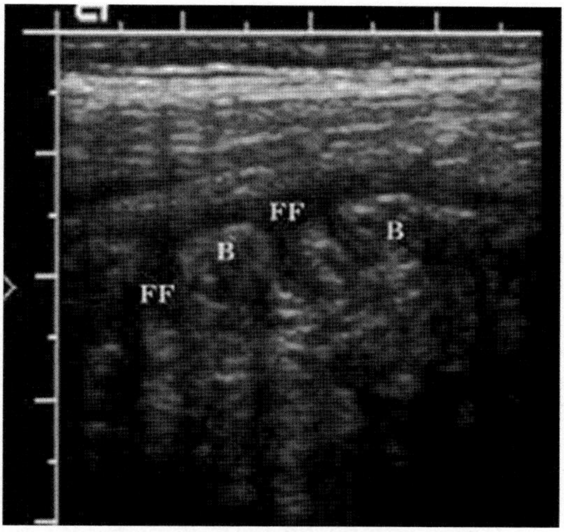

Fig. 7. FAST examination: free fluid (FF) with floating bowel (B).

DISASTER-RELATED INJURY MECHANISMS

Drowning

Drowning is defined as the process of respiratory impairment from total submersion or immersion in liquid. Submersion accidents kill more than 500.000 people per year, excluding victims of tsunamis and floods.[48,49] Drowning is subdivided into fatal and nonfatal. The term "near drowning" should be abandoned and replaced by water rescue. Drowning in fresh water produces similar degrees of damage as drowning in salt water. It induces wash out of surfactant and destabilization of alveoli. Water rescue requires rescue breathing only and should be attempted solely by trained individuals. The victim is brought ashore, placed parallel to the shoreline, and rescue breathing initiated. Hypoxia is the primary cause of cardiac arrest in drowning victims. Hence the conventional A-B-C approach should be used, but not C-A-B, as in recent ACLS guidelines. Compression-only CPR should be avoided in this group. It is recommended to start with not two but five rescue breaths.[50] Attempts to expel water from the airway with abdominal thrusts or back-blows should not be used because they are not effective and only delay initiation of rescue breathing. Abdominal thrusts may also lead to increases in intra-abdominal pressure and may induce vomiting. Chest compressions should be started if the victim has no pulse and continued as described in ACLS guidelines. Regurgitation of stomach content is very common during resuscitation of drowning victims. Suctioning and clearing of the airway should not delay resumption of ventilation.[51]

If a patient does not regain consciousness with these simple measures, ALS should be initiated. Endotracheal intubation should be done early. Supraglottic airway devices, such as LMA, are not a good choice for the drowning victim because of low pulmonary compliance and high chance of regurgitation during resuscitation. Instead, a lung-protective strategy with tidal volumes of 6 to 8 mL/kg combined with higher levels of peak end-expiratory pressure titrated to saturation of 92% to 96% should be used. Diuretics may be needed if the patient develops hypervolemia secondary to fluid absorption. Drowning frequently is associated with hypothermia. Icy water, particularly (<5°C, 41°F) may provide significant brain protection against hypoxia. Duration of resuscitative efforts lasting 2 to 2.5 hours with return of spontaneous circulation and good neurologic outcome in such circumstances has been reported.[52]

Hypothermia

Accidental hypothermia is defined as a decrease in core body temperature below 35°C. It may be underdiagnosed in multiple casualty events, especially in countries with warm climates. It always should be confirmed by measurement of core temperature with a temperature probe in the distal esophagus. A portable alternative to the esophageal temperature probe is the thermistor-based tympanic thermometer. Infrared-based techniques are not designed to accurately measure low temperatures. Hypothermic cardiac arrest calls for the most aggressive and prolonged resuscitation simultaneously with slow rewarming. Resuscitation efforts should not be discontinued until core body temperature rises to 35°C.[50] There are numerous rewarming techniques available. Osborn waves can be noticed on the electrocardiogram (ECG) and be mistaken for myocardial ischemia. Frequently, hypothermic victims have extreme bradycardia, with low blood pressure and barely palpable pulses. In this setting cardiac pacing is not required and the heart rate normalizes with increases in temperature. The metabolism of drugs in the setting of hypothermia is slowed down. Because of that there is a poor response to antiarrhythmic agents and doses should be reduced depending on the degree of hypothermia.[53]

During rewarming patients have decreases in systemic vascular resistance and relative hypovolemia, necessitating fluid resuscitation with warmed solutions. However, adjuncts used for slow rewarming, such as extracorporeal membrane oxygenation, have no practical applicability in a disaster zone.

Crush Injury

Crush injury caused by entrapment of a victim under large and heavy objects or debris is very common after earthquakes (**Fig. 8**). This may lead to crush syndrome consisting of acute renal failure, hypercalcemia, hypophosphatemia, and disseminated intravascular coagulation. The destruction of large muscle mass groups with release of intracellular components, such as myoglobin, potassium, and calcium, explains the clinical presentation. Treatment with potassium-free intravenous fluids, such as normal saline, should be initiated in the field as soon as possible, preferably before liberation of the entrapped victim. This has been shown to significantly reduce the incidence of acute renal failure and the need for renal replacement therapy, which becomes scarce in a disaster zone.[54] Initial rate of infusion should be 1000 mL/h for

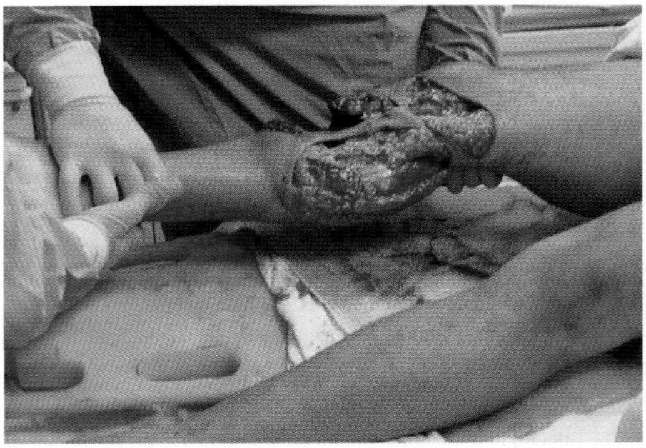

Fig. 8. Crush injury.

the first 2 hours, and decreased to 500 mL/h afterward. In children it should be started at 20 mL/kg/h and decreased to 10 mL/kg/h, respectively. Aggressive fluid therapy remains the mainstay of crush injury treatment and other methods have only a supplementary role. On-site amputation may have to be done to liberate a crushed extremity but should be a last resort and may not prevent the development of crush syndrome.[50] Ketamine in doses of 2 to 4 mg/kg can be used in the field for this procedure. Some authors have suggested prophylactic application of a tourniquet to control reperfusion of the ischemic limb to prevent crush syndrome. However, this practice is no longer recommended. Tourniquets should be used only for uncontrolled life-threatening bleeding. Urine output should be monitored as closely as conditions allow on an hourly basis for 24 hours. For anuric patients condom catheter or Foley catheters should be placed. Urine output greater than 50 mL/h or 1 mL/kg/h should be the goal of fluid therapy. Foley catheters should be removed as soon as possible to minimize the risk of urinary tract infection, ideally within 48 hours of placement. If the patient remains anuric with a Foley catheter in place and hypovolemia is excluded, then fluids should be limited to 1000 mL per 24 hours plus insensible fluid losses because acute renal failure is likely to develop and continued fluid infusion may lead to fluid overload and pulmonary edema. Intravenous hydration should be converted to oral as soon as the patient is able to maintain adequate intake. Patients who have resolution of the symptoms with initiation of intravenous fluids and cannot receive continued medical attention because of lack of human or material resources should be educated regarding signs of myoglobinuria, so they can seek medical treatment if they have a recurrence of symptoms. In general, aggressive hydration should continue until disappearance of myoglobin from the urine or normalization of urine color (as a surrogate). This usually takes 2 to 3 days. Alkalinization of the urine with intravenous sodium bicarbonate has been widely used, although evidence to prove it's efficacy is lacking, especially if the patient has adequate urine output and no signs of metabolic acidosis.

Mannitol has been used as an osmolar diuretic with additional benefits of free radical scavenging and ability to decrease intracompartmental pressures. Although it is widely used in trauma for rhabdomyolisis there is no uniform opinion regarding its role in crush injury. It is reasonable to use a "mannitol challenge" and observe the clinical response.[55] Mannitol is contraindicated in patients who are anuric or hyperosmolar.

Potassium level should be determined as soon as possible. Varieties of point-of-care devices are available on the market and may become an invaluable asset in a disaster zone.[56] ECG recording using portable monitors with attention to signs of hyperkalemia, such as peaked T waves and progressive widening of QRS complex, may be used as an alternative technique. In the hospital the patient should be monitored for signs of hyperkalemia and treated urgently for acute symptoms with calcium chloride, insulin/glucose, sodium bicarbonate, or inhaled β-agonists. Sodium polystyrene sulfonate and dialysis are second-line treatment.[57]

Blast Injury

Blast injuries may lead to organ damage through several mechanisms. Blast injury primarily affects air-filled organs: lungs, inner ear, and hollow organs of the gastrointestinal tract. Internal organ blast injuries may not be detectable on initial triage; therefore, the presence of bleeding from the ear and disruption or rupture of the tympanic membrane serves as an indicator of severe blast injury to internal organs. Subarachnoid hemorrhage, severe pulmonary contusions with pneumothorax or hemothorax, and air embolism are the most frequent causes of death in these casualties. PPV and lung-preserving ventilatory strategy should be instituted in patients with pulmonary compromise. If the patient does not require PPV then regional or neuraxial anesthesia should be used whenever possible, because general anesthesia has been linked with worse outcomes in the early postinjury period. Shrapnel and other penetrating flying debris from the blast cause secondary blast injury. Intra-abdominal injury may require exploratory laparotomy. If not recognized promptly it may lead to a delayed presentation of peritonitis.[58]

Acute Radiation Syndrome

Depending on the level of exposure to radiation acute radiation syndrome may present as a cerebrovascular syndrome and death (>20 Gy); gastrointestinal syndrome (10–20 Gy); or hematopoetic syndrome (10 Gy). Ionizing radiation leads to direct damage of DNA and death of the cells. In smaller doses it leads to inability of the victim to mount an immune response against secondary infection.[59] Administration of granulocyte colony–stimulating factor (G-CSF) is essential for prophylaxis and early treatment of acute infections and should be started promptly after acute radiation exposure. The concomitant systemic and inhalational administration of G-CSF is advocated by some authors to "seal off" alveoli from exogenous microorganisms: 250 to 400 μg granulocyte-macrophage CSF or 5 μg/kg G-CSF given systemically and corresponding inhalation of GM-CSF, 300 μg per day for at least 14 to 21 days.[60,61]

Carbon Monoxide Poisoning

Carbon monoxide poisoning can occur in the acute phase of a disaster, after entrapment inside burning buildings. More commonly it happens because of power failure in the aftermath of hurricanes, ice storms, or earthquakes. Under these circumstances people use portable generators or open fire cooking inside confined spaces. Information regarding safe use of portable generators and awareness regarding toxic products of combustion should be disseminated and emphasized in the preparation phase of disaster.

Carbon monoxide is quickly absorbed through the lungs into the bloodstream and has extremely high affinity for hemoglobin. It leads to tissue hypoxia by two mechanisms. First, it binds to hemoglobin directly, which prevents linkage of oxygen to the hemoglobin molecule. Second, there is a shift of the oxyhemoglobin dissociation curve to the left resulting in decreased release of oxygen to the tissues and tissue hypoxia. Most common symptoms include nausea, vomiting, headache, and confusion followed by cardiac dysrhythmias, altered sensorium, and coma. One-hundred percent oxygen should be given as soon as possible if carbon monoxide poisoning is suspected. The diagnosis should be confirmed with three-wavelength pulse oximetry, which monitors functional, not fractional hemoglobin oxygen saturation. Portable co-oximeters are widely available at this time. Carbon monoxide may induce symptoms of myocardial ischemia even in patients who are clinically asymptomatic. Everyone with confirmed carbon monoxide poisoning should get a 12-lead ECG. Patients with pre-existing coronary artery disease or manifestation of central nervous system symptoms should also be tested for serum cardiac troponins. Duration of supplemental oxygen therapy or need for hyperbaric oxygen should be guided by the clinical picture (symptoms of altered mental status, confusion, nausea and vomiting, chest pain, and ECG abnormalities) rather than absolute levels of carboxyhemoglobin.[62]

REFERENCES

1. Safar P, Bircher N. Cardiopulmonary: cerebral resuscitation. World Federation of Sociaties of Anesthesiologists. Philadelphia: Saunders; 1987.

2. Pretto E, Ricci E, Safar P, et al. Disaster reanimatology potentials: a structured interview study in Armenia. III. Results, conclusions, and recommendations. Prehosp Disaster Med 1992;7(4):327–38.
3. Pretto E, Safar P. National medical response to mass disasters in the United States. Are we prepared? JAMA 1991;266:1259–62.
4. Klain M, Ricchi E, Safer P, et al. Disaster reanimatology potentials: a structured interview study in Armenia. I. Methodology and preliminary results. Prehosp Disaster Med 1989;4(2):135–54.
5. Bissell R, Pretto E, Angus D, et al. Post-preparedness disaster response in Costa Rica. Prehosp Disaster Med 1994;9(2):96–106.
6. Pretto E, Angus D, Abrams JI, et al. An analysis of prehospital mortality in an earthquake. Prehosp Disaster Med 1994;9(2):107–17.
7. Angus DA, Pretto E, Abrams JI, et al. Epidemiologic assessment of building collapse pattern, mortality, and medical response after the 1992 earthquake in Erzincan Turkey. Prehosp Disaster Med 1997;12(3):222–31.
8. Aoki N, Murakawa T, Pretto EA, et al. Survival and cost analysis of fatalities of the Kobe earthquake in Japan. Prehosp Emerg Care 2004;8:217–22.
9. Crippen D. The World Trade Center attack. Similarities to the 1988 earthquake in Armenia: time to teach the public life-supporting first aid? Crit Care 2001;5(6):312–4.
10. Fleischhackl R, Nuernberger A, Sterz F, et al. School children sufficiently apply life supporting first aid: a prospective investigation. Crit Care 2009;13(4):R127.
11. Lakstein D, Blumenfeld A, Sokolov T, et al. Tourniquets for hemorrhage control on the battlefield: a 4-year accumulated experience. J Trauma 2003;54:S221–5.
12. Joffe AM, Hetzel S, Liew EC. A two-handed jaw-thrust technique is superior to the one-handed "EC-clamp" technique for mask ventilation in the apneic unconscious person. Anesthesiology 2010;113(4):873–9.
13. Gaffney FA, Bastian BC, Thal ER, et al. Passive leg raising does not produce a significant or sustained autotransfusion effect. J Trauma 1982;22(3):190–3.
14. Bridges N, Jarquin-Valdivia AA. Use of the Trendelenburg position as the resuscitation position: to T or not to T? Am J Crit Care 2005;14(5):364–8.
15. Zwingmann J, Mehlhorn A, Hammer T, et al. Survival and neurologic outcome after traumatic out-of-hospital cardiopulmonary arrest in a pediatric and adult population: a systematic review. Crit Care 2012;16(4):R117.
16. Huber-Wagner S, Lefering R, Qvick M, et al. Outcome in 757 severely injured patients with traumatic cardiorespiratory arrest. Resuscitation 2007;75(2):276–85.
17. Bullock MR, Povlishock JT. Guidelines for the management of severe traumatic brain injury 3rd edition. J Neurotrauma 2007;24. S-7.
18. Practice guidelines for management of the difficult airway. Anesthesiology 1993;78:597–602.
19. Bonanno FG. The critical airway in adults: the facts. J Emerg Trauma Shock 2012;5(2):153–9.
20. Neumar RW, Otto CW, Link MS, et al. Part 8: adult advanced cardiovascular life support: 2010 American Heart Association Guidelines for Cardiopulmonary Resuscitation and Emergency Cardiovascular Care. Circulation 2010;122(18 Suppl 3):S729–67.
21. Marini JJ. Dynamic hyperinflation and auto-positive end-expiratory pressure: lessons learned over 30 years. Am J Respir Crit Care Med 2011;184(7):756–62.
22. Brenner M, Stein D, Hu P, et al. Association between early hyperoxia and worse outcomes after traumatic brain injury. Arch Surg 2012;1–5.

23. Kilgannon JH, Jones AE, Shapiro NI, et al. Association between arterial hyperoxia following resuscitation from cardiac arrest and in-hospital mortality. JAMA 2010; 303(21):2165–71.
24. Raja AS, Jacobus CH. How accurate is ultrasonography for excluding pneumothorax? Ann Emerg Med 2012. [Epub ahead of print].
25. Ma OJ, Norvell JG, Subramanian S. Ultrasound applications in mass casualties and extreme environments. Crit Care Med 2007;35(Suppl 5):S275–9.
26. Hildebrand F, Probst C, Frink M, et al. Importance of hypothermia in multiple trauma patients. Unfallchirurg 2009;112(11):959–64.
27. Maegele M, Paffrath T, Bouillon B. Acute traumatic coagulopathy in severe injury: incidence, risk stratification, and treatment options. Dtsch Arztebl Int 2011; 108(49):827–35.
28. Bickell WH, Wall MJ Jr, Pepe PE, et al. Immediate versus delayed fluid resuscitation for hypotensive patients with penetrating torso injuries. N Engl J Med 1994; 331(17):1105–9.
29. Brown JB, Cohen MJ, Minei JP, et al. Debunking the survival bias myth: characterization of mortality during the initial 24 hours for patients requiring massive transfusion. J Trauma Acute Care Surg 2012;73(2):358–64.
30. Neal MD, Marsh A, Marino R, et al. Massive transfusion: an evidence-based review of recent developments. Arch Surg 2012;147(6):563–71.
31. Boyd JH, Walley KR. Is there a role for sodium bicarbonate in treating lactic acidosis from shock? Curr Opin Crit Care 2008;14(4):379–83.
32. Kirkpatrick AW, Holcomb JB, Stephens MH, et al. Tranexamic acid effects in trauma patients with significant hemorrhage. J Am Coll Surg 2012;215(3):438–40.
33. Raedler C, Voelckel WG, Wenzel V, et al. Treatment of uncontrolled hemorrhagic shock after liver trauma: fatal effects of fluid resuscitation versus improved outcome after vasopressin. Anesth Analg 2004;98(6):1759–66 table of contents.
34. Voelckel WG, Raedler C, Wenzel V, et al. Arginine vasopressin, but not epinephrine, improves survival in uncontrolled hemorrhagic shock after liver trauma in pigs. Crit Care 2003;31:1160–5.
35. Anand T, Skinner R. Arginine vasopressin: the future of pressure-support resuscitation in hemorrhagic shock. J Surg Res 2012;178:321–9.
36. Lienhart HG, Wenzel V, Braun J, et al. Vasopressin for therapy of persistent traumatic hemorrhagic shock: the VITRIS.at study. Anaesthesist 2007;56(2):145–8, 150.
37. Sibley A, Mackenzie M, Bawden J, et al. A prospective review of the use of ketamine to facilitate endotracheal intubation in the helicopter emergency medical services (HEMS) setting. Emerg Med J 2011;28(6):521–5.
38. Missair A, Gebhard R, Pierre E, et al. Surgery under extreme conditions in the aftermath of the 2010 Haiti earthquake: the importance of regional anesthesia. Prehosp Disaster Med 2010;25(6):494–5.
39. Kahn CA, Schultz CH, Miller KT, et al. Does START triage work? An outcomes assessment after a disaster. Ann Emerg Med 2009;54(3):424–30, 430.e1.
40. Benson M, Koenig KL, Schultz CH. Disaster triage: START, then SAVE–a new method of dynamic triage for victims of a catastrophic earthquake. Prehosp Disaster Med 1996;11(2):117–24.
41. Mariani PJ, Wittick L. Pneumothorax diagnosis by extended focused assessment with sonography for trauma. J Ultrasound Med 2009;28(11):1601 [author reply: 1602].
42. Zhou J, Huang J, Wu H, et al. Screening ultrasonography of 2,204 patients with blunt abdominal trauma in the Wenchuan earthquake. J Trauma Acute Care Surg 2012;73:890–4.

43. Bell RS, Mossop CM, Dirks MS, et al. Early decompressive craniectomy for severe penetrating and closed head injury during wartime. Neurosurg Focus 2010;28(5):E1.
44. Letoublon C, Reche F, Abba J, et al. Damage control laparotomy. J Vasc Surg 2011;148(5):e366–70.
45. Rhee PM, Acosta J, Bridgeman A, et al. Survival after emergency department thoracotomy: review of published data from the past 25 years. J Am Coll Surg 2000;190(3):288–9.
46. Harnar TJ, Oreskovich MR, Copass MK, et al. Role of emergency thoracotomy in the resuscitation of moribund trauma victims: 100 consecutive cases. Am J Surg 1981;142(1):96–9.
47. Copass MK, Oreskovich MR, Bladergroen MR, et al. Prehospital cardiopulmonary resuscitation of the critically injured patient. Am J Surg 1984;148(1):20–6.
48. Working Group, Ad Hoc Subcommittee on Outcomes, American College of Surgeons. Committee on Trauma. Practice management guidelines for emergency department thoracotomy. Working Group, Ad Hoc Subcommittee on Outcomes, American College of Surgeons-Committee on Trauma. J Am Coll Surg 2001;193(3):303–9.
49. Injuries and violence prevention: non- communicable diseases and mental health: fact sheet on drowning. Geneva: World Health Organization; 2003. Available at: http://www.who.int/violence_injury_prevention/other_injury/drowning/en/index.html.
50. Soar J, Perkins GD, Abbas G, et al. European Resuscitation Council Guidelines for Resuscitation 2010 Section 8. Cardiac arrest in special circumstances: electrolyte abnormalities, poisoning, drowning, accidental hypothermia, hyperthermia, asthma, anaphylaxis, cardiac surgery, trauma, pregnancy, electrocution. Resuscitation 2010;81(10):1400–33.
51. Manolios N, Mackie I. Drowning and near-drowning on Australian beaches patrolled by life-savers: a 10-year study, 1973–1983. Med J Aust 1988;148(4): 165–7, 170–1.
52. Deakin CD. Drowning: more hope for patients, less hope for guidelines. Resuscitation.
53. van der Ploeg G, Goslings JC, Walpoth BH, et al. Accidental hypothermia: rewarming treatments, complications and outcomes from one university medical centre. Resuscitation 2010;81(11):1550–5.
54. Aoki N, Demsar J, Zupan B, et al. Predictive model for estimating risk of crush syndrome: a data mining approach. J Trauma 2007;62(2):451–2.
55. Eneas JF, Schoenfeld PY, Humphreys MH. The effect of infusion of mannitol-sodium bicarbonate on the clinical course of myoglobinuria. Arch Intern Med 1979;139(7):801–5.
56. Vanholder R, Borniche D, Claus S, et al. When the earth trembles in the Americas: the experience of Haiti and Chile 2010. Nephron Clin Pract 2011;117(3):c184–97.
57. Sever MS, Vanholder R, RDRTF of ISN Work Group on Recommendations for the Management of Crush Victims in Mass Disasters. Recommendation for the management of crush victims in mass disasters. Nephrol Dial Transplant 2012; 27(Suppl 1):i1–67.
58. Yeh DD, Schecter WP. Primary blast injuries: an updated concise review. World J Surg 2012;36(5):966–72.
59. Saito T. Acute radiation injury. Nihon Rinsho 2012;70(3):415–20 [in Japanese].
60. Heslet L, Bay C, Nepper-Christensen S. Acute radiation syndrome (ARS): treatment of the reduced host defense. Int J Gen Med 2012;5:105–15.

61. Zane DF, Bayleyegn TM, Hellsten J, et al. Tracking deaths related to Hurricane Ike, Texas, 2008. Disaster Med Public Health Prep 2011;5(1):23–8.
62. Brooks DE, Levine M, O'Connor AD, et al. Toxicology in the ICU. Part 2. Specific toxins. Chest 2011;140(4):1072–85.

Anesthesia in an Austere Setting

Lessons Learned from the Haiti Relief Operation

Timothy E. Morey, MD[a,*], Mark J. Rice, MD[b]

KEYWORDS

• Earthquake • Triage • Regional anesthesia • Ethics • Disaster • Anesthesia

KEY POINTS

- The earthquake will leave a disorganized medical system.
- Concurrently, masses of patients will need extremity surgery for fractures, crush, and burns. These surgeries are amenable to monitored anesthesia care and regional anesthesia.
- Language barriers may become a significant challenge.
- Some patients will have nonsurvivable injuries for the local environment, but still must be cared for ethically and humanely.
- The hospital and operating room team will need leaders.
- Adjust your own mental and physical expectations for yourself and anesthetic care to that required in a disaster zone with limited resources.

OVERVIEW OF ANESTHETIC CARE IN A DISASTER ZONE

Natural disasters of many types will continue to occur and will injure people living in both the developed and the developing world. The type, scope, and location of a disaster will dictate the kind of medical support needed to care for these patients. For example, the physical injuries (eg, many limb fractures)[1,2] following an earthquake in Haiti required very different medical services than an illness sustained after a nuclear disaster in Japan.[3] In 2010, the authors journeyed to Haiti after a severe earthquake that caused widespread damage to the national infrastructure and injury to many Haitians. This article recounts some of the authors' insights that might be helpful to practitioners serving in other disaster zones.

Disclosure: Dr Morey and Dr Rice have no conflicts of interest related to disaster care.
Drug and Equipment Trademarks: The authors have taken care to use no proprietary names of drugs or equipment.

[a] Department of Anesthesiology, University of Florida, PO 100254, Gainesville, FL 32610, USA;
[b] Liver Transplantation and General Surgery Sections, Department of Anesthesiology, University of Florida, PO 100254, Gainesville, FL 32610, USA
* Corresponding author.
E-mail address: morey@ufl.edu

Anesthesiology Clin 31 (2013) 107–115
http://dx.doi.org/10.1016/j.anclin.2012.10.003 **anesthesiology.theclinics.com**
1932-2275/13/$ – see front matter

Overall, one must mentally prepare for this challenge and possibly alter one's expectations of current anesthetic practice. That is, one should be ready for massive need, which is difficult to meet with even a well-resourced health care system, for the possibility of severely limited health care resources to match this need, for alterations in anesthetic practices forced by onsite equipment and supplies, for questions about medical triage and care, and for unmitigated gratitude from injured patients and their families. As in your own practice though, all efforts should remain focused on outstanding patient care to the highest degree possible given the limitations of an environment markedly altered by the natural disaster.

ORGANIZATION AMID CHAOS AFTER AN EARTHQUAKE

Natural disaster leads to disorganization of every type: social, economic, financial, food and water supply, and others. Likewise, health care also becomes disorganized and woefully inadequate. With respect to providing anesthesia, this lack of orderliness means that scheduling governance, patients' location, and supplies require extra attention to allow surgery in a timely manner.

Governance

The type of natural disaster will modify the number of patients seeking medical care. In the event of an earthquake, many patients will likely arrive for care because of an injury from falling debris, fires, and other hazards.[1,2] Because disaster services are not immediately available, malnutrition and dehydration are almost certainly present at the time of surgical intervention.[4] In the face of this wave, governance of the surgical services is especially important to allow optimal functioning and efficiency. Societies and cultures vary on how best to achieve this task. The authors recommend a senior member of the operating room team with previous governance experience take charge of overall organization of scheduling. As in traditional hospitals, the individual is required to understand the multistep process of providing care from posting to the recovery room and must have excellent communication skills and a high degree of organized forethought. Consultation with surgeons about case postings and nursing staff is necessary to ensure that patients receive appropriate surgical triage. Successful execution of the schedule (eg, "board running") remains this individual's task in addition to providing care. Multiple changes of posting and scheduling due to new patients or patient status can be anticipated. At many current hospitals with electronic scheduling and computerized tracking, one can readily appreciate a return to former decades with an operating room schedule arranged around paper notes and a cork board (**Fig. 1**).

Patients

Because the injured may be located outside of the immediate facility (the authors used a nearby elementary school for additional patient rooms), physically locating patients can become a major challenge that may delay surgery and waste surgical resources. These patients may be found in remote, obscure hospital rooms that volunteer staff did not even know existed or distantly out of the hospital in a field, lean-to, or hut. Likewise, identification of patients in the absence of wrist bands and the presence of differing languages can become challenging. For these reasons, a native group of transporters emerges as an extremely valuable component of the team to find and transport patients to the preoperative holding area (**Fig. 2**). To allow efficient operating room service, it may be advisable to queue all patients for the operating room the night before surgery. Likewise, knowledge of and fasting of several other "back-up" patients

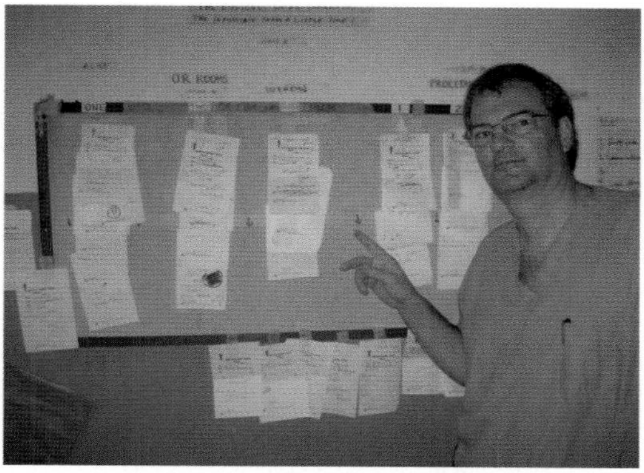

Fig. 1. Dr Mark J. Rice organizes the operating suite scheduling board. Shown are case postings on paper slips with patient name, surgeon name, and procedure. Those notes taped to the bottom of the corkboard frame indicate patients posted for surgery that could never be found.

requiring surgery may be advisable given the limited nature of operating room resources to allow maximal use of surgical resources.

Supplies

If fortunate, medical supplies will stream into the natural disaster site, although a wise clinician will attempt to bring his own provisions. Supplies may arrive in containers of every shape and material and identified in many languages. The onslaught of materials may lead to great disorganization of the anesthesia workroom, if one is even fortunate enough to have such a protected environment for supplies (**Fig. 3**). In the absence of supply organization, the services provided by anesthesia technicians, pharmacists, and pharmacy technicians in the home countries become much more appreciated during these times. For this reason, anesthetists can reliably plan on needing extra time to actually find drugs and supplies for any particular case. Likewise, nonclinical time (ie, late nights) can be valuably spent organizing supplies for yourself and colleagues, even if only in the most rudimentary manner. Alternatively, one should

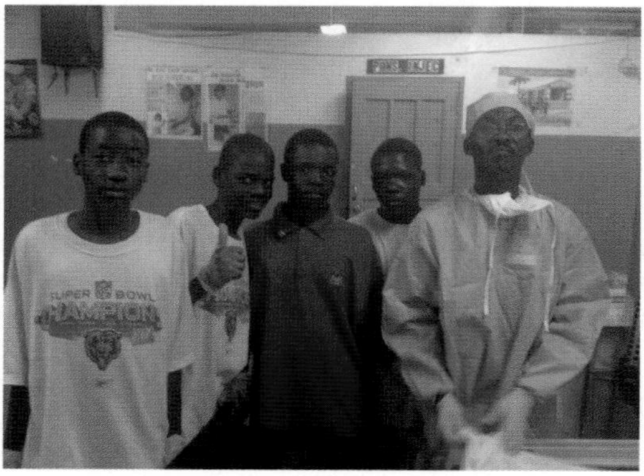

Fig. 2. Invaluable native citizens who provided translation services, located patients, and transported patients for surgery to the preoperative holding area.

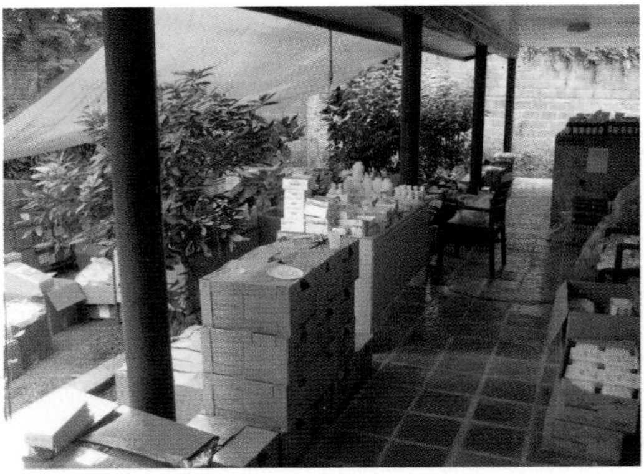

Fig. 3. Combined surgery and anesthesia supply area from supplies donated to the hospital for medical and surgical services.

consider bringing an anesthesia technician to assist with these duties. In addition, many of the supplies donated from distant locations may be unfamiliar to even experienced clinicians. That is, supplies delivered from around the globe may have different names for the same pharmaceutical (eg, lidocaine, lignocaine) or perhaps different concentrations (eg, 1 mg/mL or 10 mg/mL midazolam). Proper care to understand what medicine is actually being used requires additional effort, especially when anesthetists are fatigued, distracted, hungry, or working in poor lighting. In addition to supplies, previously donated anesthesia equipment may not be completely functional. Simple assessments and fixes can be attempted and achieved to enable fully functional equipment. For example, the authors reactivated an anesthesia machine simply by replacing an electrical fuse scavenged from an automobile. Simple tools (eg, multifunctional utility hand tool, fuses, electrical multimeter) can be uncommonly useful.

TRIAGE ETHICS IN A DISASTER

Natural disasters will mean a triage of patients and forced decisions about the use of medical resources. For example, which patients will receive care in an operating room when there are masses of patients needing limb amputation or incisional debridement? Likewise, with limited oxygen cylinders and a single working ventilator on only one of the anesthesia machines, is it wise to chronically ventilate a patient with such pressing needs before other injured patients in the community? In the presence of diabetic coma, which patients will receive extremely limited supplies of insulin, a drug that needs refrigeration, when the electrical supply (and local batteries) may be disrupted? Whatever your own personal choices, medical ethics at any particular disaster site will reflect the morals and religions of the local society. These local ethics may be quite different from physicians visiting from other locations, but are just as valid and locally in force. During one's visit to care for natural disaster patients, the local and guest values may well conflict. Successful resolution of this conflict relies on clear communication and mutual respect between local leaders (eg, native physicians, hospital director, priest, mayor) and those of the guest health care providers. Some starting points for resolution may include the formation of a local ethics committee that is charged with understanding the position of all parties, such as the hospital administration, guest anesthetists, local religious leaders and physicians, and the patient's family. Indeed, one of the authors (MJR) served on such an emergency committee to assist in developing appropriate choices for the discontinuance of ventilation in a patient with nonsurvivable injuries. In additional, this committee can obtain information from outside sources. For example, a Catholic hospital and community may well be attuned to church doctrine for the faithful that can be learned by communicating with global centers such as the National Catholic Bioethics Center (NCBC, Philadelphia, PA, USA). This organization is "...committed to applying the moral teachings of the Catholic Church to ethical issues arising in health care and the life sciences. The NCBC provides consultations to individuals and institutions seeking its opinion on the appropriate application of Catholic moral teaching to these ethical issues."[5] Given the authors'deployment to a Catholic hospital, the services rendered by the NCBC were extremely valuable to address when the aforementioned situations were encountered (**Fig. 4**). In any event, no visiting anesthetist should be compelled to commit acts that violate his own personal medical ethics.

PERSONAL HEALTH OF VOLUNTEERS IN A DISASTER ZONE

Finding a Way There

The authors worked at the Hôpital Sacré Coeur, which is about 16 km south of the Cap Haitien International Airport. This airport is the second largest in Haiti and serves the city of Cap Haitien, with a population of 180,000. Like the surrounding city, the airport is destitute without runway lighting (ie, no night flights) or fuel depot. Because pilots must bring their own fuel, they pay scrupulous attention to weight limits, with all passengers and supplies carefully weighed. When necessary, medical supplies and equipment are abandoned to achieve a safe weight before takeoff. Indeed, the large trailer of medical supplies donated by the authors' hospital was decimated to only what could physically be carried in a single knapsack at the expense of valuable supplies and personal items. At the Haitian airport, people and various animals were observed, including goats and dogs, on the runway both when the authors arrived and when the authors departed. The authors also took a letter of authorization from their sponsor, the CRUDEM (Center for the Rural Development of Milot) Foundation, which the authors were told would be required to pass through customs, although the officials never asked for this letter. It is not possible to know how the earthquake affected immigration and customs services. Several airlines serve Cap Haitien Airport, with flights to Fort Lauderdale, Florida and several Caribbean destinations, such as the Bahamas and

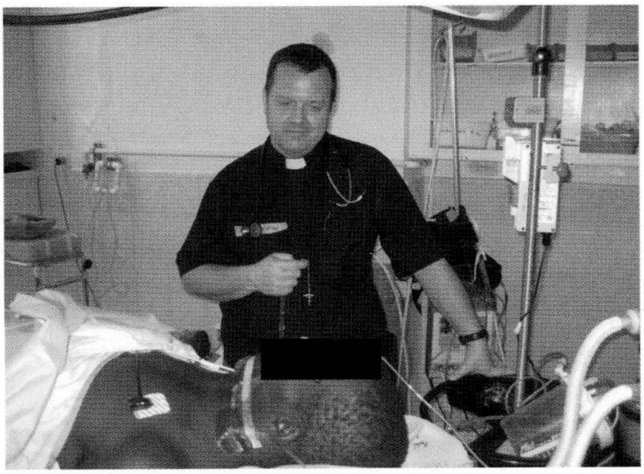

Fig. 4. A patient receives the Sacrament of Anointing of the Sick from a priest in an operating room.

Turks. Following the earthquake, the majority of medical personnel flying in and out of Haiti arrived via private aircraft. Hundreds of nongovernmental organizations and private individuals donated their airplanes, pilots, fuel, and maintenance to fly medical staff and supplies to Haiti. Given the private nature of flights, however, schedules can be chaotic and unpredictable. Prudent travelers will plan appropriately. The hospital provided ground transportation down a 9-mile, mostly dirt road littered with large potholes, people, goats, cows, and pigs. There was no organized traffic pattern of any kind.

Living in a Natural Disaster

In Milot, local citizens obtain water from a small river flowing through the town, which they also use to bathe and wash clothes. Fortunately, engineers constructing the Crudem Compound drilled a large well and installed a purification system to provide potable water in small quantities for cooking and washing clothes. Bottled water was used for drinking and brushing teeth. Meals were prepared from food bought locally, with all preparation and cooking performed by locals employed by the CRUDEM Foundation. Meals consisted of eggs, bread, lettuce, rice, beans, squash, and carrots with meat, such as chicken, goat, and ox tail, served every other day. The food was served in small quantities by American standards, but was delicious and wholesome.

A large gas generator and 24-lead-acid batteries provided electricity for the residential compound. Electricity at the hospital was supplied by 2 smaller gas generators; routine transfer of power from one to the other required a "blackout" twice daily for 30 to 60 seconds. Initially, Digicel, one of the largest mobile carriers in Haiti, was nonfunctional for several days following the earthquake; there are no landlines and no power grids in this area. At the compound and hospital, intramedical staff communications was limited to 20 two-way radios with just 1 band, which created issues with personnel "stepping" on one another and at night for staff "on call" who had to listen to the constant chatter. Cell phones worked intermittently and were highly position dependent as was the compound's only satellite phone, reminiscent of an archaic military handset. Internet using a satellite high-speed system was set up by a local compound engineer. The access was 5 Ethernet stations hooked up to a variety of computers. The signal was intermittent and with so many trying to communicate back to their homes, access was quite limited. The Internet became a very important source of information, with searches ranging from treating an unfamiliar disease, such as tetanus, to the volume of oxygen in an H cylinder that allowed the authors to calculate their available oxygen supply.

Bedding was of a variable nature. Most of the workers were relegated to either an outdoor tent, sleeping on a mattress on the floor, a small couch, military cots in a hallway, or, if fortunate, a bed with mosquito netting treated with insecticides such as permethrin or deltamethrin. Because the netting was not available for all, high doses of DEET-containing insect spray was applied before sleeping. In addition, sleep deprivation was a major problem for some and resulted from the emotionally charged environment, uncomfortable accommodations, overcrowding, and lack of uninterrupted sleep from buzzing mosquitoes, boisterous crowing and clucking of several roosters, and multiple visits from the occasional large insect. Most laundry was done by Sisters from the local convent, using an industrial washer and dryer, providing the workers with clean scrubs and usually 1 small towel each day.

Staying Healthy

Tropical diseases are a fact of life in Haiti, the poorest country in the Western hemisphere, but receiving the appropriate immunizations and arranging for prophylaxis before traveling was straightforward. Assuming that hepatitis B and tetanus immunizations are current, additional prophylaxis was required for hepatitis A and typhoid. Because malaria is common in Haiti, the authors' group members took doxycycline, starting 2 days before departure and continuing for 1 month after leaving the island. Tuberculosis is also endemic in Haiti. Although there is no prophylaxis, the authors were advised to take N95 masks. Finally, because approximately 2.0% to 3.5% of the Haitian population is HIV positive, universal precautions are necessary to avoid contact with body fluids, just as in any other nation.[6,7] In addition to physical health, the mental health of volunteers is important to sustain daily care to patients. For the authors, 2 elements contributed to their own mental health. First, the authors went with a well-known, long-standing partner (one another) that allowed each to discuss the day's events, provide mutual support, and consultation. Second, the director of the health care relief effort arranged nightly debriefing sessions of approximately 30 minutes, where problems of the day were openly discussed and solutions suggested. The authors think that it is important to stay healthy not only for one's own sake, but to avoid burdening the already overtaxed health care system.

Security

During the authors' stay at Hôpital Sacré Coeur, they felt perfectly safe. Even the women in the authors' group felt safe enough to walk the short distance from the CRUDEM residential compound where they lived to the hospital, even at night. However, in the course of the week the authors provided service, there was a noticeable increase in the people living in the streets, most of whom had moved the 90 miles from the earthquake zone. Patients were not happy to be discharged from the hospital, which was their only known safe environment, along with their only source of daily meals. The security environment was unknown and dependent on the United Nations troops, Haitian military and police, and nongovernmental organizations. In a different situation of mounting desperation for food and shelter, it is unknown how secure these health care facilities might have been. Compound security was provided by the occasionally seen United Nations peacekeepers from Chile and Nepal, using armored vehicles and the sparse local police force. During the authors' stay, they had only 1 intrusion by a group of local citizens looking for supplies.

ANESTHETIC PRACTICE IN AN EARTHQUAKE ZONE

Organizing this article, the authors left the nature of anesthetic practice as a last topic of discussion because one's previous experience, nature of the natural disaster, and equipment or supplies currently available will focus on the anesthetic. Almost all surgeries consisted of limb amputation, incision and debridement, or burn care. Many of the more severely injured patients, mostly with chest or abdominal injuries, likely were immediately killed or died in the aftermath of the earthquake. In addition to physical traumatic injury, many may also have suffered from mental disease because of the stress of the event. From the patient's point of view, an injured patient may have been trapped under rubble in Port-au-Prince, had one or more limbs amputated several days after the earthquake by search and rescue teams who have less than 60 seconds to spend on each patient, been evacuated to Milot by helicopter, been admitted to a new hospital without family members whose fate was unknown, without funds, without clothes, and without identity papers. For these reasons, the health care team tried to provide the most gentle and humane care possible.

In the authors' own practice in the aftermath of the Haitian earthquake, their limitations revolved around minimal preoperative or postoperative care. For that reason,

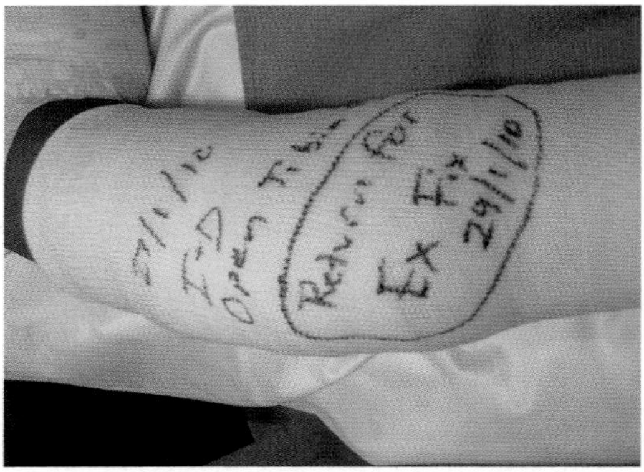

Fig. 5. Medical records for a patient with a previous open fracture of the tibia sustained in Port-au-Prince. Follow-up directions on his medical record were written on his cast, "27/1/10. I&D Open Tibia. Return for Ex Fix 29/1/10."

the authors took steps to alter their patient's native physiology as little as possible. Preoperatively and with the help of a translator, an anesthetic assessment consisted of fasting status, allergies, and past medical history (almost none of the authors' patients had ever had any health care). Medical records during this tumultuous time were disorganized and often had to be co-located with the patient (eg, written on dressing or casts, **Fig. 5**). Without routine care, almost all past medical history dated to January 12, 2010, when the earthquake occurred. Intraoperatively, the authors' focus was to cause as little physiologic perturbation as possible while rendering sufficient anesthesia. For that reason, the authors' primary anesthetic technique relied on intravenous midazolam and ketamine with appropriate local anesthetic use by the surgeon, while minimizing the need for oxygen (**Fig. 6**). This technique was useful to fully use all 3 operating rooms (with a single fully functional anesthesia machine) and to convert 3 examination rooms into operating rooms to allow a 6-room surgical suite. Moreover, the continuation of spontaneous ventilation allowed only a brief stay in the 5-bed

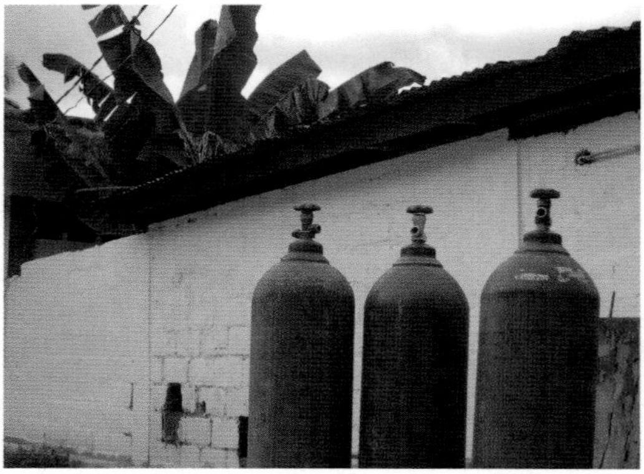

Fig. 6. A week's supply of oxygen for the entire hospital composed of three H cylinders. A full H cylinder contains about 7000 L of oxygen. A patient on 2 L/min nasal cannula oxygen for 3 days would consume 8640 L of oxygen, over a third of the weekly oxygen allocation for all patients.

recovery room that was severely strained because of understaffing and co-location of critically ill patients with medical conditions, such as unremitting diabetic coma in the absence of insulin and fulminant tetanus. If monitored anesthesia care was insufficient, then a regional anesthetic was the next preferred technique with common techniques being brachial plexus from multiple approaches, femoral nerve and popliteal nerve block, or intrathecal anesthesia for the lower extremities. Given the lack of any oral analgesics in the hospital and surrounding community, regional anesthesia also provided some benefit for immediate postoperative analgesia. The authors discussed the creation of an acute regional pain treatment team using regional anesthesia, but the scope of the disaster, lack of supplies, and sheer provider exhaustion precluded this event. Authors participating in the Haitian earthquake relief independently reached similar conclusions.[1,4,8,9] For example, a French team in Port-au-Prince conducted 92% of their anesthetics with conscious sedation or regional anesthesia in patients who suffered most of the time (79%) with limb injuries.[8]

General anesthesia was possible, although supplies of oxygen and volatile agents were limited. In the authors' cases, they recall only a single general anesthetic for a woman hit in the face by a falling roof truss who sustained a Lefort type III injury. In the absence of maxillofacial surgeons, the team was limited to the placement of a gastrostomy tube to facilitate nutrition until a definitive resolution could be arranged. In any event, anesthetic care that allows rapid throughput in the operating and recovery rooms is essential to care for large populations.

REFERENCES

1. Rice MJ, Gwertzman A, Finley T, et al. Anesthetic practice in Haiti after the 2010 earthquake. Anesth Analg 2010;111:1445–9.
2. Chen G, Lai W, Liu F, et al. The dragon strikes: lessons from the Wenchuan earthquake. Anesth Analg 2010;110:908–15.
3. Fushiki S. Radiation hazards in children—lessons from Chernobyl, Three Mile Island and Fukushima. Brain Dev 2012. [Epub ahead of print].
4. Jiang J, Xu H, Liu H, et al. Anaesthetic management under field conditions after the 12 May 2008 earthquake in Wenchuan, China. Injury 2010;41:e1–3.
5. National Catholic Bioethics Center. Consultation. 2012. Available at: http://www.ncbcenter.org/page.aspx?pid=1170. Accessed October 14, 2012.
6. Halperin DT, de Moya EA, Perez-Then E, et al. Understanding the HIV epidemic in the Dominican Republic: a prevention success story in the Caribbean? J Acquir Immune Defic Syndr 2009;51(Suppl 1):S52–9.
7. Figueroa JP. The HIV epidemic in the Caribbean: meeting the challenges of achieving universal access to prevention, treatment and care. West Indian Med J 2008;57:195–203.
8. Benner P, Stephan J, Renard A, et al. Role of the French Rescue Teams in Diquini Hospital: Port-au-Prince, January 2010. Prehosp Disaster Med 2012;1–5. [Epub ahead of print].
9. Osteen KD. Orthopedic anesthesia in Haiti. Ochsner J 2011;11:12–3.

Anesthesia Department Preparedness for a Multiple-Casualty Incident

Lessons Learned from the Fukushima Earthquake and the Japanese Nuclear Power Disaster

Masahiro Murakawa, MD

KEYWORDS

• Great East Japan Earthquake • Fukushima nuclear power plant • Giant tsunami

KEY POINTS

- The earthquake-resistant design of the hospital and the stock of oxygen and the other utilities are essential.
- Disaster prevention drills, especially independent for the operating rooms are important.
- Radioactive contamination of filtered oxygen and environment in hospital was also minimal and was not problematic.

INTRODUCTION

A huge earthquake off the coast of Sanriku, the Great East Japan Earthquake, occurred at 14:46 on March 11, 2011, and many lives were lost in the accompanying giant tsunami. Fukushima prefecture was widely contaminated with radioactive substances emitted by the accident at the Fukushima Dai-ichi nuclear power plant, and residents around the nuclear power plant had to evacuate. In this article, we describe the actions taken by the Fukushima Medical University Hospital, as a logistic support hospital, during the disaster, and discuss the role of anesthesiologists at university hospitals in the actions taken following a widespread disaster.

GREAT EAST JAPAN EARTHQUAKE AND ACTIONS TAKEN

Overview of the Hospital and the First Actions

The Fukushima Medical University Hospital is the only medical school–affiliated hospital in the prefecture. It is a general hospital with 778 beds and 30 departments in a 10-story building that was completed in 1987. The hospital deals with about

Department of Anesthesiology, Fukushima Medical University School of Medicine, 1 Hikariga-oka, Fukushima City, Fukushima 960-1295, Japan
E-mail address: murakawa@fmu.ac.jp

Anesthesiology Clin 31 (2013) 117–125
http://dx.doi.org/10.1016/j.anclin.2012.11.007 **anesthesiology.theclinics.com**
1932-2275/13/$ – see front matter

630 inpatients and 1500 outpatients per day. The hospital is also specified as an emergency medical care center and is the only one equipped with a helicopter for emergency medical care in the Tohoku region. It is located in the north central part of Fukushima prefecture; 57 km distant from the Fukushima Dai-ichi nuclear power plant (**Fig. 1**). The surgical department is located on the third floor of a 3-story outpatient/central ward building adjacent to the 10-story building. There are 12 operating rooms, in which about 5500 surgeries are performed annually; about 4000 of these are performed under general or spinal anesthesia, and are managed by the anesthesiologists. The intensive care unit has 8 beds and is located on the same floor, adjacent to the surgical department, and can accommodate about 600 patients per year, mainly those after surgery.

The magnitude of the earthquake was 9.0 on the Richter scale, and the maximum intensity was measured 7 in Kurihara, Miyagi prefecture. In Fukushima prefecture, the intensity was measured as upper 6 in the southern region and eastern Pacific coast, and as a lower 6 in the central northern region, where this hospital is located, and in the western region.[1] The magnitudes and maximum intensities of the Great Hanshin-Awaji Earthquake in 1995, Chuetsu Earthquake in 2004, and Niigata-ken Chuetsu-oki Earthquake in 2007, were 7.3 and 7, 6.8 and 7, and 6.8 and upper 6, respectively, showing that the intensities were similar to that of this earthquake; however, the day of the week and time of occurrence were 5:46 AM on Tuesday, 17:56 on Saturday, and 10:13 AM on Monday, a public holiday, respectively, showing that these earthquakes occurred on holidays or in the early morning before clinic hours. This earthquake was the first large-scale earthquake to have occurred during working hours on a weekday in modern Japan.

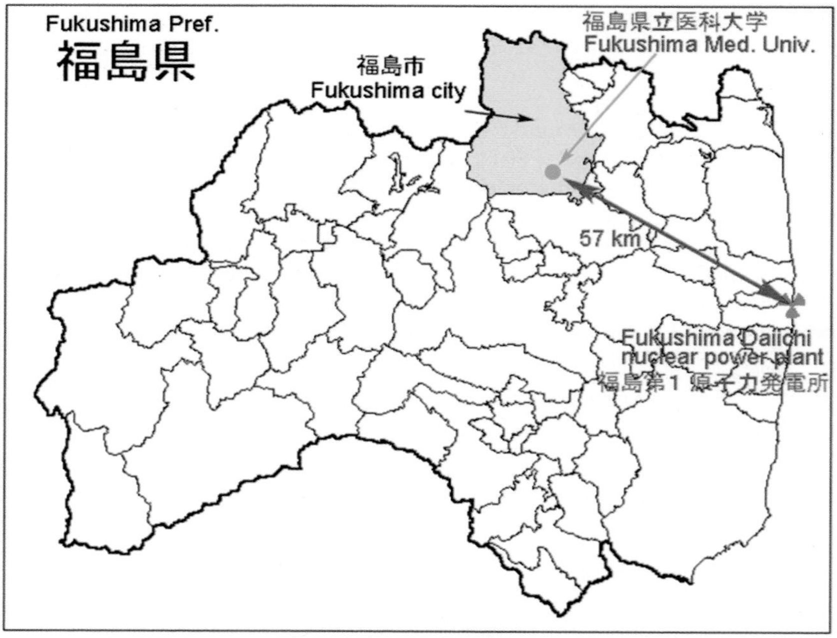

Fig. 1. Map of Fukushima prefecture. Fukushima Medical University Hospital is located in the north central part of Fukushima prefecture; 57 km distant from the Fukushima Dai-ichi nuclear power plant. (*Data from* Available at: http://www.fmu.ac.jp/home/lib/radiation/. Accessed December, 2012.)

On the day of the Great East Japan Earthquake, 1345 outpatients visited our hospital and there were 642 inpatients. It is unclear how many outpatients still remained after the earthquake, but outpatients were evacuated to the main entrance. After confirming their safety, we quickly let them go home because of the frequent occurrence of strong aftershocks. It was difficult to move many of the inpatients despite the continued aftershocks. Excluding the patients who were undergoing surgery, we allowed the inpatients to return to their rooms and confirmed their safety. It was necessary to carry patients present in the outpatient and rehabilitation departments (first and second floors) up to higher floors on stretchers because elevators had stopped (the elevators stop automatically at an earthquake intensity of 5 or more, and a safety inspection is necessary to restart). One patient, who had been riding in an elevator, after completion of cardiac catheterization in the radiology department on the first floor, had to get out of the elevator at the second floor, instead of the intended 10th floor, because the elevator had stopped automatically. Because carrying the patient up to a higher floor was considered difficult, the patient was accommodated in the Class I infectious disease facility equipped with same monitoring devices on the intended floor.

These first actions were taken under the judgment of the persons in charge of each department, and the condition in each department was reported to the nursing supervisory office through the chief nurse for each department. At the same time, a disaster countermeasures office was established under the leadership of the university president in the office of the director of the hospital. Information was collected from each of the hospital departments, and commands were issued.

Actions Taken for Patients Undergoing Surgery or in the Intensive Care Unit

At the time of the earthquake, 9 patients were present in the surgical department, including those under local anesthesia. The surgeries were stopped because of the strong shaking. The surgical lights were removed from the surgical fields, and the surgical fields and instrument tables were covered with drapes because of the significant amount of dust and dirt falling from the ceiling. To secure an evacuation route, the entrances to the operating rooms and doors of the rooms were left open. The air-conditioning stopped, but there were no problems in the electrical system or oxygen and air supply. Some electronic medical record displays fell, but none of the biologic information monitors, anesthesia apparatuses, or devices of electric scalpels tumbled or fell. Later, commands were integrated by the manager of the anesthesiology department, and stretchers, bag valve masks, circulatory agents, and sedatives were prepared in each room in preparation for moving. No steps toward immediate emergency evacuation were taken, but whether or not surgery should be continued was determined for each case because of the frequent aftershocks. At about 15:30, 40 minutes after the earthquake, the order came through to suspend any surgeries that could be suspended, and the patients were transported to the intensive care unit on the same floor. Removal of all patients from the surgical department was completed by 16:42, 2 hours after the earthquake.

Six patients were located in the intensive care unit at that time, and normal treatment could be continued because there were no problems in maintaining electricity or the supply of oxygen and air. In addition, 2 patients were accommodated per booth after completion of surgery under general anesthesia, and these patients were returned to the general ward after weaning from a respirator on or after the following day.

Emergency System

In the hospital, beds were prepared in the reception hall in the hospital entrance and the adjacent training rooms of the School of Nursing. Triage decisions were made in the lobby in front of the clinical lecture building adjacent to the emergency medical care center, and a system was established to treat the primary, secondary, and tertiary priority cases at the orthopedic outpatient clinic, general internal medical outpatient clinic, and emergency center, respectively.

Thirty-five disaster medical assistance teams (DMAT), composed of about 180 members, assembled on the day of the earthquake. Physicians from our hospital (including trainees) treated patients in cooperation with student volunteers. The number of emergency patients who visited the hospital within 3 days was 168, and 30 of these patients were severe and required admission.[2]

In the surgical department, 5 rows of operating rooms were prepared, and 5 anesthesiologists, 6 staff from the surgical department, and 2 clinical engineers sufficient to handle operations were ready 24 hours a day. Twenty-five patients were surgically treated (eg, for reduction of fracture and caesarean delivery), within 10 days after the earthquake.

Utilities and Restoration

Regarding access to utilities at the hospital, there were no problems in the supply of electricity or gas, but the water service stopped for 8 days. The water tank volume is 700 tons, which corresponds to only 1 day of consumption for normal practice. We attempted to save water as of the following day (ie, we canceled the outpatient clinic and did not perform elective surgeries, and discharged inpatients as much as possible to about 70% of the normal number). More than 100 tons of water was supplied by the water wagons daily, but the supply was mostly exhausted after 1 week.

Oxygen is provided from a stationary cryogenic liquefied oxygen storage system with a volume of 8600 m^3, which is sufficient for more than 14 days for normal consumption (at about 600 m^3 per week day). Normally, the oxygen store is supplemented once a week, and reserve cylinders are available for 0.75 days (7000 L $\times$ 72 cylinders = 453 m^3). On the day of the earthquake, there was sufficient liquefied oxygen for about 10 days, which was not damaged by the earthquake, and the oxygen was supplied normally. There was no problem in the provision of air supply because compressed air was used; however, the potential for radioactive contamination was of concern, as described later in this article. No problems occurred with the small oxygen cylinders.

Three days of reserved food was on hand for patients, along with about 7 days of reserved drugs and reagents for tests. Because medical service was limited, there were no shortages of food, drugs, or oxygen, but reagents for tests were slightly short, because production plants was also affected. Modification of food service was necessary (ie, cooking rice with bottled drinking water and putting cling wrap on the work surface to reduce the necessity for cleaning) because of the suspension of the water supply.

Water service was resumed 8 days after the earthquake. Outpatient services were re-initiated for outpatients with appointments and inpatient surgeries, beginning with scheduled surgeries that had been suspended. About 3 weeks were required to resume normal hospital function. The gasoline shortage became serious at that time, and it was difficult to ensure reliable methods for the staff to commute because of the location of the hospital in the suburbs.

NUCLEAR POWER PLANT ACCIDENT AND ACTIONS TAKEN

Radiation Emergency Medicine

There were 6 power generators in the Fukushima Dai-ichi nuclear power plant at the time of the earthquake. Commercial operation of nuclear reactor No. 1 started in

March 1971, and the reactor had been in operation for nearly 40 years. External power facilities were damaged by the giant tsunami caused by the earthquake. The reactor became uncontrollable, and core meltdown occurred in reactor Nos. 1 to 3. Hydrogen explosions occurred in the No. 1 reactor on March 12, the day following the earthquake, and in the No. 3 reactor on March 14. The vent was opened to prevent elevation of pressure in the containment vessel, thus dispersing radioactive substances in the air. An evacuation order was issued for the surrounding area on the day of earthquake, and was expanded to a 30-km radius area after 4 days.

Our hospital is accredited as a medical institution for secondary radiation medicine and accepted exposed sick and injured patients associated with the nuclear power plant accident from the day following the earthquake. Eight injured patients were sent to our hospital, but the exposures were not severe, and they were transferred to the National Institute of Radiological Sciences after decontamination and wound treatment. Work aimed at restoration of the nuclear power plant continued after the accident, and our hospital remained prepared 24 hours a day for the occurrence of sickness and injury by contamination. We prepared for surgery of contaminated patients through simulations of large-scale disasters and preparing the operating rooms (ie, covering and sanitizing the patient areas) (**Fig. 2**). Fortunately, medical facilities were already in place at the nuclear power plant and in the neighboring region, and no cases requiring decontamination occurred.

Relay Transport of Evacuated Patients

More than 1300 inpatients in medical institutions in the area were ordered to evacuate at that time, and a government-led evacuation occurred.[3] Patients were initially transferred to the western region of Fukushima prefecture, but the capacity reached the limit, and others were transferred outside the prefecture. Our hospital could not accept many patients because of the suspension of the water supply, as described previously, and functioned as a transit point for relay inside and outside the prefecture. Many patients who were transported en masse by helicopters, ambulances, and buses of the Japan Self-Defense Forces and the fire brigade were accepted temporarily, screened for radiation, and underwent assessment of their general condition. Patients who were judged as not being capable of surviving transport were admitted.

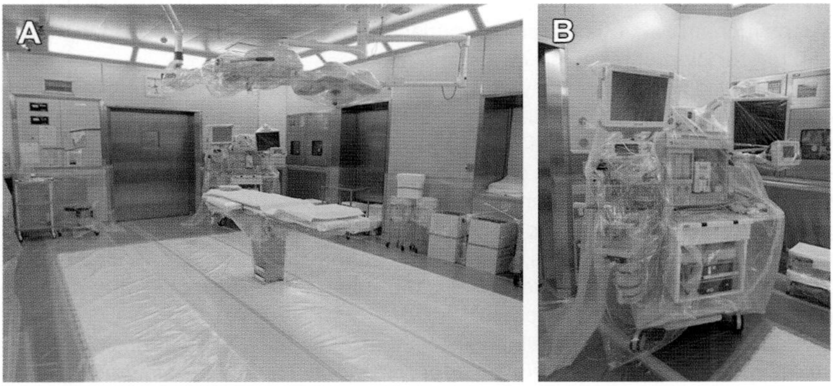

Fig. 2. Preparing the operating room for surgery of contaminated patients by radioactive agents. The patient area (*A*) and anesthesia machine (*B*) were covered and sanitized by polychoride vinyl.

Within several days, 175 patients were accepted, and 125 were admitted and treated, although the duration of stay varied. However, none of the patients required surgery or intensive care.

Medical Support for the Evacuated Residents

A traveling clinic was started at shelters after completion of the first stage of inpatient transport in the evacuated area, and water service to the hospital resumed. Many physicians from medical associations nationwide and the Japanese Red Cross Society were already working to provide support. In cooperation with these groups, our hospital performed pediatric, otolaryngologic, and ophthalmologic treatments, infection control, mental care, and screening of deep vein thrombosis and heart disease using ultrasonography throughout the prefecture, for which international assistance was also provided by Jordan and Thailand.

Radioactive Contamination of the Hospital Environment

After the nuclear power plant accident, the environmental radiation level rose in the hospital, and the value, as measured by our university, reached 7 μSv/h.[4,5]

When the indoor air dose rate was measured, the value in the intensive care unit was about 0.1 μSv/h (the maximum value in the open air during the same period was 4.5 μSv/h). Because compressed air was used, the dose rate in the gas supplied by this means was measured, and it was 0.1 to 0.2 μSv/h, similar to the indoor rate. Because it was possible that radioactive substances could accumulate somewhere in the open air, the air conditioning machine room was inspected closely. The air dose rate in the machine room was 0.2 to 0.4 μSv/h, which was higher than that in the hospital rooms (<0.1 μSv/h at that time), and the rate in the air-inlet filter was 4.0 to 7.0 μSv/h, suggesting that radioactive substances in the open air were captured by the filter, and most were absent in hospital rooms and in the air inhaled by patients.

FUTURE ISSUES

Disaster Measures in the Hospital

Although direct damage by this earthquake was not as severe as that by the Great Hanshin-Awaji Earthquake; damage as a result of the tsunami was serious.[6] From this experience, the tasks of anesthesiologists include (1) establishment of a patient safety-securing system in disaster, (2) improvement of infrastructure, such as provision of oxygen and air, (3) provision of patient transport and accommodation facilities, and (4) preparation of reserved drugs and food.

Hospital buildings are unlikely to collapse if they meet the earthquake-resistance standards, but protection of patients and staff from falling items in the surgical department is necessary. Shelves and surgical devices that are likely to fall should be sufficiently reinforced, glass bottles should be abandoned, as much as possible, to avoid cuts and tears, and medicine shelves should be replaced with cabinets. Anesthesia apparatuses and endoscope racks should be anchored because these may fall or move. Wheels, such as casters, should also be locked in place. It is also necessary to remove items that are located above the patients (ie, surgical lights and microscopes) when an earthquake occurs.

Oxygen supply is the very lifeline for anesthesiologists, and anesthesiologists must make every effort to keep a sufficient supply in stock. Regarding the storage of liquefied oxygen, two-thirds of the maximum amount stored would last for 10 days, and the reserve cylinder capacity lasts for more than 1 day. We had no problem in the liquefied oxygen store, but the reserve capacity was inadequate. This earthquake damaged some of the production plants of suppliers, but oxygen was supplied to the affected area without delay as a result of strenuous efforts.

Regarding surgery during the suspension of water service, prolongation of the water storage period could have a negative influence on hand-washing and cleaning of the surgical instruments. Washer disinfectors also could not be used, resulting in insufficient cleaning of instruments, which is unfavorable for infection control. Elective surgeries should inevitably be limited during suspension of water service. Securing a reliable water source is an urgent need for our hospital, and preparation of a well, regulating reservoir, and water-purifying devices are being considered.

There were no power outages in our hospital, because electricity was supplied through a system that is independent from that used for the residential district, but this required private power generation and fuel storage. Because the supply of electricity and the duration of the supply to the hospital by a private power generator are limited, it is necessary to stop surgeries as soon as possible. When surgeries that cannot be stopped are under way, such as open heart surgery, supply of electricity to that surgery is prioritized. Laminar flow from air conditioning ceases, and the amount of floating dust increases. Therefore, prevention of turbulence is important (ie, avoidance of opening and shutting doors as much as possible and minimizing the number of persons entering the operating rooms). It is also desirable to clean wounds frequently. Among the countermeasures against a power outage, it is necessary to consider how to transport patients and food in the event that elevator operation ceases. In our situation, elevator operation stopped as a result of aftershocks at mealtime, and all staff delivered the meals via the stairs, like a bucket brigade. It is also difficult to transport patients, particularly surgically treated patients and patients in intensive care. Because there are not a sufficient number of recovery rooms in the surgical department and the intensive care unit is located on the same floor in our hospital, patients were transported to the intensive care unit; however, it could be better to take care of surgical patients in the recovery or operating rooms without moving them. It has also been proposed to establish a server that could allow sharing of electronic medical records among hospitals as a countermeasure for the loss of power supply.

Consideration of the food for staff is also necessary, in addition to storage of drugs and food for patients. When the distribution system is paralyzed, it is difficult to ensure provision of food to the staff. It is also necessary to secure places for staff to stay and to prepare a medical service system for conditions in which the number of staff is reduced.

Anesthesiologists at a University Hospital in a Widespread Disaster

As described previously, the tsunami damage was enormous in this earthquake, but not many patients required emergency surgery or intensive care. Because the condition was similar in facilities related to this hospital, no dispatch of anesthesiologists or provision was demanded immediately after the earthquake during the acute phase; however, transport of a large number of patients requiring surgery or dispatch of physicians may be requested from university hospitals serving as disaster base hospitals from the affected area in an earthquake. In these cases, it is necessary to confirm the capability of related hospitals to deal with it, to efficiently and cooperatively accept patients and dispatch physicians, for which additional considerations are necessary (ie, avoidance of surgery for mild cases by high-level hospitals, such as university hospitals).

To understand the conditions of the affected area and related facilities and cooperate with them, it is also important to prepare a means of communication. After the

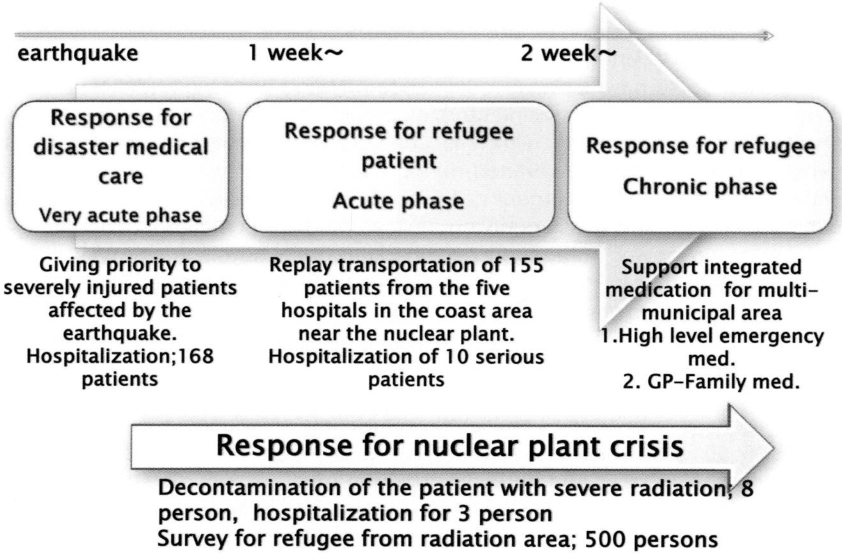

Fig. 3. Fukushima Medical University's response to the Great East Japan earthquake and subsequent disasters.

Niigata-ken Chuetsu Earthquake, 3 days were required to identify any road damage and passable routes, and to mobilize and operate rescue helicopters.[7] In this earthquake, communication and cooperation among helicopters for emergency medical care, the Japan Self-Defense Forces, and fire brigade functioned from a relatively early phase, but there was no functional communication network, and it was difficult to clarify the situation. Preparation of a satellite phone network that is less likely to be influenced by congestion in a disaster is desired. Mutual understanding of the needs of the affected area and equipment available on the support side, including manpower, may facilitate achieving appropriate and rapid responses.

Disaster Prevention Drills

In general, disaster prevention drills may be performed by the entire hospital, but independent drills for operating rooms are not performed widely. Periodic evacuation drills on the assumption of the potential for a disaster improves antidisaster consciousness. At our hospital, in addition to the drills throughout the entire hospital, operating rooms have independently performed disaster evacuation drills annually. In addition, learning a lesson from the Niigata-ken Chuetsu-oki Earthquake, we had performed a DMAT assembling drill about 6 months before the earthquake, which may have been why we were able to rapidly take action in this earthquake. This re-confirms the importance of manual preparation and routine drills.

SUMMARY

The actions taken by our hospital against the earthquake and nuclear power plant accident are summarized in **Fig. 3**. The scale of this earthquake was large, but there were no problems in the supply of oxygen or electricity, suggesting that the earthquake-resistant design of the hospital building was effective. Accordingly, there were no direct injuries among the patients undergoing surgery or those in the intensive care unit, but surgeries were stopped and performed at a later date. Only a small number of trauma and emergency patients were brought to our hospital by ambulance, and an unexpectedly small number of emergency surgeries were performed. This may have been because enormous damage was caused by the giant tsunami. Regarding the nuclear power plant accident, there were patients with radiation-induced sickness and injury, but no cases of severe exposure requiring surgery or intensive care have occurred so far. We prepared for and simulated these cases to respond to any such occurrence. Radioactive contamination of medical gas and hospital environment was also minimal and was not problematic.

REFERENCES

1. Japan Meteorological Agency. Available at: http://www.jma.go.jp/jma/en/2011_Earthquake/Information_on_2011_Earthquake.html. Accessed December, 2012.
2. Fukushima Medical University. Available at: http://cbbstoday.org/images/nolletprs/fmu_pr14mar11.pdf. Accessed December, 2012.
3. Yanagawa Y, Miyawaki H, Shimada J, et al. Medical evacuation of patients to other hospitals due to the Fukushima I nuclear accidents. Prehosp Disaster Med 2011;26(5):391–3.
4. Kobayashi T. Radiation measurements at the campus of Fukushima medical university through the 2011 off the Pacific Coast of Tohoku earthquake and subsequent nuclear power plant crisis. Fukushima J Med Sci 2011;57(2):70–4.
5. Tsuji M, Kanda H, Kakamu T, et al. An assessment of radiation doses at an educational institution 57.8 km away from the Fukushima Daiichi nuclear power plant 1 month after the nuclear accident. Environ Health Prev Med 2012;17(2):124–30.
6. Nakahara S, Ichikawa M. Mortality in the 2011 tsunami in Japan. J Epidemiol. http://dx.doi.org/10.2188/jea.JE20120114.
7. Satomi S. The great east Japan earthquake: Tohoku University Hospital's efforts and lessons learned. Surg Today 2011;41:1171–81.

Trauma in the Elderly
Considerations for Anesthetic Management

Shawn E. Banks, MD[a,*], Michael C. Lewis, MD[b]

KEYWORDS

• Geriatric trauma • Physiology of aging • Geriatric anesthesia • Hip fracture
• Pulse pressure variation • Systolic pressure variation • Regional anesthesia

KEY POINTS

- The volume of geriatric trauma patients is expected to increase significantly in coming years.
- Recognition of severe injuries may be delayed because they are less likely to mount classic symptoms of hemodynamic instability.
- Anesthetic medications and opiates will require reductions in doses for elderly patients.
- Monitoring pulse pressure and systolic pressure variations can provide an accurate assessment of volume status in mechanically ventilated patients.
- Regional anesthesia for hip fractures may offer better patient outcomes than general anesthesia.

INTRODUCTION

Geriatric patients comprise a rapidly expanding age segment of the population of developed countries. It is the fastest growing population segment in the United States. Individuals older than 65 years of age currently represent 13% of the US population, but the US Census Bureau projects that by 2050, they will represent more than 21%.[1] Accidental injury was the fifth most frequent cause of mortality among the elderly in 2009 and 2010,[2] and utilization of trauma care services is expected to increase significantly among older age groups. It is projected that geriatric patients will account for almost 39% of trauma admissions by 2050.[3] Our understanding of best practices in geriatric trauma and anesthesia care continues to expand, as it does in all other areas of medicine.

DEFINITIONS OF AGING

Aging is a progressive process depicted as maintenance of life with a diminishing capability for adjustment.[4] Senescence results in a progressive decline in cellular

[a] Ryder Trauma Center, University of Miami Miller School of Medicine, Miami, FL, USA;
[b] University of Miami Miller School of Medicine, Miami, FL, USA
* Corresponding author. 1611 Northwest 12th Avenue Suite SW303, Miami, FL 33136.
E-mail address: sbanks2@med.miami.edu

Anesthesiology Clin 31 (2013) 127–139
http://dx.doi.org/10.1016/j.anclin.2012.11.004 **anesthesiology.theclinics.com**
1932-2275/13/$ – see front matter

function, resulting in a loss of organ performance. Cells lose their capacity to respond to injury and eventually die. Senescence is associated with impaired adaptive and homeostatic mechanisms, resulting in an increased susceptibility to the effects of stress. Function may seem to be unchanged, yet physiologic reserve diminishes. Any disruption of homeostasis that is well tolerated by younger adults might precipitate functional decline in the elderly population. The situation is further compounded by variable response to medications and comorbidity.

A standard age-based definition for the term "geriatric" does not exist. Most researchers have used the breakpoint of 65 years of age and more, perhaps somewhat arbitrarily. Geriatric trauma has historical roots in the establishment of the social security system in the United States. Using a strict age-based criterion is also difficult because it is generally believed that aging adults will be entering their "geriatric" years in better health that they did in preceding generations and that preinjury function may significantly influence recovery from injury.

PHYSIOLOGIC CHANGES IN THE ELDERLY POPULATION

As a result of the aging process, there is a wide set of physiologic changes each of which result in a decreased ability to maintain homeostasis during stress.

Between the ages of 20 and 80 years there is a progressive decline in cardiac function, estimated to be as great as 50%. The progressive stiffening of the arterial tree and resultant adaptations of the aging myocardium can result in ventricular hypertrophy as shown in **Fig. 1**. This impaired cardiac function, paired with decreased sensitivity to catecholamines, complicates the management of the hemodynamically compromised older patient.

Above the age of 50 years, renal mass is lost, with a corresponding fall in glomerular filtration rate.[5,6] Renal tubular function is also compromised. These changes decrease the ability of the elderly to cope with large volume resuscitation.

Respiratory function is also compromised in the elderly population. There is an observed loss of lung elastic recoil and significant reduction of the vital capacity. Moreover, there is impaired mucociliary clearance of bacteria, dependence on diaphragmatic breathing, and reduced ability to cough.[7] There is a disruption of the normal matching of ventilation and perfusion. Forced expiratory volume in 1 second, forced vital capacity, and peak expiratory flow rate are decreased.[8] Such changes in diffusion capacity, ventilation-perfusion mismatch,[9] and closing volumes mean that there is a decrease in baseline arterial oxygen tension with age.[10] Alterations in compliance result in an increased work of breathing.[11] The combination of these factors means that there is an increased risk of respiratory failure in the elderly patient, resulting in a higher incidence of mechanical ventilation,[12] acute lung injury, and ventilation-associated pneumonia as a consequence of longer intensive care unit stay and high morbidity.

There are age-related changes of endocrine function. The tissue responsiveness to thyroxin and its production is reduced with aging.[13] Secretion of cortisol does not seem to change with aging.[14]

FUNCTIONAL RESERVE

When an organism maintains a steady state in the face of increased physiologic demand, it is said to demonstrate a good functional reserve. **Fig. 2** illustrates this divergence between "baseline" and "stress" situations. Imbalance within the system therefore results in a breakdown of homeostatic compensation. A decline in functional

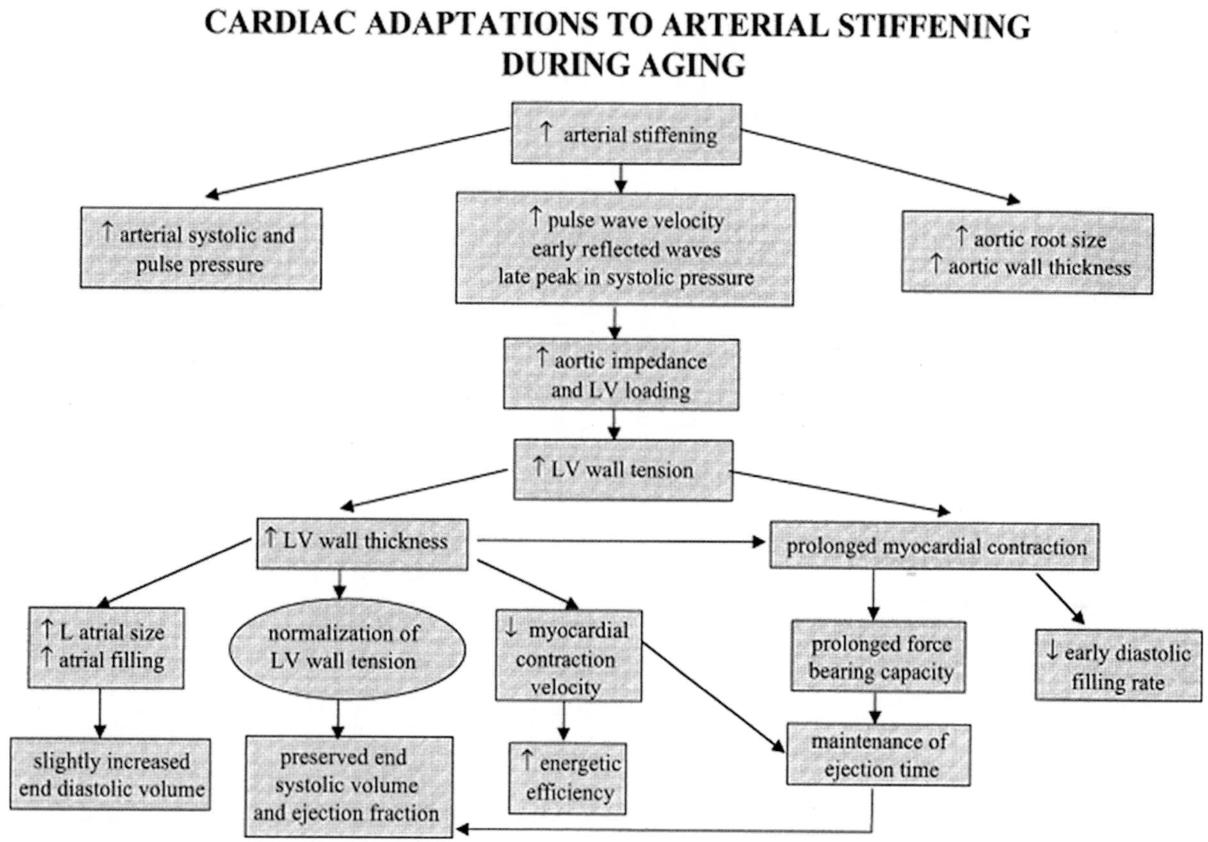

Fig. 1. Loss of elasticity in the arterial tree is thought to be responsible for increasing left ventricular (LV) afterload. The resulting ventricular hypertrophy may lead to diastolic dysfunction. (*Reprinted from* Lakatta EG, Sollott SJ. Perspectives on mammalian cardiovascular aging: humans to molecules. Comp Biochem Physiol A Mol Integr Physiol 2002;132(4):699–721. Elsevier, with permission.)

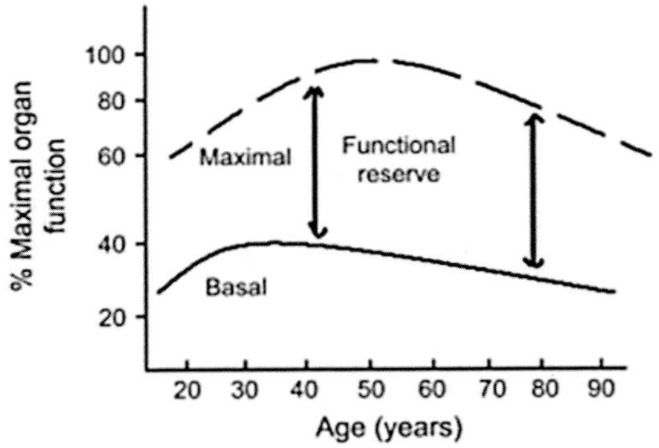

Fig. 2. The functional reserve is the difference between basal function (solid line) and maximal function (broken line). Even in healthy individuals, this functional reserve is reduced. (*From* Muravchick S. Geroanesthesia: principles for management of the elderly patient. St Louis (MO): Mosby 1997; with permission.)

reserve may in the elderly patient precipitate a serious decline in performance when the elderly patient is exposed to stress and increases the risk of age-related disease.

Because of decreasing functional reserve, the older patient is less able to preserve homeostasis in face of such a physical insult.[15] Fortunately, this functional decline does not occur in all individuals at the same pace. A significant amount of variability occurs. This unevenness is rooted within lifestyle choices, environmental factors, genetics, and the presence of age-related disease. Older trauma victims do not cope as well as younger adults.[16,17] After injury, elderly patients are more likely to arrive in the emergency department in hypotensive shock and to be hypothermic, 2 factors that portend worse outcomes at any age. Decreased functional reserve contributes to the higher percentage of the geriatric trauma victims that appear in the early trauma mortality statistics. It affects infection-related deaths and multiple organ dysfunction syndromes. Diminished reserve, manifested as comorbid disease states, seems to have a negative predictive value for outcome.[18] However, when aggressive treatment is initiated, the outcome difference between younger and older adult decreases.[19]

PREINJURY MEDICAL CONDITIONS AND THERAPIES

As the risk of cardiovascular disease increases with age, so does the prevalence of β-blockade and oral anticoagulation therapies. These therapies may have direct impact on evaluation and early management of traumatically injured patients. A retrospective study across ten years at one Level I trauma center demonstrated that preinjury β-blocker therapy was associated with an odds ratio for mortality of 2.1 when head injuries were excluded. β-Blocker therapy was also positively associated with the incidence of other coexisting diseases like diabetes, hypertension, renal failure, and dyslipidemia.[20] Recognition of injury severity and appropriate resuscitation may be delayed if the classic symptom of tachycardia is blunted.

Head-injured patients on preinjury warfarin therapy have demonstrated significantly worse outcomes in multiple studies; the risk of mortality is more than doubled.[21,22]

MECHANISMS OF INJURY

Elderly patients are victim to many of the same injury mechanisms as their younger counterparts (**Table 1**). Low-energy falls remain the most common mechanism for

Table 1
Leading causes of injuries for persons older than 65 years of age in the United States in 2009

Rank	Nonfatal Injuries	Fatal Injuries
1	Fall	Fall
2	Struck by/against object	Motor vehicle traffic
3	Overexertion	Suicide firearm
4	Motor vehicle occupant	Unintentional unspecified
5	Cut/penetrating injury	Unintentional suffocation

Data from Centers for Disease Control and Prevention National Center for Injury Prevention and Control. Available at: http://www.cdc.gov/injury/wisqars/LeadingCauses.html. Accessed August 29, 2012.

traumatic injury in the elderly.[23,24] Various factors predispose elderly persons to falls, such as unsteady gait, orthostatic hypotension, and slow reaction time.[25] Falls can lead to significant injuries,[26] even if from standing height. It has been estimated that falls can account for more than 50% of eventual trauma-related deaths.[27] Minor mechanisms of injury may lead to severe injury with much greater frequency as age increases from 55 years,[28] and the death rate is especially high in octogenarians.[29]

Traffic accidents involving drivers or pedestrians are also leading causes of injuries in the elderly population.[23] Underlying diseases, decreased hearing or vision, muscle weakness, and reduced reaction times[30] are contributing factors.[31]

Thermal injuries occur more frequently in the elderly population. This increased risk could be attributable to a reduced sense of smell, impaired hearing or vision, or reduced mobility and reaction time. These injuries are inclined to be more serious in terms of surface area and depth.[32] The propensity to more severe thermal injury may be attributable to age-related alterations in skin morphology and diminished visual, olfactory, and auditory senses.

Elder mistreatment should be considered when evaluating the injured older patient. Investigations suggest that excess of 2% of elders are abused or neglected.[33,34]

INITIAL PREHOSPITAL EVALUATION: TRIAGE AND TREATMENT

Limited physiologic reserve means that the prognosis of the elderly injured patient is much better when the patient is rapidly transported to a trauma center.[35,36] Patient outcomes may be improved when care is provided by higher-volume trauma centers with broader experience in care of the elderly.[3] One Level II trauma center demonstrated improved patient outcomes with regard to infections, respiratory failure, and overall survival by creating a designated trauma care team for the elderly.[37] Despite this observation, there is a continuing phenomenon of under-triaging the elderly to trauma centers. One review of a statewide trauma network showed that the elderly were significantly less likely to receive trauma team activation when compared to younger patients with similar injuries. The under-triaged elderly patients were found to have 4 times the risk of mortality and disability compared to their younger counterparts.[38]

INJURY ASSESSMENT AND RESUSCITATION

Airway and Breathing

In conscious patients, initial airway assessment can begin by asking questions as simple as “What is your name?” A clear, appropriate response indicates that the airway is patent and that the brain is adequately perfused. Unconscious or obtunded patients require further attention.

Laryngeal reflexes may be diminished or absent. Because of a widespread loss of all muscular and neural elements, laryngeal structures undergo a gradual deterioration in function. Older patients may also exhibit a decrease in protective airway reflexes.[39] Edentulous patients may suffer from oropharyngeal obstruction when maintained in a mandatory supine position. In addition, the airway can be physically obstructed as a result of direct injury, edema, or foreign bodies. There is increased concern for cervical spine injuries in elderly patients suffering from blunt mechanism of injury. Fractures of the first and second cervical vertebrae are more common in geriatric patients.[40]

Pulmonary contusion is one of the most common blunt thoracic injuries. Rib fractures are expected to occur with greater frequency than in younger patients. Noninvasive ventilation via a continuous positive airway pressure mask has been described in the literature for the management of hypoxemia caused by lung contusion and for other medical conditions.[26] This effect may serve as a pathophysiology-directed therapy for hypoxemic patients who have blunt chest injury in whom endotracheal intubation is not required. The use of thoracic epidural analgesia has not been consistently shown to influence the rates of pulmonary complications but provides analgesia that is superior to other modes. It should be considered early in the pain management plan.

Orotracheal intubation under anesthesia with planned neuromuscular blockade and manual in-line stabilization remains the safest and most effective method for airway control in the severely injured patient.[41] Confirmation of intubation should be established with capnography or capnometry, and continuous pulse oximetry should be used. Recommendations concerning the doses of medications used to facilitate intubation are shown in **Table 2**. In the older adult, the doses of many of the sedative agents used to facilitate intubation may have to be further altered. Their pharmacokinetics could be altered due to the trauma[42] or to physiologic changes associated with aging.[10,43,44]

To avoid hypotension in the elderly trauma patient, the doses of the etomidate,[45] barbiturates,[46] and benzodiazepines[47,48] should be reduced. For example, an 80-year-old trauma patient needs less than half the amount of etomidate to reach the same electroencephalographic endpoint as a 22-year-old patient.[45] This reduction of blood pressure in the elderly patient is especially marked when the patient is hypovolemic. Ketamine is commonly used in the trauma scenario. In the geriatric patient, this drug has a reduced clearance and is expected to have a longer duration of action.

The opioids have an increased activity or alterations in pharmacokinetics in the elderly patient. A reduction in the dosage of morphine,[49] alfentanil, fentanyl,[50] and remifentanil[51] is recommended. The only exception to this rule is meperidine, for which no changes in clearance rate or terminal elimination half-time value have been

Table 2
Dosage alteration for the anesthetic drugs used to facilitate intubation in the elderly patient

Class of Medication	Change of Dose in the Elderly Patient
Sedatives	Reduction of 50% of bolus dose
Depolarizing neuromuscular blocking agent (succinylcholine)	No reduction in bolus dose
Nondepolarizing neuromuscular blocking agents	No reduction in bolus dose
Opioids	Reduction of 50% of bolus dose

shown.[52] However, because of its central nervous system–active toxic metabolite, normeperidine, its use is not advocated in elderly patients.

In the geriatric population, a reduction in physical activity theoretically should result in a reduction in sensitivity because of up-regulation to neuromuscular blockers. In contrast, augmented exercise increases sensitivity to neuromuscular blocking drugs receptors.[53] Clinical doses of neuromuscular blockers are usually unchanged.[54]

Circulation

Significant reductions in coronary blood flow can occur in the absence of known coronary artery disease.[55] The aging myocardium is also less able to respond to circulating catecholamines.[41] Therefore, the geriatric patient may not develop tachycardia in the presence of hypovolemia. Elderly patients may also be taking medications such as β-blockers that alter their heart rate response. Often, geriatric patients have hypertension; therefore, a normal or borderline blood pressure should be treated with a degree of suspicion.

In recent years, it has been suggested that the minimum acceptable systolic blood pressure (SBP) during initial evaluation of geriatric patients should be significantly higher than the acceptable limits for younger adults. Similarly, a lower threshold for the definition for tachycardia may be warranted. Advanced Trauma Life Support guidelines from the American College of Surgeons classify severe hemorrhage (Class 3 or 4) when the SBP is less than 90 mm Hg and heart rate is greater than 120 bpm. It has been suggested that these thresholds may not reliably indicate severe hemorrhage in the elderly. Investigators have suggested hypotension be defined as SBP less than 100 to 110 mm Hg and tachycardia greater than 90 bpm.[56,57] Along those lines, it has also been proposed that the definition of hypotension continues to change with age, with 120 mm Hg for ages 50 to 69 years and 140 mm Hg for ages 70 years and greater as cutoff points for minimum acceptable SBPs.[58] Severely elevated SBP in younger patients without significant head injuries has been associated with worse outcomes, but this trend does not seem to hold in the geriatric population. Elevations in SBP have actually been associated with improved outcomes in the elderly.[59] Despite these findings, there is still an insufficient amount of data to warrant changes to existing evaluation criteria from specialty organizations.

Given the challenges of interpreting vital signs, it is important to measure other markers of perfusion as early as possible. Lactic acid levels and base deficit calculations are particularly useful. One center reported that 42% of its elderly trauma admissions were found to have significant alteration of lactate levels or base deficits, despite “normal” vital signs.[57] In patients who are “normotensive” by standard definitions, elevated serum lactate levels are associated with increased mortality. One investigator showed that lactate levels in excess of 4 mmol/L resulted in a mortality rate near 40% for patients older than 65 years of age. The mortality rate for younger patients with similar lactate levels was 12%. Base deficits greater than 6 were associated with similar outcomes.[60]

The elderly trauma victim as compared with their younger counterpart may be less able to compensate for changing oxygen demands by increasing cardiac output. It has been proposed that oxygen carrying capacity of blood should be optimized by maintaining adequate hemoglobin levels at all times.[16]

Monitoring

Early invasive monitoring with hemodynamic optimization has been associated with improved survival in the geriatric trauma patient.[55] Primarily based on these findings, the Eastern Association for the Surgery of Trauma (EAST) 2001 guidelines for resuscitation state that any severely injured geriatric patient should undergo invasive monitoring.[61] This study has not been duplicated and the topic has not been reviewed in more recent guideline updates from EAST, and the extent to which routine invasive monitoring is applied in geriatric trauma patients is not known.

In recent years, there has been a renewed focus on measurement of dynamic parameters of hemodynamics including pulse pressure variation (PPV), systolic pressure variation (SPV), and stroke volume variation (SVV) as indicators of fluid responsiveness in mechanically ventilated patients. Although SVV will require additional equipment that may not be available in many hospitals, SPV and PPV can be followed via arterial blood pressure catheters alone. There are no prospective trials focused on the geriatric population in trauma. However, meta-analysis of available literature from 1998 to 2008 demonstrated that the accuracy of these variables is significantly better at determining volume responsiveness in the critically ill than central venous pressure or indices of the left ventricular end-diastolic area and global end-diastolic volume. Among the 3, PPV was shown to have the greatest accuracy.[62]

COMMON SPECIFIC INJURIES OF THE ELDERLY

Hip Fractures

Osteoporosis and tendency to fall increase the incidence of hip fractures, which is the most common cause of traumatic injury in geriatric patients, mainly in women. Hip fracture can occur as part of a multitrauma or as an isolated injury. Hip fracture in multitrauma is associated with other bone and soft-tissue injuries, intra-abdominal and intrapelvic injuries, major blood loss, head and neck injuries, and other extremity injuries. Overall, an inability to return to a preinjury level of mobility results in precipitous functional decline, a loss of independence, quality-of-life reduction, and depression in older persons. There are data to suggest that outcome in these patients is superior when they are managed by a specialized multidisciplinary team.[63]

The timing of hip surgery in the elderly may play a significant role in morbidity and mortality. Numerous small studies have produced mixed findings, but larger analyses have provided some clarification. This finding was demonstrated in a 2008 meta-analysis that reported both an increased 30-day and 1-year mortality (odds ratio 1.41 and 1.32, respectively) for delays greater than 48 hours.[64] Looking more closely, the investigators commented that early surgery was probably of greatest benefit to younger patients and those with a low baseline risk of mortality in one year. Patients with higher baseline risk did not necessarily receive benefit from earlier surgery. A more recent prospective cohort study of patients found that mortality was not increased by delays up to 120 hours, when adjusted for severity of comorbid disease.[65] Decisions about timing should therefore be made with regard to a patient's baseline risk and comorbidities. In patients without significant comorbid conditions, there is a definite benefit to early operation within the first 24 to 48 hours after injury. Although there is evidence that patients with uncontrolled comorbid conditions may not fare worse after up to 5 days of delay, efforts should be directed at timely optimization to allow the earliest possible surgical correction of the hip fracture.

Early ambulation and daily physical therapy after hip fracture surgery should be encouraged. Delayed ambulation after hip fracture surgery is related to the development of new-onset delirium, postoperative pneumonia, and increased length of hospital stay.[66]

The best choice of anesthetic technique for hip fracture surgery has been debated for quite some time, with small studies resulting in mixed findings. The most recent, and possibly best, study was a large retrospective analysis of hip fracture patients from 126 New York hospitals. This finding indicated that regional anesthesia was associated with a 29% reduction in mortality and 25% reduction in pulmonary complications while in hospital.[67] These data are similar to data that were published earlier in the veteran population.[68] Based on these findings, it is most likely appropriate to choose regional techniques for hip fracture surgeries when feasible. There appears to be no significant difference in postoperative cognitive functioning between the 2 techniques.[69]

Head Injuries

Head injuries of any severity have a worse prognosis in the geriatric population. The risks of mortality and poor functional outcomes increase progressively with age. Researchers have also consistently found that higher severity injuries, lower Glasgow Coma Scale (GCS) scores on admission, preinjury anticoagulant therapies are all associated with poor neurologic outcomes in this population. Increased vascular vulnerability is characteristic of the aging brain. Subdural hematoma can result in changes in mental status, headache, disturbances in ambulation, or nonfocal neurologic findings.

One meta-analysis of 5600 severe head-injured patients treated in the late 1980s to 1990s demonstrated a risk of poor outcome that increased 40% to 50% per decade of life. At that time, the 6-month mortality for those aged more than 65 years was around 72%.[70] Outcomes have not necessarily improved over the years. In a more recent report from one state trauma network, geriatric patients with moderate to severe brain injury had an overall in-hospital mortality rate approaching 30%, and no patient with an admission GCS score less than 9 had good outcomes; the mortality for that subgroup was 80%.[71]

Even those patients with mild head injury are expected to fare worse than their younger counterparts, as mortality rates are elevated[72] and postdischarge function is reduced. Although better outcomes were associated with increased use of specialty consults and multidisciplinary care, it has also been reported that older patients tend to receive lower-intensity care for their injuries.[73]

Anesthetic management for the head-injured older patient follows the same general principles applied to younger patients. Etomidate hydrochloride and propofol are used to induce anesthesia before intubation; no single agent has been shown to be superior. Each decreases the systemic response to intubation, blunts intracranial pressure changes, and decreases the cerebral metabolic rate for oxygen.[74]

The ability of the aging brain to autoregulate blood flow may be similar to that of younger patients under normal conditions.[75] Autoregulation is often severely impaired after head injury in any patient, but this impairment may be exaggerated in the old. It is unclear if this is related purely to age or the presence of comorbid conditions.[76] Maintenance of adequate cerebral perfusion pressure (CPP) should be a priority during anesthetic care, but there is currently no recommendation to adjust CPP based on age. Current recommendations indicate that CPP should be maintained at least 60 mm Hg. There is no evidence that artificially elevating it greater than 70 mm Hg is beneficial.[77]

SUMMARY

Elderly patients represent the most rapidly expanding segment of our population, and a significant portion will rely on trauma care services during their lives. The progressive functional decline that occurs with normal aging, especially when chronic disease states are superimposed, makes these patients more physiologically fragile. They are less capable of sustaining the stresses of traumatic injury and their injuries are often much worse than those sustained by younger patients via similar mechanisms. Geriatric patients have been shown to benefit from focused, intensive care and from multidisciplinary teams with geriatric experience. Despite these facts, the geriatric population in developed countries may be the least likely to be triaged into trauma care systems that can best deal with their injuries.

Routinely administered anesthetic medications should be adjusted appropriately for age, often being reduced by as much as half. Volume resuscitative therapies should be directed to maintain cardiac output and oxygen carrying capacity, and a lower threshold for conducting invasive cardiac monitoring is recommended. Normal-appearing vital signs may not indicate occult hypoperfusion.

Hip fractures are among the most common injuries sustained by elderly patients. There is reasonable evidence that the surgical repair of such fractures should be achieved as soon as possible to minimize risks for mortality. The use of regional anesthesia for such cases may significantly reduce morbidity and mortality. Head injuries of any severity may place geriatric patients at increased risk of mortality, but there are currently no geriatric-specific treatment recommendations that differ from usual adult guidelines.

REFERENCES

1. United States Census Bureau. Projected population of the United States, by age and sex: 2000 to 2050. Available at: http://www.census.gov/population/www/projections/usinterimproj/natprojtab02a.pdf. Accessed August 29, 2012.
2. Murphy SL, Xu J, Kochanek KD. Deaths: preliminary data for 2010. Natl Vital Stat Rep 2012;60:1–52.
3. Pandya SR, Yelon JA, Sullivan BS, et al. Geriatric motor vehicle collision survival: the role of institutional trauma volume. J Trauma 2011;70:1326–30.
4. Travis KW, Mihevc NT, Orkin FK, et al. Age and anesthetic practice: a regional perspective. J Clin Anesth 1999;11:175–86.
5. Muhlberg W, Platt D. Age-dependent changes of the kidneys: pharmacological implications. Gerontology 1999;45:243–53.
6. Buemi M, Nostro L, Aloisi C, et al. Kidney aging: from phenotype to genetics. Rejuvenation Res 2005;8:101–9.
7. Janssens JP. Aging of the respiratory system: impact on pulmonary function tests and adaptation to exertion. Clin Chest Med 2005;26:469–84.
8. Williams JM, Evans TC. Acute pulmonary disease in the aged. Clin Geriatr Med 1993;9:527–45.
9. Cardus J, Burgos F, Diaz O, et al. Increase in pulmonary ventilation-perfusion inequality with age in healthy individuals. Am J Respir Crit Care Med 1997;156: 648–53.
10. Nickalls RW, Mapleson WW. Age-related iso-MAC charts for isoflurane, sevoflurane and desflurane in man. Br J Anaesth 2003;91:170–4.
11. Thompson LF. Failure to wean: exploring the influence of age-related pulmonary changes. Crit Care Nurs Clin North Am 1996;8:7–16.
12. Chalfin DB. Outcome assessment in elderly patients with critical illness and respiratory failure. Clin Chest Med 1993;14:583–9.
13. Mooradian AD. Normal age-related changes in thyroid hormone economy. Clin Geriatr Med 1995;11:159–69.
14. Barton RN, Horan MA, Clague JE, et al. The effect of aging on the metabolic clearance rate and distribution of cortisol in man. Arch Gerontol Geriatr 1999; 29:95–105.

15. Frankenfield D, Cooney RN, Smith JS, et al. Age-related differences in the metabolic response to injury. J Trauma 2000;48:49–56.
16. Demarest GB, Osler TM, Clevenger FW. Injuries in the elderly: evaluation and initial response. Geriatrics 1990;45:36–8.
17. Scwab C, Shapiro M, Kauder D. Geriatric trauma: patterns, care and outcomes. In: Mattox K, Feliciano D, Moore E, editors. Trauma. New York: McGraw-Hill; 2000. p. 1099–113.
18. Gubler KD, Davis R, Koepsell T, et al. Long-term survival of elderly trauma patients. Arch Surg 1997;132:1010–4.
19. DeMaria EJ, Kenney PR, Merriam MA, et al. Aggressive trauma care benefits the elderly. J Trauma 1987;27:1200–6.
20. Neideen T, Lam M, Brasel KJ. Preinjury beta blockers are associated with increased mortality in geriatric trauma patients. J Trauma 2008;65:1016–20.
21. Franko J, Kish KJ, O'Connell BG, et al. Advanced age and preinjury warfarin anticoagulation increase the risk of mortality after head trauma. J Trauma 2006;61:107–10.
22. Lavoie A, Ratte S, Clas D, et al. Preinjury warfarin use among elderly patients with closed head injuries in a trauma center. J Trauma 2004;56:802–7.
23. Pudelek B. Geriatric trauma: special needs for a special population. AACN Clin Issues 2002;13:61–72.
24. Wofford JL, Moran WP, Heuser MD, et al. Emergency medical transport of the elderly: a population-based study. Am J Emerg Med 1995;13:297–300.
25. McMahon DJ, Shapiro MB, Kauder DR. The injured elderly in the trauma intensive care unit. Surg Clin North Am 2000;80:1005–19.
26. Hurst JM, DeHaven CB, Branson RD. Use of CPAP mask as the sole mode of ventilatory support in trauma patients with mild to moderate respiratory insufficiency. J Trauma 1985;25:1065–8.
27. Mosenthal AC, Livingston DH, Elcavage J, et al. Epidemiology and strategies for prevention. J Trauma 1995;38:753–6.
28. Velmahos GC, Jindal A, Chan LS. "Insignificant" mechanism of injury: not to be taken lightly. J Am Coll Surg 2001;192:147–52.
29. Lambert DA, Sattin RW. Death from falls, 1978-1984. MMWR CDC Surveill Summ 1998;37:S21–6.
30. Ruhle R, Wolff H. Psychological aspects of traffic fitness of aging car drivers. Z Gesamte Hyg 1990;3:346–50 [in German].
31. Sjogren H, Eriksson A, Ostrom M. Role of disease in initiating the crashes of fatally injured drivers. Accid Anal Prev 1996;28:307–14.
32. Linn BS. Age differences in the severity and outcome of burns. J Am Geriatr Soc 1980;28:118–23.
33. Kennedy RD. Elder abuse and neglect: the experience, knowledge, and attitudes of primary care physicians. Fam Med 2005;37:481–5.
34. Elder abuse and neglect: council on scientific affairs. JAMA 1987;257:966–71.
35. Finelli FC, Jonsson J, Champion HR, et al. A case control study for major trauma in geriatric patients. J Trauma 1989;29:541–8.
36. Phillips S, Rond PC, Kelly SM, et al. The failure of triage criteria to identify geriatric patients with trauma: results from the Florida Trauma Triage Study. J Trauma 1996;40:278–83.
37. Mangram AJ, Mitchell CD, Shifflette MD, et al. Geriatric trauma service: a one-year experience. J Trauma 2011;72:119–22.
38. Lehmann R, Beekley A, Casey L, et al. The impact of advanced age on trauma triage decisions and outcomes: a statewide analysis. Am J Surg 2009;197:571–4.

39. Pontoppidan H, Beecher HK. Progressive loss of protective reflexes in the airway with the advance of age. JAMA 1960;174:2209–13.
40. Lomoschitz FM, Blackmore CC, Mirza SK, et al. Cervical spine injuries in patients 65 years old and older: epidemiologic analysis regarding the effects of age and injury mechanism on distribution, type, and stability of injuries. Am J Roentgenol 2002;178:573–7.
41. Adnet F, Lapostolle F, Ricard-Hibon A, et al. Intubating trauma patients before reaching hospital—revisited. Crit Care 2001;5:290–1.
42. Berkenstadt H, Mayan H, Segal E, et al. The pharmacokinetics of morphine and lidocaine in nine severe trauma patients. J Clin Anesth 1999;11:630–4.
43. Eilers H, Niemann C. Clinically important drug interactions with intravenous anaesthetics in older patients. Drugs Aging 2003;20:969–80.
44. Vuyk J. Pharmacodynamics in the elderly. Best Pract Res Clin Anaesthesiol 2003; 17:207–18.
45. Arden JR, Holley FO, Stanski DR. Increased sensitivity to etomidate in the elderly: initial distribution versus altered brain response. Anesthesiology 1986;65:9–27.
46. Homer TD, Stanski DR. The effect of increasing age on thiopental disposition and anesthetic requirement. Anesthesiology 1985;62:714–24.
47. Reves JG, Fragen RJ, Vinik HR, et al. Midazolam: pharmacology and uses. Anesthesiology 1985;62:310–24.
48. Smith MR, Bell GD, Quine MA, et al. Small bolus injections of intravenous midazolam for upper gastrointestinal endoscopy: a study of 788 consecutive cases. Br J Clin Pharmacol 1993;36:573–8.
49. Kaiko RF, Wallenstein SL, Rogers AG, et al. Narcotics in the elderly. Med Clin North Am 1982;66:1079–89.
50. Shafer SL. The pharmacology of anesthetic drugs in the elderly patients. Anesthesiol Clin North America 2000;18:1–29.
51. Minto CF, Schnider TW, Egan TD, et al. Influence of age and gender on the pharmacokinetics and pharmacodynamics of remifentanil: I. Model development. Anesthesiology 1997;86:10–23.
52. Herman RJ, McAllister CB, Branch RA, et al. Effects of age on meperidine disposition. Clin Pharmacol Ther 1985;37:19–24.
53. Martyn JA, White DA, Gronert GA, et al. Up and down regulation of skeletal muscle acetylcholine receptors. Anesthesiology 1992;76:822–43.
54. Rupp SM, Castagnoli KP, Fisher DM, et al. Pancuronium and vecuronium pharmacokinetics and pharmacodynamics in younger and elderly adults. Anesthesiology 1987;67:45–9.
55. Scalea TM, Simon HM, Duncan AO, et al. Geriatric blunt multiple trauma: improved survival with early invasive monitoring. J Trauma 1990;30:129–34.
56. Heffernan DS, Thakkar RK, Monaghan SF, et al. Normal presenting vital signs are unreliable in geriatric blunt trauma victims. J Trauma 2010;69:813–20.
57. Martin J, Alkhoury F, O'Connor J, et al. 'Normal' vital signs belie occult hypoperfusion in geriatric trauma patients. Am Surg 2010;76:65–9.
58. Edwards M, Ley E, Mirocha J, et al. Defining hypotension in moderate to severely injured trauma patients: raising the bar for the elderly. Am Surg 2010; 76:1035–8.
59. Ley EJ, Singer MB, Gangi A, et al. Elevated systolic blood pressure after trauma: tolerated in the elderly. J Surg Res 2012;177(2):326–9.
60. Callaway DW, Shapiro NI, Donnino MW, et al. Serum lactate and base deficit as predictors of mortality in normotensive elderly blunt trauma patients. J Trauma 2009;66:1040–4.

61. Jacobs DG, Plaisier BR, Barie PS, et al. Practice management guidelines for geriatric trauma: the EAST practice management guidelines work group. J Trauma 2003;54:391–416.
62. Marik PE, Cavallazzi R, Vasu T, et al. Dynamic changes in arterial waveform derived variables and fluid responsiveness in mechanically ventilated patients: a systematic review of the literature. Crit Care Med 2009;37:2642–7.
63. Khasraghi FA, Christmas C, Lee EJ, et al. Effectiveness of a multidisciplinary team approach to hip fracture management. J Surg Orthop Adv 2005;14:27–31.
64. Shiga T, Wajima Z, Ohe Y. Is operative delay associated with increased mortality of hip fracture patients? Systematic review, meta-analysis, and meta-regression. Can J Anaesth 2008;55:146–54.
65. Vidan MT, Sanchez E, Gracia Y, et al. Causes and effects of surigical delay in patients with hip fracture: a cohort study. Ann Intern Med 2011;155:226–33.
66. Kamel HK, Iqbal MA, Mogallapu R, et al. Time to ambulation after hip fracture surgery: relation to hospitalization outcomes. J Gerontol A Biol Sci Med Sci 2003;58:1042–5.
67. Neuman MD, Silber JH, Elkassabany NM, et al. Comparative effectiveness of regional versus general anesthesia for hip fracture surgery in adults. Anesthesiology 2012;117:72–92.
68. Radcliff TA, Henderson WG, Stoner TJ, et al. Patient risk factors, operative care, and outcomes among older community-dwelling male veterans with hip fracture. J Bone Joint Surg Am 2008;90:34–42.
69. Berggren D, Gustafson Y, Eriksson B, et al. Postoperative confusion after anesthesia in elderly patients with femoral neck fractures. Anesth Analg 1987;66:497–504.
70. Hukkelhoven CW, Steyerberg EW, Rampen AJ, et al. Patient age and outcome following severe traumatic brain injury: an analysis of 5600 patients. J Neurosurg 2003;99:666–73.
71. Utomo WK, Gabbe BJ, Simpson PM, et al. Predictors of in-hospital mortality and 6-month functional outcomes in older adults after moderate to severe traumatic brain injury. Injury 2011;40:973–7.
72. Susman M, DiRusso SM, Sullivan T, et al. Traumatic brain injury in the elderly: increased mortality and worse functional outcome at discharge despite lower injury severity. J Trauma 2002;53:219–23.
73. Thompson HJ, Rivara FP, Jurkovich GJ, et al. Evaluation of the effect of intensity of care on mortality after traumatic brain injury. Crit Care Med 2008;36:282–90.
74. Unni VK, Johnston RA, Young HS, et al. Prevention of intracranial hypertension during laryngoscopy and endotracheal intubation. Br J Anaesth 1984;56:1219–23.
75. Yam AT, Lang EW, Lagopoulos J, et al. Cerebral autoregulation and ageing. J Clin Neurosci 2005;12:643–6.
76. Thompson HJ, McCormick WC, Kagan SH. Traumatic brain injury in older adults: epidemiology, outcomes, and future implications. J Am Geriatr Soc 2006;54:1590–5.
77. Bratton SL, Chestnut RM, Ghajar J, et al. Guidelines for the management of severe traumatic brain injury. IX. Cerebral perfusion thresholds. J Neurotrauma 2007;24:S59–64.

Management and Outcomes of Trauma During Pregnancy

Sharon Einav, MD[a,*], Hen Y. Sela, MD[b], Carolyn F. Weiniger, MBChB[c]

KEYWORDS

- Pregnancy • Wounds and injuries • Multiple trauma • Anesthesia and analgesia
- Therapeutics • Education • Outcome and process assessment (health care)
- Pregnancy outcome

KEY POINTS

- Approximately 1% to 4% of pregnant women are evaluated in emergency/delivery rooms because of traumatic injury.
- Pregnancy should be sought in all trauma cases involving women of childbearing age.
- Use of illicit drugs and alcohol, domestic abuse, and depression contribute to maternal trauma; thus a high index of suspicion should be maintained when treating injured young women.
- If pregnancy is confirmed, gestational age should be assessed while providers adhere to the advanced trauma life support (ATLS) guidelines.
- Fetal viability should be assessed after maternal stabilization.
- Pregnancy-related morbidity occurs in approximately 25% of cases and may include placental abruption, uterine rupture, preterm delivery, and the need for cesarean delivery (CD).

EPIDEMIOLOGY

The rate of maternal death due to penetrating trauma, suicide, homicide, and motor vehicle accidents (MVAs) is increasing,[1] whereas the rate of maternal death from direct causes is decreasing. This seemingly increased mortality may be the result of

---

Prior presentations: None.
Funding sources: None.
Acknowledgments: None.
Disclosures: None.

[a] Hebrew University School of Medicine, Shaare Zedek Medical Centre, POB 3235, Samuel Byte 12, Jerusalem 91031, Israel; [b] Allen Hospital MFM Ultrasound & Consult Services, Division of Maternal Fetal Medicine, Department of Obstetrics and Gynecology, Columbia University Medical Center, 622 West 168th Street, PH-16, New York, NY 10032, USA; [c] Department of Anesthesiology and Critical Care Medicine, Hadassah Hebrew University Medical Center, Ein Kerem, Jerusalem 91120, POB 12000, Israel
* Corresponding author.
E-mail address: einav_s@szmc.org.il

Anesthesiology Clin 31 (2013) 141–156
http://dx.doi.org/10.1016/j.anclin.2012.10.002 **anesthesiology.theclinics.com**
1932-2275/13/$ – see front matter

improved ascertainment of death during pregnancy.[2] Population-based studies show that approximately 1% to 4% of pregnant women are admitted for medical treatment because of traumatic injury,[3–5] the predominant cause of external injury during pregnancy being falls.[3,4] Although MVAs, domestic and/or nondomestic violence, and self-inflicted injury are less common than falls, they are associated with a higher likelihood of severe injury and death[3] and are perceived to be within societal responsibility.[6–9]

Pregnancy-related death is defined as the death of a woman while pregnant or within 42 days of termination of pregnancy, irrespective of the cause of death. Contrary to maternal death, accidental or incidental causes are included in the definition of pregnancy-related death. The definition of pregnancy-related death was introduced at the time of change from ICD9 to ICD10 coding and facilitated the identification of maternal deaths not directly associated with the pregnant state, in circumstances in which the cause of death was incidental.[10] Before this change, no code existed for incidental cause of death during pregnancy. Hence the cause of death was frequently misclassified as pregnancy related. Many trauma databases still lack fields for data regarding pregnancy. Because registry data on maternal trauma remains deficient, most publications constitute retrospective analyses of causes of maternal deaths in single institutions rather than prospective analyses of maternal injury across multiple medical centers.

The case fatality rate of MVAs during pregnancy remains relatively low compared with the case fatality rates from causes such as maternal cardiovascular diseases[11] and thromboembolic phenomena during pregnancy.[12,13] However, because the average person has a 1:200 lifetime risk for being involved in a fatal MVA and a 57% lifetime risk of being injured in an MVA,[14] it is not surprising that MVAs constitute a significant cause of maternal, fetal, and neonatal death in North America and Europe. Worldwide, data from the Global Burden of Disease study of mortality among adolescents and young adults (ages 10–24 years) showed that within the category of deaths from injury, MVAs constituted the most significant cause of death and accounted for 5% of female deaths among women of childbearing age regardless of the existence of a pregnancy at the time of trauma.[15]

Several variables have been associated with maternal injury and death from trauma. Data from the American College of Surgeons National Trauma Data Bank associate 19.6% of pregnancy-related traumas with the use of illicit drugs and 12.9% of pregnancy-related traumas with the use of alcohol.[16] Poor compliance with the use of restraints during pregnancy is not a major issue. Use of restraints is generally similar to that of the general MVA population in the United States,[17] although it is highly dependent on the region.[16,18,19] Intimate partner abuse is an important contributor to maternal trauma.[20] Unwanted pregnancy may play a substantive role in this type of violence,[21] and pregnancy during adolescence is associated with a higher-than-usual likelihood of both violence and suicide.[22–24] Because homicide and suicide-related maternal deaths are often underreported[25,26] and both could be associated with MVA injury, one should bear in mind that nonfatal violence and suicide attempts may also be associated with pregnancy and a high index of suspicion should be maintained when treating young women thus injured.[27]

THE PRIMARY AND SECONDARY SURVEYS AND SURGICAL TREATMENT

The ATLS guidelines provide a framework for rapid assessment and management of the injured patient and have been demonstrated to improve patient outcomes.[28,29] Implementation of the ATLS guidelines deflects needless deaths during the first stage of resuscitation.[30] Although a multidisciplinary team approach is recommended for the treatment of pregnant trauma patients,[28,31] all providers caring for such patients should follow the ATLS guidelines.[28]

All women of childbearing age should be assessed for possible pregnancy. If pregnancy is confirmed, estimation of the gestational age has implications for fetal viability and adds to the complexity of the decision-making process. Gestational age may be assessed either through patient history or by physical examination of the pelvis and abdomen; the uterine fundus is palpable above the pubic crest from the second trimester of gestation.

The ATLS guidelines should be adhered to despite the distracting presence of the fetus.[32] Treating the mother appropriately is beneficial for both the mother and the fetus.[31] The modifications to ATLS guidelines that may be considered for the pregnant casualty are provision of supplemental oxygen (because of maternal susceptibility to hypoxia and desaturation, see "Section on anesthetic management"),[33] preference for establishment of intravenous access above the diaphragm,[34] and left lateral positioning of the patient as soon as possible[35] (because of the possibility of reduced venous return secondary to uterine pressure on the vena-cava [aortocaval syndrome]).

Notwithstanding the presence of a pregnancy, the secondary survey should include the usual in-depth physical assessment of injuries. In addition, an obstetrician should conduct a proper pelvic examination to ascertain fetal position and should perform an examination for cervical dilation/effacement and the presence of blood and/or amniotic fluid leakage.[28] Placenta previa must be excluded before sterile vaginal examination of a pregnant patient with vaginal bleeding because bleeding may be provoked/exacerbated by the examination.[36] Previous publications examining the quality of maternal care after an MVA suggest that the presence of a pregnancy may distract the trauma team's attention away from the mother.[32,37] Because both maternal and fetal survival are primarily dependent on maternal well-being, assessment of fetal viability should be withheld until both the primary and secondary surveys of the mother have been performed and a formal pelvic examination has been performed in full.

In cases of massive transfusion, general trauma protocols should be adhered to; obstetric transfusion guidelines have recently adopted the transfusion protocols used in trauma.[38] Blood testing should also be in accordance with the regular trauma protocol[28,31] with the addition of a Kleihauer–Betke (KB) test (see "Section on Obstetric workup and treatment"). Radiographic examinations and computed tomography should be performed according to routine indications (see "Diagnostic Imaging").[39,40] The accuracy of focused abdominal sonography for trauma during pregnancy is almost comparable to that observed in nonpregnant women.[41–44] The indications for surgery are similar in pregnant and nonpregnant patients, and urgent maternal surgery should not be delayed for the purpose of assessing fetal viability. It is prudent to add an obstetrician to the surgical team in cases requiring abdominal/pelvic surgery.

OBSTETRIC WORKUP AND TREATMENT

Maternal Assessment

Clinical examination during the secondary survey constitutes the first step in assessing the risk for obstetric complications such as placental abruption, uterine rupture, preterm delivery, and need for CD. Further workup includes monitoring of the fetal heart rate (FHR) and uterine activity, ultrasonographic evaluation of the fetus and the pregnancy, further imaging modalities, and laboratory studies. Obstetric ultrasonography should be used to ascertain the gestational age, confirm the presence of a FHR, identify multifetal pregnancy, and seek placental abruption.[45] The clinician should, however, keep in mind the low sensitivity of ultrasound testing for this indication; thus a negative result for placental abruption does not exclude this possibility.[46,47] Placental abruption complicates 1.7% of maternal traumas and is significantly more common after blunt trauma (4.4%–6.8%).[48–50] Although placental abruption is more likely with increasing severity of maternal injury, it may occur and thus should be considered, even with mild trauma.[49] Signs and symptoms include abdominal pain, contractions with pain that is disproportionate to the degree of cervical dilation, and/or vaginal bleeding. Physical examination reveals a tender and rigid uterus. Hemorrhage may be occult even when significant and may lead to coagulopathy and hemodynamic instability. Appropriate therapies consist of correction of hematological abnormalities in mild cases and prompt delivery in severe cases.

Uterine rupture is often associated with other severe injuries. Maternal death may be caused by massive hemorrhage from the ruptured uterus or from the associated injuries, and fetal/neonatal death occurs in up to 17.5% of the cases.[13]

Amniotic fluid embolus is a rare event specifically after trauma.[51] The presenting signs and symptoms may vary, including respiratory distress, shock or severe hypertension, coma, seizure, disseminated intravascular coagulation, cardiac arrest, or other coagulation disorders. All these presentations contribute to the high reported maternal mortality of 30% to 50%. Thus these clinical situations, which may be associated with amniotic fluid embolism, warrant prompt recognition and appropriate supportive care, to optimize outcomes.[52]

Fetal assessment should be performed only after maternal stability has been established.[31] Uterine activity should be monitored when the gestational age is greater than 20 weeks, and FHR should be monitored when the gestational age is greater than 24 weeks.[28,31] Recurrent uterine contractions suggest premature labor if accompanied by cervical change.[28] Excess uterine activity (>4 contractions per hour) suggests either placental abruption, which may jeopardize both maternal and fetal life, or preterm contractions, which too may lead to premature labor.

Early recognition of fetal distress may improve fetal outcome. The optimal length of continuous FHR monitoring is not well established, but most authorities concur on an initial 2 to 6 hours.[31] Monitoring for at least 24 hours may be indicated for both obstetric and trauma-associated reasons (**Box 1**).[28,31] Abnormal FHR observed during

Box 1
Indications for prolonged obstetric monitoring (ie, beyond the initial period of 2–6 hours)

Obstetric findings[a]

Suspected placental abruption

Suspected preterm labor

Evidence of uterine contractions

Evidence of vaginal bleeding

Any sign of fetal distress

Trauma-associated findings

Maternal injuries requiring admission in accordance with trauma guidelines (unrelated to pregnancy)

Requires general anesthesia

Severe head injury

[a] Observed within the initial 2- to 6-hour monitoring period.

continuous monitoring best recognizes fetal distress[53] but may also be the first sign of maternal hemodynamic compromise because of blood shunting from the uterus.[54,55] If a nonreassuring FHR pattern is detected, with no evidence of maternal compromise, "in utero resuscitation" should be attempted (ie, provision of supplemental oxygen and fluids to the mother and left lateral decubitus positioning).[56] Lack of improvement should lead to expedited delivery, most likely through CD.

Fetal–maternal hemorrhage may complicate 10% to 30% of maternal traumas.[57] The KB test detects fetal blood cells in the maternal circulation, and in Rh-negative mothers, this test can provide a rough estimate of the volume of maternal–fetal hemorrhage. Rh-negative pregnant patients should receive Rh-D immunoglobulin within 72 hours of injury to prevent future Rh alloimmunization.

DIAGNOSTIC IMAGING

Plain radiographs of the cervical spine, chest, and pelvis are the recommended ATLS adjuncts to the primary survey. The trauma team should be acquainted through institution-specific drills with local guidelines regarding management of maternal trauma. A priori training will enable diagnostic imaging to be performed without delay despite diagnosis of a pregnancy at the critical time that the medical team is attempting to save the life of the trauma patient.[58] Without advance training, delays may transpire as physicians ponder the balance between maternal benefit and potential fetal harm. This situation is complicated further by the fact that diagnostic guidelines are not always evidence based.

Two variables determine the type and severity of damage caused during fetal exposure to radiation: the gestational age (ie, the developmental stage of the fetus) and the radiation dose. At a gestational age of 4 to 10 weeks (ie, the period of organogenesis), radiation is most likely to cause congenital malformations. The fetus is most susceptible to radiation-induced mental retardation at a gestational age of 10 and 17 weeks,[59] but there have been reports of developmental injury with fetal exposure up to 25 weeks.[60] The risk of noncancer biologic injury caused by exposure to diagnostic imaging levels of radiation diminishes with increasing gestational age and reaches a minimum by a gestational age greater than 26 weeks.[59] In contrast, childhood leukemia has been associated with fetal exposure to radiation at any stage.[59]

Although natural ionized radiation is a constant daily occurrence, the American College of Radiologists Practice Guidelines recommend that diagnostic imaging for pregnant patients be minimized if possible.[61] A radiation dose less than 50 mSv is not likely to increase the risk of fetal malformation or childhood cancer. Medical diagnostic imaging techniques use less than this dose, even when pelvic or whole body computed tomography is performed (these imaging procedures entail the highest exposure).[62,63] The dose of radiation associated with neonatal death or miscarriage (even during late pregnancy) is far higher than that used in diagnostic radiology (>1 Gy). Nonetheless, the possibility that in utero exposure to radiation may be associated with an increased risk of childhood leukemia (absolute risk ~1:2000) should guide physicians to maintain exposure to the lowest possible level.[39,64] Several possibilities exist for reducing the radiation dose in emergency trauma cases complicated by pregnancy; Use of a posteroanterior exposure method can increase the distance from the anterior uterus.[59] Computed tomography can be performed with increased slice depth, reduced current, or increased pitch. Internal shielding[65] and lead apron shielding[62] have been advocated where possible.[61]

Abortion is not recommended in cases of fetal exposure to diagnostic radiation[66] because it is unlikely that the dose administered during a diagnostic procedure will harm the fetus.[67,68] After maternal trauma issues have been resolved, the parents should be informed regarding fetal exposure to radiation. This information should be accompanied by suitable explanation of the inclusive nature of reports of childhood cancer after in utero exposure to radiation.

Contrast media, lipid-soluble solutions, and small-molecular-weight solutions easily penetrate the placental barrier[69] and are potentially teratogenic.[63] Use of radioiodine isotopes is contraindicated during pregnancy because of concerns regarding the likelihood of inducing thyroid cancer in the fetus.[66] Nonionic iodinated agents and gadolinium do cross the barrier but their movement is restricted because of high water solubility and larger molecular weights. Despite this, it is recommended to avoid using gadolinium where possible because there is little data regarding the long-term effect of such exposure.[69,70]

ANESTHETIC MANAGEMENT

Anesthetic management should be directed toward achievement and maintenance of maternal oxygenation and perfusion. Optimization of both will provide the best in utero conditions.[71] The pregnant patient is at increased risk for airway complications because of pregnancy-induced weight gain, breast tissue hypertrophy, and respiratory tract mucosal edema.[72] The incidence of difficult/failed intubation in obstetric anesthesia is 4 times higher than that in the surgical nonobstetric population.[73] The pregnant patient should be considered at risk for aspiration because of a full stomach from the second trimester. In the situation of trauma, a full stomach should always be considered. This consideration requires the use of rapid sequence induction and cricoid pressure for intubation. However, the use of cricoid pressure has been recently questioned because of both potential nonefficacy and distortion of laryngoscope view.[74] Guidelines recommend pharmacologic therapies to reduce acid aspiration,[75] but these are less suited to the emergency maternal trauma scenario. It is thus sensible to use methods to prevent clinically significant aspiration when possible, seek expert help before advanced airway management, and insert a tracheal tube of 0.5 to 1 mm internal diameter smaller than that used for nonpregnant woman of similar size.

Minute ventilation is approximately 30% higher in healthy women with singleton and twin pregnancies compared with nonpregnant women, and already during the first trimester, functional reserve capacity and expiratory reserve volume are lower by about 20% to 30%.[33] Because the pregnant trauma patient has lower respiratory reserves and the fetus can suffer easily from maternal hypoxia, early tracheal intubation has been advocated, with consideration for normal physiologic $Pa\small{CO}_2$ in pregnancy.[76] Induction drugs should be used with care to minimize vasodilation and hypotension. Propofol or ketamine are suitable, although both cross the placenta and can cause fetal depression.[77] Suxamethonium may be used to provide conditions for rapid intubation, and muscle relaxants do not cross the placenta in clinically relevant concentrations.[71] If suxamethonium is contraindicated (eg, with burns) rocuronium is also suitable.[78] The intubating dose of rocuronium is 1.2 mg/kg; however, the duration of action is relatively long.[79,80] Sugammadex (currently not licensed in the United States), which may be used to rapidly reverse rocuronium in cases of failed intubation, has been used in induction for CD but not for cases with ongoing pregnancy such as some maternal trauma situations.[81] The pediatrician caring for the neonate should be notified if drugs that traverse the placenta have been used (eg, opiates); temporary neonatal respiratory depression and flaccidity may occur.

RESCUE THERAPIES

Cesarean Delivery

About 2.4% to 7.2% of maternal trauma cases require CD shortly after trauma.[82–84] One study found that these cases have notably higher mortality rates than the general maternal trauma population (28.1%).[84]

In these cases maternal life may be at risk due to both obstetric and nonobstetric hemorrhage (ie, associated injuries).[84] Resuscitation and obstetric guidelines suggest that perimortem cesarean Delivery (PMCD) be considered within 4 minutes of maternal collapse for any cause, provided there is no evidence of return of spontaneous circulation.[85–87] This recommendation is based on physiologic evidence that compression of the vena cava by the gravid uterus may compromise maternal hemodynamics.[86,88] The concept of PMCD within 4 minutes of maternal arrest was introduced by Katz and colleagues.[89,90] In the first article discussing a possible time limit to good maternal and fetal outcomes, trauma constituted the cause of the arrest in less than 10% of the cases.[89] In 2 later articles, trauma was the most common cause of maternal death and accounted for about 20% of PMCD cases.[90,91] The paucity of reported cases prevents association between the cause of arrest and the likelihood of successful maternal return of spontaneous maternal circulation after PMCD. The role of PMCD for maternal salvage in traumatic cardiac arrest thus remains controversial. PMCD should, however, be considered for fetal salvage, that is, when maternal resuscitation efforts have been futile for 5 to 10 minutes and the fetus is likely to be viable (gestational age $\geq$23 weeks).

Extracorporeal Membranous Oxygenation

Use of extracorporeal membranous oxygenation (ECMO) for treatment of refractory hypoxemia or cardiac support in trauma has been limited by the difficulties of emergency vascular access, risk of hemorrhage, and lack of proof regarding benefit. Several investigators have suggested that ECMO therapy may be beneficial during pregnancy/in the early postpartaum period in H1N1-related hypoxemia,[92,93] massive thrombotic/amniotic fluid embolism,[94,95] and peripartum cardiomyopathy.[96] Only 1 case of successful ECMO therapy for maternal trauma has been reported.[97] This therapeutic option should thus be considered rescue therapy in the setting of maternal trauma with refractory hypoxemia.

MATERNAL OUTCOMES AND THE IMPACT OF PREGNANCY ON TRIAGE

Triage and Trauma Team Activation

Recommendations for field triage of injured patients cite pregnancy with a gestational age greater than 20 weeks as a criterion for patient transport to a Level I trauma center.[98] Recent assessment of the yield of these prehospital trauma triage guidelines through review of hospital discharge records revealed that major trauma was confirmed in only 1.5% (2 of 129) of the injured women transferred to Level I trauma centers because of pregnancy.[99] Many hospitals include pregnancy as a sole criterion for trauma team activation (TTA). For example, a survey of practice in the metropolitan Sydney area showed that 71% (5 of 7) of hospitals surveyed used this criterion, the only difference being slightly different gestational age cutoffs for TTA.[100] The presence of pregnancy is also a trigger for patient admission; pregnant women admitted for observation after trauma would not have been admitted in the absence of pregnancy.[16,32,101] Overtriage and overadmission because of the existence of a pregnant state may be the reasons for the low case fatality rates observed after maternal MVA. For example, one study found that among 188 of 352 pregnant trauma patients in whom pregnancy was the sole indication for TTA (58%), none were admitted to the surgical service[102] and that among the pregnant patients with a gestational age less than 20 weeks, 94% (33 of 35) were not admitted.[102] Another study demonstrated that when pregnancy was the sole criterion for TTA, the mean injury severity score (ISS) of this population was 1.053 (range 1–4) and the only required surgical intervention was CD, which was performed in 3.5% of the patients (2 of 57).[83] If a decision is made to activate the trauma team based on pregnancy as the sole criterion, a 2-tiered system or reduced team approach may be suitable. This approach would take into consideration the erosion of adherence to trauma protocol because of low rates of significant injury.

Maternal Outcomes

Population-based studies show that among the women admitted to hospital after an MVA, about 0.003% are admitted to an intensive care unit and less than 0.01% die.[5,13] Deaths usually occur in the subgroup of women that have sustained bruising injuries to the abdomen, pelvis or lower back, pelvic fractures and/or intra-abdominal injuries and in the subgroup of women who deliver during the index admission.[5] Thus, the overall maternal mortality rates after trauma are not high (0%–3.8%),[18,19,48,82,103] but the clinician should be aware that there are certain factors associated with increased mortality rates. These include the need for CD shortly after trauma, penetrating trauma,[84] and lack of restraints during involvement in an MVA.[104] Head injuries,[16] lower GCSs,[84,105] higher ISSs,[49] associated internal injuries,[49] and shock on admission[84] are also associated with poorer maternal outcomes, as is greater maternal age.[49] Despite this, a study from the National Trauma Data Bank (2001–2005) suggests that mortality among pregnant women is overall lower than that among matched nonpregnant women. This difference has been attributed to protective hormonal and physiologic effect of pregnancy.[106] Cesarean delivery is more common in pregnant women who had been injured during pregnancy than among those who had not been injured (odds ratio, 1.27; 95% confidence interval [CI], 1.19–1.36).[50] The average time elapsing between the index trauma hospital arrival and CD is 5.6 hours.[84] Severely injured pregnant casualties have a significantly higher likelihood of CD than those with milder injury or control population (71.4% vs 18% and 18.9%, respectively, risk ratio, 3.8; 95%CI, 2.1–6.9).[107]

Between 9.2% and 16.2% of maternal trauma cases who are admitted to hospital are severely injured (ISS >8).[48,108,109] The severity of injury described in pregnancy is diverse and similar to those described in the nonpregnant population.[13] Pregnancy-related morbidity after trauma occurs in about 25% of maternal injury and may include placental abruption, uterine rupture, and CD despite prematurity, as described earlier.[110]

FETAL/NEONATAL OUTCOMES

Maternal trauma may affect fetal survival in the immediate posttrauma period, eventual pregnancy outcome, and later neonatal development. Early articles focused on describing the outcome of the pregnancy of interest; retrospective chart review included follow up until neonatal delivery or termination of the pregnancy.[104,111,112] More recent papers are population based and thus better reflect the true effect of maternal trauma on neonatal outcomes.[3,13,50]

According to hospital-based studies, the rate of fetal loss after maternal trauma ranges between 4.7% and 19.1%.[18,102,111,113] Rates of fetal loss described in this type of literature are biased by differing case mixes (ie, database, trauma center, and nontrauma center), loss to follow-up, and case selection methods. Population-based studies suggest that there are 3.7 cases of fetal/neonatal loss directly due to maternal trauma per 100,000 live births.[13,114] MVAs are by far the most common known cause of trauma-associated fetal/neonatal loss and constitute more than 80% of cases,[114] but maternal injury resulting from domestic violence may also lead to poor fetal outcomes.[3,115] In addition to fetal loss, there may be an increased incidence of preterm birth and low birth weight among women injured during pregnancy,[50,116] although this finding is controversial.[4]

High maternal ISS is the only factor consistently associated with acute termination of pregnancy and/or fetal mortality after trauma (**Table 1**).[16,17,103,111–113,117] This association is highly sensitive but very nonspecific.[103] Several case reports suggest that 3-point restraints and deployed air bags caused direct fetal injury.[118–120] In larger studies, lack of restraints was associated with poorer neonatal outcomes.[17] Cohort studies also found no increased risk of adverse pregnancy outcomes with air bag deployment, but these studies may have been limited by the small number of cases.[121,122]

EDUCATION AND TRAINING

There is a dearth of educational strategies targeted toward prevention of maternal trauma (among the general public) and toward management of maternal trauma (among medical professionals). This paucity is likely due to lack of data regarding the process issues requiring address and the public health and economic implications of resultant maternal debilitation and/or pediatric critical illness.[123] Public education is beyond the scope of this article. Within the medical profession, there is evidence that practice simulations of obstetric catastrophes are beneficial to clinical performance.[124] Courses intended to develop and update (through simulation and assessment) the emergency skill set of the medical professionals who treat pregnant women do exist.[125,126] These MOET courses (Managing Obstetric Emergencies and Trauma),

Table 1
Studies of variables potentially associated with trauma-associated fetal loss

Variables Found Associated with Fetal Loss		Variables Found not to be Associated with Fetal Loss	
Variable	**Source**	**Variable**	**Source**
Severe hemorrhage and DIC Shock (lactic acidosis)	113 111,117	Maternal hemodynamic parameters	103,111,113
Loss of consciousness	18	Head injury	16,113,117
Low GCS	112	Low GCS	117
Pelvic injury Abdominal injury	18 16,111,117	Abdominopelvic injury	113
Gestational age Nonviable pregnancy (<23 wk)	49 103	Gestational age	18
Older maternal age	18		
Hypoxia	111	Use of restraints	18
Lower extremity injury	16	Position in vehicle Ejection from vehicle Speed	18 18 18
Vaginal bleeding	117	Abnormal uterine activity Abnormal FHR	117 117

originally developed in the United Kingdom, have been taught around the world but are not mandatory and not widely available. At present, the simulations and clinical drills that are recommended in the maternal safety educational program initiated by the American College of Obstetricians and Gynecologists (ACOG) include maternal cardiac arrest and perimortem CD but not maternal trauma.[127–129] It may be wise to consider adopting a similar educational route for management of maternal trauma. Importantly, if a decision is taken to pursue such a route, knowledge should be reinforced periodically; retention usually does not extend beyond 12 months.[130]

REFERENCES

1. Desjardins G. Management of the injured pregnant patient. Available at: http://www.trauma.org/archive/resus/pregnancytrauma.html. Accessed July 20, 2012.
2. Chang J, Elam-Evans LD, Berg CJ, et al. Pregnancy-related mortality surveillance–United States, 1991–1999. MMWR Surveill Summ 2003;52(2):1–8.
3. Fischer PE, Zarzaur BL, Fabian TC, et al. Minor trauma is an unrecognized contributor to poor fetal outcomes: a population-based study of 78,552 pregnancies. J Trauma 2011;71(1):90–3.
4. Virk J, Hsu P, Olsen J. Socio-demographic characteristics of women sustaining injuries during pregnancy: a study from the Danish National Birth Cohort. BMJ Open 2012;2(4). pii: e000826.
5. Vivian-Taylor J, Roberts CL, Chen JS, et al. Motor vehicle accidents during pregnancy: a population-based study. BJOG 2012;119(4):499–503.
6. Elliott DC, Rodriguez A. Cost effectiveness in trauma care. Surg Clin North Am 1996;76(1):47–62.
7. Prada SI, Salkever D, Mackenzie EJ. Level-I trauma center effects on return-to-work outcomes. Eval Rev 2012;36(2):133–64.
8. Palladino CL, Singh V, Campbell J, et al. Homicide and suicide during the perinatal period: findings from the National Violent Death Reporting System. Obstet Gynecol 2011;118(5):1056–63.
9. Sharps PW, Koziol-McLain J, Campbell J, et al. Health care providers' missed opportunities for preventing femicide. Prev Med 2001;33(5):373–80.
10. Hoyert DL. Maternal mortality and related concepts. National Center for Health Statistics. Vital Health Stat 3 2007;(33). Available at:. http://www.cdc.gov/nchs/data/series/sr_03/sr03_033.pdf. Accessed July 20, 2012.
11. Lisonkova S, Liu S, Bartholomew S, et al, Maternal Health Study Group of the Canadian Perinatal Surveillance System. Temporal trends in maternal mortality in Canada II: estimates based on hospitalization data. J Obstet Gynaecol Can 2011;33(10):1020–30.
12. Liu S, Rouleau J, Joseph KS, et al, Maternal Health Study Group of the Canadian Perinatal Surveillance System. Epidemiology of pregnancy-associated venous thromboembolism: a population-based study in Canada. J Obstet Gynaecol Can 2009;31(7):611–20.
13. Kvarnstrand L, Milsom I, Lekander T, et al. Maternal fatalities, fetal and neonatal deaths related to motor vehicle crashes during pregnancy: a national population-based study. Acta Obstet Gynecol Scand 2008;87(9):946–52.
14. Redelmeier DA, Bayoumi AM. Time lost by driving fast in the United States. Med Decis Making 2010;30:E12e9.
15. Patton GC, Coffey C, Sawyer SM, et al. Global patterns of mortality in young people: a systematic analysis of population health data. Lancet 2009;374(9693):881–92.

16. Ikossi DG, Lazar AA, Morabito D, et al. Profile of mothers at risk: an analysis of injury and pregnancy loss in 1195 trauma patients. J Am Coll Surg 2005;200: 49–56.
17. Klinich KD, Flannagan CA, Rupp JD, et al. Fetal outcome in motor-vehicle crashes: effects of crash characteristics and maternal restraint. Am J Obstet Gynecol 2008;198(4):450.e1–9.
18. Aboutanos MB, Aboutanos SZ, Dompkowski D, et al. Significance of motor vehicle crashes and pelvic injury on fetal mortality: a five-year institutional review. J Trauma 2008;65(3):616–20.
19. Patteson SK, Snider CC, Meyer DS, et al. The consequences of high-risk behaviors: trauma during pregnancy. J Trauma 2007;62(4):1015–20.
20. Martin SL, Macy RJ, Sullivan K, et al. Pregnancy-associated violent deaths: the role of intimate partner violence. Trauma Violence Abuse 2007;8(2):135–48.
21. Gazmararian JA, Adams MM, Saltzman LE, et al. The relationship between pregnancy intendedness and physical violence in mothers of newborns. The PRAMS Working Group. Obstet Gynecol 1995;85(6):1031–8.
22. Ronsmans C, Khlat M. Adolescence and risk of violent death during pregnancy in Matlab, Bangladesh. Lancet 1999;354(9188):1448.
23. Campero L, Walker D, Hernández B, et al. The contribution of violence to maternal mortality in Morelos, Mexico. Salud Publica Mex 2006;48(Suppl 2): S297–306 [in Spanish].
24. Krulewitch CJ, Pierre-Louis ML, de Leon-Gomez R, et al. Hidden from view: violent deaths among pregnant women in the District of Columbia, 1988-1996. J Midwifery Womens Health 2001;46(1):4–10.
25. Dannenberg AL, Carter DM, Lawson HW, et al. Homicide and other injuries as causes of maternal death in New York City, 1987 through 1991. Am J Obstet Gynecol 1995;172(5):1557–64.
26. Christiansen LR, Collins KA. Pregnancy-associated deaths: a 15-year retrospective study and overall review of maternal pathophysiology. Am J Forensic Med Pathol 2006;27(1):11–9.
27. Moracco KE, Runyan CW, Butts JD. Female intimate partner homicide: a population-based study. J Am Med Womens Assoc 2003;58(1):20–5.
28. By the American College of Surgeons Committee on Trauma. Chapter 12: "Trauma in women". In: Advanced trauma life support for doctors: Student Course Manual. 8th edition. Chicago: American College of Surgeons; 2008. p. 259–68.
29. Van Olden GD, Meeuwis JD, Bolhuis HW, et al. Clinical impact of advanced trauma life support. Am J Emerg Med 2004;22(7):522–5.
30. Shackford SR, Hollingworth-Fridlund P, Cooper GF, et al. The effect of regionalization upon the quality of trauma care as assessed by concurrent audit before and after institution of a trauma system: a preliminary report. J Trauma 1986;26(9):812–20.
31. ACOG educational bulletin. Obstetric aspects of trauma management. Number 251, September 1998. American College of Obstetricians and Gynecologists. Int J Gynaecol Obstet 1999;64:87–94.
32. Sela HY, Weiniger CF, Hersch M, et al. The pregnant motor vehicle accident casualty: adherence to basic workup and admission guidelines. Ann Surg 2011;254(2):346–52.
33. McAuliffe F, Kametas N, Costello J, et al. Respiratory function in singleton and twin pregnancy. BJOG 2002;109(7):765–9.
34. Bieniarz J, Gulin L, Arnt IC, et al. Aortoiliac compression by uterus containing hydrocephalic fetus. Obstet Gynecol 1968;31(1):90–6.

35. Kinsella SM, Lohmann G. Supine hypotensive syndrome. Obstet Gynecol 1994; 83(5 Pt 1):774–88.
36. Oyelese Y, Smulian JC. Placenta previa, placenta accreta, and vasa previa. Obstet Gynecol 2006;107(4):927–41.
37. Bowman M, Giles W, Deane S. Trauma during pregnancy-a review of management. Aust N Z J Obstet Gynaecol 1989;29:389–93.
38. Saule I, Hawkins N. Transfusion practice in major obstetric haemorrhage: lessons from trauma. Int J Obstet Anesth 2012;21(1):79–83.
39. Austin LM, Frush DP. Compendium of national guidelines for imaging the pregnant patient. AJR Am J Roentgenol 2011;197(4):W737–46.
40. ACOG Committee on Obstetric Practice. ACOG Committee Opinion. Number 299. Guidelines for diagnostic imaging during pregnancy. ACOG Committee on Obstetric Practice. Obstet Gynecol 2004;104:647–51.
41. Goodwin H, Holmes JF, Wisner DH. Abdominal ultrasound examination in pregnant blunt trauma patients. J Trauma 2001;50(4):689–94.
42. Sirlin CB, Casola G, Brown MA, et al. Us of blunt abdominal trauma: importance of free pelvic fluid in women of reproductive age. Radiology 2001;219(1):229–35.
43. Brown MA, Sirlin CB, Farahmand N, et al. Screening sonography in pregnant patients with blunt abdominal trauma. J Ultrasound Med 2005;24(2):175–81.
44. Richards JR, Ormsby EL, Romo MV, et al. Blunt abdominal injury in the pregnant patient: detection with US. Radiology 2004;233(2):463–70.
45. Houston LE, Odibo AO, Macones GA. The safety of obstetrical ultrasound: a review. Prenat Diagn 2009;29(13):1204–12.
46. Masselli G, Brunelli R, Di Tola M, et al. MR imaging in the evaluation of placental abruption: correlation with sonographic findings. Radiology 2011;259(1):222–30.
47. Baughman WC, Corteville JE, Shah RR. Placenta accreta: spectrum of US and MR imaging findings. Radiographics 2008;28(7):1905–16.
48. Schiff MA, Holt VL. Pregnancy outcomes following hospitalization for motor vehicle crashes in Washington State from 1989 to 2001. Am J Epidemiol 2005;161(6):503–10.
49. El-Kady D, Gilbert WM, Anderson J, et al. Trauma during pregnancy: an analysis of maternal and fetal outcomes in a large population. Am J Obstet Gynecol 2004;190(6):1661–8.
50. Weiss HB, Sauber-Schatz EK, Cook LJ. The epidemiology of pregnancy-associated emergency department injury visits and their impact on birth outcomes. Accid Anal Prev 2008;40(3):1088–95.
51. Ellingsen CL, Eggebø TM, Lexow K. Amniotic fluid embolism after blunt abdominal trauma. Resuscitation 2007;75(1):180–3.
52. Conde-Agudelo A, Romero R. Amniotic fluid embolism: an evidence-based review. Am J Obstet Gynecol 2009;201(5):445.e1–13.
53. Capogna G. Effect of epidural analgesia on the fetal heart rate. Eur J Obstet Gynecol Reprod Biol 2001;98(2):160–4.
54. Chandraharan E, Arulkumaran S. Prevention of birth asphyxia: responding appropriately to cardiotocograph (CTG) traces. Best Pract Res Clin Obstet Gynaecol 2007;21(4):609–24.
55. Grivell RM, Alfirevic Z, Gyte GM, et al. Antenatal cardiotocography for fetal assessment. Cochrane Database Syst Rev 2010;(1):CD007863.
56. Garite TJ, Simpson KR. Intrauterine resuscitation during labor. Clin Obstet Gynecol 2011;54(1):28–39.
57. Wylie BJ, D'Alton ME. Fetomaternal hemorrhage. Obstet Gynecol 2010;115(5): 1039–51.

58. Shetty MK. Abdominal computed tomography during pregnancy: a review of indications and fetal radiation exposure issues. Semin Ultrasound CT MRI 2010;31:3–7.
59. Nguyen CP, Goodman LH. Fetal risk in diagnostic radiology. Semin Ultrasound CT MRI 2012;33:4–10.
60. Schull WJ, Otake M. Cognitive function and prenatal exposure to ionizing radiation. Teratology 1999;59(4):222–6.
61. Wagner LK, Applegate K. ACR practice guideline for imaging pregnant or potentially pregnant adolescents and women with ionizing radiation. In: American College of Radiology Practice guidelines & technical standards 2008 (resolution 26). Available at: http://www.who.int/tb/advisory_bodies/impact_measurement_taskforce/meetings/prevalence_survey/imaging_pregnant_arc.pdf.
62. Lockwood D, Einstein D, Davros W. Diagnostic imaging: radiation dose and patients' concerns. Cleve Clin J Med 2006;73(6):583–6.
63. Tremblay E, Thérasse E, Thomassin- Naggara I, et al. Quality initiatives. Guidelines for use of medical imaging during pregnancy and lactation. Radiographics 2012;32:897–912.
64. Wakeford R. Childhood leukaemia following medical diagnostic exposure to ionizing radiation in utero or after birth. Radiat Prot Dosimetry 2008;132(2):166–74.
65. Yousefzadeh D, Ward M, Reft C. Internal barium shielding to minimize fetal irradiation in spiral chest CT: a phantom simulation experiment. Radiology 2006;239:751–8.
66. ACOG Committee on Obstetric Practice. ACOG Committee Opinion, no. 299, September 2004 (replaces no. 158, September 1995): guidelines for diagnostic imaging during pregnancy. Obstet Gynecol 2004;104(3):647–51.
67. Brent RL. Saving lives and changing family histories: appropriate counseling of pregnant women and men and women of reproductive age, concerning the risk of diagnostic radiation exposures during and before pregnancy. Am J Obstet Gynecol 2009;200(1):4–24.
68. Wall BF, Meara JR, Muirhead CR, et al. Protection of pregnant patients during diagnostic medical exposures to ionising radiation: advice from the Health Protection Agency, the Royal College of Radiologists and the College of Radiographers. Documents of the Health Protection Agency: radiation, chemical and environmental hazards. United Kingdom, 2009.
69. Webb JA, Thomsen HS, Morcos SK, Members of Contrast Media Safety Committee of European Society of Urogenital Radiology (ESUR). The use of iodinated and gadolinium contrast media during pregnancy and lactation. Eur Radiol 2005;15(6):1234–40.
70. Medical Devices Agency. Guidelines for magnetic resonance diagnostic equipment in clinical use. London, England: Medicines and Healthcare products Regulatory Agency; 2002.
71. Weinberg L, Steele RG, Pugh R, et al. The pregnant trauma patient. Anaesth Intensive Care 2005;33(2):167–80.
72. Kuczkowski KM, Reisner LS, Benumof JL. Airway problems and new solutions for the obstetric patient. J Clin Anesth 2003;15:552–63.
73. Suresh M, Wali A. Failed intubation in obstetrics: airway management strategies [guest editorial]. Anesthesiol Clin North Am 1998;16:477–98.
74. De Souza DG, Doar LH, Mehta SH, et al. Aspiration prophylaxis and rapid sequence induction for elective cesarean delivery: time to reassess old dogma? Anesth Analg 2010;110(5):1503–5.

75. American Society of Anesthesiologists Task Force on Obstetric Anesthesia. Practice guidelines for obstetric anesthesia. An updated report by the American Society of Anesthesiologists Task Force on Obstetric Anesthesia. Anesthesiology 2007;106:843–63.
76. Meroz Y, Elchalal U, Ginosar Y. Initial trauma management in advanced pregnancy. Anesthesiol Clin 2007;25(1):117–29.
77. Van de Velde M, Teunkens A, Kuypers M, et al. General anaesthesia with target controlled infusion of propofol for planned caesarean section: maternal and neonatal effects of a remifentanil-based technique. Int J Obstet Anesth 2004; 13(3):153–8.
78. Abu-Halaweh SA, Massad IM, Abu-Ali HM, et al. Rapid sequence induction and intubation with 1 mg/kg rocuronium bromide in cesarean section, comparison with suxamethonium. Saudi Med J 2007;28(9):1393–6.
79. Pühringer FK, Sparr HJ, Mitterschiffthaler G, et al. Extended duration of action of rocuronium in postpartum patients. Anesth Analg 1997;84(2): 352–4.
80. Gin T, Chan MT, Chan KL, et al. Prolonged neuromuscular block after rocuronium in postpartum patients. Anesth Analg 2002;94(3):686–9.
81. Williamson RM, Mallaiah S, Barclay P. Rocuronium and sugammadex for rapid sequence induction of obstetric general anaesthesia. Acta Anaesthesiol Scand 2011;55(6):694–9.
82. Rogers FB, Rozycki GS, Osler TM, et al. A multi-institutional study of factors associated with fetal death in injured pregnant patients. Arch Surg 1999; 134(11):1274–7.
83. Aufforth R, Edhayan E, Dempah D. Should pregnancy be a sole criterion for trauma code activation: a review of the trauma registry. Am J Surg 2010; 199(3):387–90.
84. Morris JA Jr, Rosenbower TJ, Jurkovich GJ, et al. Infant survival after cesarean section for trauma. Ann Surg 1996;223(5):481–91.
85. Soar J, Perkins GD, Abbas G, et al. European Resuscitation Council Guidelines for Resuscitation 2010 Section 8. Cardiac arrest in special circumstances: Electrolyte abnormalities, poisoning, drowning, accidental hypothermia, hyperthermia, asthma, anaphylaxis, cardiac surgery, trauma, pregnancy, electrocution. Resuscitation 2010;81(10):1400–33.
86. Vanden Hoek TL, Morrison LJ, Shuster M, et al. Part 12: cardiac arrest in special situations: 2010 American Heart Association Guidelines for cardiopulmonary resuscitation and emergency cardiovascular care. Circulation 2010;122(18 Suppl 3): S829–61.
87. RCOG, maternal collapse in pregnancy and the puerperium green-top guideline no. 56. 2011. p. 24. Available at: http://digitalrepository.e-medicinafetal.org/bitstream/10615/261/1/Maternal%20collapse%20in%20pregnancy%20and%20the%20puerperium%20RCOG%202011-3.pdf. Accessed February 9, 2011.
88. Ueland K, Novy MJ, Peterson EN, et al. Maternal cardiovascular dynamics, IV: the influence of gestational age on the maternal cardiovascular response to posture and exercise. Am J Obstet Gynecol 1969;104:856–64.
89. Katz VL, Dotters DJ, Droegemueller W. Perimortem caesarean delivery. Obstet Gynecol 1986;68(4):571–6.
90. Katz V, Balderston K, DeFreest M. Perimortem caesarean delivery: were our assumptions correct? Am J Obstet Gynecol 2005;192(6):1916–21.
91. Einav S, Kaufman N, Sela HY. Maternal cardiac arrest and perimortem caesarean delivery: evidence or expert-based? Resuscitation 2012;83(10):1191–200.

92. Nair P, Davies AR, Beca J, et al. Extracorporeal membrane oxygenation for severe ARDS in pregnant and postpartum women during the 2009 H1N1 pandemic. Intensive Care Med 2011;37(4):648–54.
93. Dubar G, Azria E, Tesnière A, et al, French Registry on 2009 A/H1N1v during pregnancy. French experience of 2009 A/H1N1v influenza in pregnant women. PLoS One 2010;5(10). pii: e13112.
94. Ho CH, Chen KB, Liu SK, et al. Early application of extracorporeal membrane oxygenation in a patient with amniotic fluid embolism. Acta Anaesthesiol Taiwan 2009;47(2):99–102.
95. Weinberg L, Kay C, Liskaser F, et al. Successful treatment of peripartum massive pulmonary embolism with extracorporeal membrane oxygenation and catheter-directed pulmonary thrombolytic therapy. Anaesth Intensive Care 2011;39(3):486–91.
96. Smith IJ, Gillham MJ. Fulminant peripartum cardiomyopathy rescue with extracorporeal membranous oxygenation. Int J Obstet Anesth 2009;18(2):186–8.
97. Plotkin JS, Shah JB, Lofland GK, et al. Extracorporeal membrane oxygenation in the successful treatment of traumatic adult respiratory distress syndrome: case report and review. J Trauma 1994;37(1):127–30, 7.
98. Sasser SM, Hunt RC, Sullivent EE, et al, National Expert Panel on Field Triage, Centers for Disease Control, Prevention (CDC). Guidelines for field triage of injured patients. Recommendations of the National Expert Panel on Field Triage. MMWR Recomm Rep 2009;58(RR-1):1–35.
99. Cox S, Smith K, Currell A, et al. Differentiation of confirmed major trauma patients and potential major trauma patients using pre-hospital trauma triage criteria. Injury 2011;42(9):889–95.
100. Smith J, Caldwell E, Sugrue M. Difference in trauma team activation criteria between hospitals within the same region. Emerg Med Australas 2005; 17(5–6):480–7.
101. Drost TF, Rosemurgy AS, Sherman HF, et al. Major trauma in pregnant women: maternal/fetal outcome. J Trauma 1990;30(5):574–8.
102. Greene W, Robinson L, Rizzo AG, et al. Pregnancy is not a sufficient indicator for trauma team activation. J Trauma 2007;63(3):550–5.
103. Theodorou DA, Velmahos GC, Souter I, et al. Fetal death after trauma in pregnancy. Am Surg 2000;66(9):809–12.
104. Esposito TJ, Gens DR, Smith LG, et al. Trauma during pregnancy. A review of 79 cases. Arch Surg 1991;126(9):1073–8.
105. Corsi PR, Rasslan S, de Oliveira LB, et al. Trauma in pregnant women: analysis of maternal and fetal mortality. Injury 1999;30(4):239–43.
106. John PR, Shiozawa A, Haut ER, et al. An assessment of the impact of pregnancy on trauma mortality. Surgery 2011;149(1):94–8.
107. Schiff MA, Holt VL, Daling JR. Maternal and infant outcomes after injury during pregnancy in Washington State from 1989 to 1997. J Trauma 2002;53(5): 939–45.
108. Curet MJ, Schermer CR, Demarest GB, et al. Predictors of outcome in trauma during pregnancy: identification of patients who can be monitored for less than 6 hours. J Trauma 2000;49(1):18–25.
109. Aboutanos SZ, Aboutanos MB, Dompkowski D, et al. Predictors of fetal outcome in pregnant trauma patients: a five-year institutional review. Am Surg 2007;73(8): 824–7.
110. Trivedi N, Ylagan M, Moore TR, et al. Predicting adverse outcomes following trauma in pregnancy. J Reprod Med 2012;57(1–2):3–8.

111. Hoff WS, D'Amelio LF, Tinkoff GH, et al. Maternal predictors of fetal demise in trauma during pregnancy. Surg Gynecol Obstet 1991;172(3):175–80.
112. Kissinger DP, Rozycki GS, Morris JA Jr, et al. Trauma in pregnancy. Predicting pregnancy outcome. Arch Surg 1991;126(9):1079–86.
113. Ali J, Yeo A, Gana TJ, et al. Predictors of fetal mortality in pregnant trauma patients. J Trauma 1997;42(5):782–5, 19.1%.
114. Weiss HB, Songer TJ, Fabio A. Fetal deaths related to maternal injury. JAMA 2001;286(15):1863–8.
115. Tinker SC, Reefhuis J, Dellinger AM, et al. Maternal injuries during the periconceptional period and the risk of birth defects, National Birth Defects Prevention Study, 1997-2005. Paediatr Perinat Epidemiol 2011;25(5):487–96.
116. Shah PS, Shah J, Knowledge Synthesis Group on Determinants of Preterm/LBW Births. Maternal exposure to domestic violence and pregnancy and birth outcomes: a systematic review and meta-analyses. J Womens Health (Larchmt) 2010;19(11):2017–31.
117. Shah KH, Simons RK, Holbrook T, et al. Trauma in pregnancy: maternal and fetal outcomes. J Trauma 1998;45(1):83–6.
118. Bard MR, Shaikh S, Pestaner J, et al. Direct fetal injury due to airbag deployment and three-point restraint. J Trauma 2009;67(4):E98–101.
119. Nguyen CS, Chase DM, Wing DA. Severe fetal skull fracture and death subsequent to a motor vehicle crash with frontal airbag deployment. J Trauma 2009; 67(6):E220–1.
120. Schultze PM, Stamm CA, Roger J. Placental abruption and fetal death with airbag deployment in a motor vehicle accident. Obstet Gynecol 1998;92(4 Pt 2): 719.
121. Schiff MA, Mack CD, Kaufman RP, et al. The effect of air bags on pregnancy outcomes in Washington State: 2002-2005. Obstet Gynecol 2010;115(1):85–92.
122. Metz TD, Abbott JT. Uterine trauma in pregnancy after motor vehicle crashes with airbag deployment: a 30-case series. J Trauma 2006;61(3):658–61.
123. Shudy M, de Almeida ML, Ly S, et al. Impact of pediatric critical illness and injury on families: a systematic literature review. Pediatrics 2006;118(Suppl 3): S203–18.
124. Cass GK, Crofts JF, Draycott TJ. The use of simulation to teach clinical skills in obstetrics. Semin Perinatol 2011;35(2):68–73.
125. Johanson RB, Menon V, Burns E, et al. Managing obstetric emergencies and trauma (MOET) structured skills training in Armenia, utilising models and reality based scenarios. BMC Med Educ 2002;2:5.
126. Jyothi NK, Cox C, Johanson R. Management of obstetric emergencies and trauma (MOET): regional questionnaire survey of obstetric practice among career obstetricians in the United Kingdom. J Obstet Gynaecol 2001;21(2):107–11.
127. American College of Obstetricians, Gynecologists. ACOG Practice Bulletin: Clinical Management Guidelines for Obstetrician-Gynecologists Number 76, October 2006: postpartum hemorrhage. Obstet Gynecol 2006;108(4):1039–47.
128. Argani CH, Eichelberger M, Deering S, et al. The case for simulation as part of a comprehensive patient safety program. Am J Obstet Gynecol 2012;206(6): 451–5.
129. Lipman SS, Daniels KI, Arafeh J, et al. The case for OBLS: a simulation-based obstetric life support program. Semin Perinatol 2011;35(2):74–9.
130. Yang CW, Yen ZS, McGowan JE, et al. A systematic review of retention of adult advanced life support knowledge and skills in healthcare providers. Resuscitation 2012;83(9):1055–60.

Use of Video-assisted Intubation Devices in the Management of Patients with Trauma

Michael Aziz, MD

KEYWORDS

• Video laryngoscopy • Trauma • Airway • Manual in-line stabilization
• Cervical immobilization • Fiberoptic intubation • Flexible fiberoptic

KEY POINTS

- Because the risk of cervical spine injury is high in the patient with associated head trauma, airways are often managed to maintain cervical immobilization.
- The application of manual in-line stabilization facilitates safe intubation, but makes direct laryngoscopy more difficult.
- The use of video laryngoscopy for the management of the patient with cervical spine immobilization is growing because the techniques are easy to learn and video laryngoscopes facilitate a better laryngeal view.
- Although cervical spine motion may or may not be reduced by using video laryngoscopes compared with direct laryngoscopes, the improvement of the laryngeal view seems to translate into higher intubation success rates.

INTRODUCTION

Patients with trauma present unique airway management concerns. Because the patients are unfasted and may have impaired oxygen delivery, airway management is more challenging. Furthermore, conditions common to trauma medicine, such as active regurgitation, abnormal patient position, and cervical spine immobilization, are factors that are known to increase the risk of difficult intubation. Patients with these conditions may benefit from newer airway technologies. This article focuses on airway management tools as they pertain to the patient with trauma.

THE UNSTABLE CERVICAL SPINE: TRAUMATIC INJURY EVALUATION

The incidence of injury to the cervical spine in patients with blunt trauma is estimated to be 1.8%.[1] The most common level of injury is the C2 vertebra, followed by the

---

Disclosures: None.

Department of Anesthesiology & Perioperative Medicine, Oregon Health & Science University, Mail Code KPV 5A, 3181 SW Sam Jackson Park Rd, Portland, OR 97239, USA
E-mail address: azizm@ohsu.edu

Anesthesiology Clin 31 (2013) 157–166
http://dx.doi.org/10.1016/j.anclin.2012.10.001 **anesthesiology.theclinics.com**
1932-2275/13/$ – see front matter

C6 and C7 levels.[2] The patient with head trauma is more likely to have a cervical spine injury than the patient experiencing blunt trauma without associated head injury.[3–6] Guidelines are established within emergency medicine and trauma care to screen for cervical spine trauma and take appropriate precautions until cervical spine trauma is ruled out. The patient with trauma should not require further evaluation or care of the cervical spine if (1) there is no midline cervical tenderness; (2) there is no focal neurologic deficit; (3) the patient is alert; and (4) the patient has no distracting injuries. computed tomography scanning is appropriate for those patients at increased risk who cannot be cleared by these standard criteria, because plain radiographs cannot rule out ligamentous injury.

THE UNSTABLE CERVICAL SPINE: CLINICAL PRECAUTIONS AND MANUAL IN-LINE STABILIZATION

The patient who cannot be cleared should be maintained in cervical spine precautions early in their care. Insertion of airway devices and laryngoscopy become more challenging as the cervical collar limits mouth opening.[7] Manual in-line stabilization (MILS) has been adopted as a practice to immobilize the spine when the cervical collar needs to be removed for situations such as airway management.[8] Gerling and colleagues[9] compared cervical immobilization techniques in destabilized human cadavers and found that cervical motion is less and glottis visualization better with MILS compared with leaving the cervical collar in place alone. Soft collars alone insufficiently mobilize the cervical spine during airway management.[10] Correct application of MILS involves a second provider fixing the head in a neutral position and applying countertraction to any suspension forces that may be applied during laryngoscopy. The motion of the cervical spine is limited by various airway maneuvers when MILS is applied.[9,11–14] The exclusion of this practice in patients with recognized or unrecognized cervical spine injury has been associated with catastrophic neurologic events.[15–18] Therefore, MILS remains a low-cost critical intervention for airway management in the patient with potential cervical spine instability.

THE UNSTABLE CERVICAL SPINE: IMPLICATIONS FOR AIRWAY INTERVENTIONS

Flexible Fiberoptic Intubation

Indirect laryngoscopy techniques have been studied to try to balance the need to limit cervical motion and overcome the difficulty of obtaining laryngeal views when MILS is applied. Intubating supraglottic airways have been studied, but their failure rate may be high in routine clinical practice.[19–21] Furthermore, cervical flexion is realized across the C0 to C5 segments during intubation with these devices.[22] Flexible fiberoptic techniques may also be difficult for inexperienced providers to perform but flexible nasal fiberoptic intubation results in less cervical motion to destabilized cadavers than the use of a supraglottic airway, direct laryngoscopy, intubating supraglottic airway, or even mask ventilation with chin lift and jaw thrust.[13]

Rigid Video Laryngoscopy

Video laryngoscopy has grown in popularity over the past 10 years. Evidence suggests benefit for intubation of patients predicted to be more difficult to intubate.[23–29] Several studies have now addressed the scenario of cervical spine immobilization by artificially applying MILS in testing models. These studies are further summarized in **Table 1**. Laryngeal view is consistently improved using video laryngoscopy compared with direct laryngoscopy in the setting of MILS.[30–33] Furthermore, a broader assessment of intubation difficulty, the Intubation Difficulty Scale Score,[34] is improved with video laryngoscopy compared with direct laryngoscopy.[28,31–33,35] In one of these studies, intubation success rate was improved with video laryngoscopy compared with direct laryngoscopy in the setting of artificially applied MILS.[30] However, video laryngoscopy still carries limitations for the patient with restricted neck movement. In our study of 1 video laryngoscope, the presence of limited cervical spine motion either from the application of MILS or existing abnormality independently predicted video laryngoscopy failure (relative risk 1.76; 95% confidence interval [CI] 1.01, 3.06).[23] Therefore, although these devices provide benefit in terms of ease of intubation and may improve intubation success compared with direct laryngoscopy, they are still prone to failure in the patient with cervical spine abnormality or precautions.

Several studies have tested the extent of cervical motion while using rigid video laryngoscopes compared with direct laryngoscopy by evaluating fluoroscopic images during the intubation procedure (**Table 2**). Without the application of MILS, less cervical extension (as assessed by fluoroscopy) may be necessary with video laryngoscopes compared with direct laryngoscopy.[36–38] When MILS is applied, the findings are inconsistent. In some studies, isolated segments of the cervical spine may realize less cervical extension compared with direct laryngoscopy,[39–41] but another study shows no difference in cervical motion between video laryngoscopy and direct laryngoscopy when MILS is applied.[42]

The studies of various airway device approaches to limited cervical spine motion have yet to show any alterations in neurologic outcomes. As such, the application of techniques with the highest likelihood of success while maintaining MILS is the best approach. Although flexible fiberoptic intubation may expose the cervical spine to the least traction, this procedure requires significant skill and a cooperative patient if it is to be performed on an awake patient. For the anesthetized patient, this procedure still often requires jaw thrust, which may expose the patient to cervical traction. Video laryngoscopes may be easier to learn than flexible fiberoptic intubation and offer improvement in terms of intubation difficulty compared with direct laryngoscopy. As such, their use has grown for the management of the patient with cervical spine precautions. Until further evidence guides care, expert opinion continues to encourage the application of MILS with an intubation technique that is familiar to the laryngoscopist.

PREHOSPITAL AIRWAY MANAGEMENT

Patients with trauma who initially present to emergency medical services are exposed to the most difficult intubation conditions. Difficult patient positions, blood, and aspirate compromise intubation performance. Furthermore, providers are exposed to stressful and urgent conditions with variable training in intubation. Compared with direct laryngoscopy, video laryngoscopy offers benefits for the untrained paramedic in controlled operating room conditions.[43] Therefore, prehospital providers with variable training and experience may perform better with video laryngoscopy compared with direct laryngoscopy; however, these outcome studies have so far been difficult to perform.

Several observational studies of prehospital video laryngoscopy have been performed. In a European medical system, the C-MAC (Karl Storz, Tuttlingen, Germany) video laryngoscope was successful in 80 tracheal intubations either when used with

Table 1
Studies of video laryngoscopy on intubation performance for the patient maintained in MILS

Author	Device	Control	Sample	Outcome Assessed	Major Findings
Malik et al[31]	GlideScope (Verathon, Bothell, WA) AWS (Pentax, Hoya, Japan)	DL	120	Laryngeal view IDS Intubation time Success rate	Improved laryngeal view and IDS Slower intubation time No difference in success
Maharaj et al[26]	Airtraq (Prodol, Vizcaya, Spain)[a]	DL	40	IDS Intubation attempts Laryngeal view	Reduced number of intubation attempts. Improved IDS, improved laryngeal view
Smith et al[33]	WuScope (Pentax, Orangeburg, NY)	DL	87	IDS Laryngeal view, intubation attempts	Improved IDS and laryngeal view. No difference in success or number of attempts
Malik et al[28]	AWS	DL	90	IDS, laryngeal view	Improved IDS and laryngeal view
Enomoto et al[30]	AWS	DL	203	Laryngeal view, intubation time, success rate	Improved laryngeal view, increased success rate, faster intubation time
Liu et al[56]	AWS	GlideScope	70	IDS, Intubation time, success rate within a defined time interval	Faster intubation time, lower IDS, improved laryngeal view, and higher intubation success with AWS
McElwain and Laffey[35]	Airtraq C-MAC (Karl Storz, Tuttlingen, Germany)	DL	90	IDS Success rate Laryngeal view Hemodynamic stability	Reduced IDS, improved laryngeal view with Airtraq

Abbreviations: DL, direct laryngoscopy; IDS, Intubation Difficulty Scale score.
[a] Not a video laryngoscope, but often included in this category.

video assistance or as a direct laryngoscope when lens contamination occurred.[44] In a before-and-after study of a busy air medical unit in the United States, the GlideScope (Verathon, Bothell, WA) video laryngoscope offered faster intubation times with fewer intubation attempts than direct laryngoscopy, although with similarly high

Table 2
Studies of cervical motion while using video laryngoscopes

Study	Device	Control	Cervical Precautions	Fluoroscopy	Major Findings
Hastings et, al[38]	Bullard (Circon ACMI, Stamford, CT)	DL	None	In selected patients (C0–C4). Angle finder used in the entire sample	Reduced extension across (C0–C4)
Robitallie et al[42]	GlideScope	DL	MILS	Continuous C0–C5 during several time points	No decrease in cervical movement
Maruyama et al[36]	AWS	DL and McCoy	None	C1/C2, C3/C4	Reduced extension at adjacent vertebra
Hirabayashi et al[37]	AWS	DL	None	C0–C4	Reduced extension at all segments
Turkstra et al[40]	GlideScope Lightwand (Trachlight, Laerdal, Armonk, NY)	DL	MILS	C0–C5	Reduced C2–C5 motion with Glidescope. Reduced motion across all segments with Lightwand
Watts et al[57]	Bullard	DL	One arm with MILS One arm without	C0–C5	Reduced cervical extension in the Bullard + MILS arm
Maruyama et al[39]	AWS	DL	MILS	C0–C4	Reduced cumulative cervical motion
Turkstra et al[41]	Airtraq[a]	DL	MILS	C0–thoracic	No difference at C1–C2 segment, less extension at C2–C5, and C5–thoracic

[a] Not a video laryngoscope, but often included in this category.

success rates. Carlson and colleagues[45] analyzed metrics of successful prehospital video laryngoscopy and determined that successful intubations were associated with improved laryngeal views and faster times to laryngeal view than unsuccessful video attempts.

Prospective randomized data are limited, but 1 such study has been conducted in a European medical system. Trimmel and colleagues[46] enrolled 212 prehospital patients into a randomized comparison of direct laryngoscopy versus Airtraq

(Prodol Meditec, Vizcaya, Spain). The success rate for direct laryngoscopy was 99% versus 47% in the Airtraq group. This poor performance of the optical laryngoscope is interesting. In controlled operating room settings, this device performs well compared with direct laryngoscopy, even in the setting of cervical spine mobilization or other predictors of difficult intubation.[26,32] This device design does not use video-empowered optics, but uses prisms with a light source to reflect an anterior laryngeal view through an eyepiece. The unique situations of prehospital emergency care may have resulted in excessive lens contamination. Furthermore, ambient natural light with difficult provider orientation to the optical piece may have compromised the providers' capacity to visualize the airway. Prehospital randomized controlled trials are difficult to conduct, but the existing data are inadequate to guide care. Well-designed studies of commonly used video laryngoscopes used by the routine prehospital providers are urgently needed to determine whether this technology can improve the care of patients with trauma.

USE OF VIDEO-ASSISTED DEVICES IN THE EMERGENCY DEPARTMENT

Airway management in the emergency department represents unique concerns because of both challenging patient conditions and provider variability with exposure to certain techniques. Flexible fiberoptic intubation is used in some academic emergency departments, but 1 survey reports that only 64% of emergency departments carry a dedicated bronchoscope.[47] Therefore, the skill of community emergency physicians with the technique is likely to be similarly variable. Flexible fiberoptic intubation has been used by emergency physicians as a primary device and to rescue failed alternate techniques.[48] However, surgical approaches to rescue techniques may be used more frequently than fiberoptic techniques.[49] These data may represent the extreme urgency of the patient with trauma, but may also reflect inadequate skill acquisition with the common anesthesiologists' approach to the difficult airway.

More recently, the use of rigid video laryngoscopy has grown for emergency medicine use. Patients with cervical spine abnormalities or reduced mouth opening from trismus may benefit from the augmented laryngeal view afforded by video laryngoscopy. Early observational studies reported less frequent use of video laryngoscopy compared with direct laryngoscopy and similar success rates when the techniques were compared.[50–52] However, these studies did not evaluate the nature of patient selection for the various techniques studied. In more recent observational studies, video laryngoscopy seems to be used more frequently overall, and with the greatest frequency in the patient predicted to be difficult to intubate by direct laryngoscopy. For patients with predictors of difficult direct laryngoscopy, success rates seem to be higher for video laryngoscopy compared with direct laryngoscopy across multiple institutions.[51] In a study by Sakles and colleagues,[53] 38% of patients were intubated with video laryngoscopy to achieve a higher first-attempt success rate than direct laryngoscopy. In another study by Sakles and colleagues,[54] a different video laryngoscope was used in 34% of emergency intubations to show a higher overall intubation success rate with video laryngoscopy compared with direct laryngoscopy. Mosier and colleagues[55] similarly showed a higher success rate with video laryngoscopy (78%) compared with direct laryngoscopy (68%) for emergency airway management even when video laryngoscopy was used more frequently in those with predictors of difficult direct laryngoscopy. It seems that the use of video laryngoscopy for airway management of the patient with trauma in the emergency department is growing in frequency. Furthermore, these data suggest that more frequent use of these new devices by emergency medicine providers can translate to increased intubation success compared with direct laryngoscopy. However, video laryngoscopy has been inadequately tested in a prospective randomized fashion for the emergency medicine patient with trauma.

SUMMARY

The patient with trauma presents unique challenges for airway management. Because the risk of cervical spine injury is high in the patient with associated head trauma, airways are often managed to maintain cervical immobilization. The application of MILS facilitates safe intubation, but makes direct laryngoscopy more difficult. The use of video laryngoscopy for the management of the patient with cervical spine immobilization is growing because the techniques are easy to learn and video laryngoscopes facilitate a better laryngeal view. Although cervical spine motion may or may not be reduced while using video laryngoscopes compared with direct laryngoscopes, the improvement of the laryngeal view seems to translate into higher intubation success rates. More research is needed to validate preliminary data on intubation performance in the operating room. Furthermore, well-conducted randomized controlled trials are needed to show the benefit of video laryngoscopy compared with direct laryngoscopy for the patient with trauma treated in the prehospital environment or emergency medicine setting.

REFERENCES

1. Crosby ET, Lui A. The adult cervical spine: implications for airway management. Can J Anaesth 1990;37:77–93.
2. Goldberg W, Mueller C, Panacek E, et al, NEXUS Group. Distribution and patterns of blunt traumatic cervical spine injury. Ann Emerg Med 2001;38:17–21.
3. Blackmore CC, Emerson SS, Mann FA, et al. Cervical spine imaging in patients with trauma: determination of fracture risk to optimize use. Radiology 1999;211: 759–65.
4. Demetriades D, Charalambides K, Chahwan S, et al. Nonskeletal cervical spine injuries: epidemiology and diagnostic pitfalls. J Trauma 2000;48:724–7.
5. Hackl W, Hausberger K, Sailer R, et al. Prevalence of cervical spine injuries in patients with facial trauma. Oral Surg Oral Med Oral Pathol Oral Radiol Endod 2001;92:370–6.
6. Holly LT, Kelly DF, Counelis GJ, et al. Cervical spine trauma associated with moderate and severe head injury: incidence, risk factors, and injury characteristics. J Neurosurg 2002;96:285–91.
7. Goutcher CM, Lochhead V. Reduction in mouth opening with semi-rigid cervical collars. Br J Anaesth 2005;95:344–8.
8. Grande CM, Barton CR, Stene JK. Appropriate techniques for airway management of emergency patients with suspected spinal cord injury. Anesth Analg 1988;67:714–5.
9. Gerling MC, Davis DP, Hamilton RS, et al. Effects of cervical spine immobilization technique and laryngoscope blade selection on an unstable cervical spine in a cadaver model of intubation. Ann Emerg Med 2000;36:293–300.
10. Aprahamian C, Thompson BM, Finger WA, et al. Experimental cervical spine injury model: evaluation of airway management and splinting techniques. Ann Emerg Med 1984;13:584–7.
11. Lennarson PJ, Smith D, Todd MM, et al. Segmental cervical spine motion during orotracheal intubation of the intact and injured spine with and without external stabilization. J Neurosurg 2000;92:201–6.

12. Lennarson PJ, Smith DW, Sawin PD, et al. Cervical spinal motion during intubation: efficacy of stabilization maneuvers in the setting of complete segmental instability. J Neurosurg 2001;94:265–70.
13. Brimacombe J, Keller C, Kunzel KH, et al. Cervical spine motion during airway management: a cinefluoroscopic study of the posteriorly destabilized third cervical vertebrae in human cadavers. Anesth Analg 2000;91:1274–8.
14. Majernick TG, Bieniek R, Houston JB, et al. Cervical spine movement during orotracheal intubation. Ann Emerg Med 1986;15:417–20.
15. Muckart DJ, Bhagwanjee S, van der Merwe R. Spinal cord injury as a result of endotracheal intubation in patients with undiagnosed cervical spine fractures. Anesthesiology 1997;87:418–20.
16. Redl G. Massive pyramidal tract signs after endotracheal intubation: a case report of spondyloepiphyseal dysplasia congenita. Anesthesiology 1998;89:1262–4.
17. Farmer J, Vaccaro A, Albert TJ, et al. Neurologic deterioration after cervical spinal cord injury. J Spinal Disord 1998;11:192–6.
18. McLeod AD, Calder I. Spinal cord injury and direct laryngoscopy–the legend lives on. Br J Anaesth 2000;84:705–9.
19. Martel M, Reardon RF, Cochrane J. Initial experience of emergency physicians using the intubating laryngeal mask airway: a case series. Acad Emerg Med 2001;8:815–22.
20. Joo HS, Kapoor S, Rose DK, et al. The intubating laryngeal mask airway after induction of general anesthesia versus awake fiberoptic intubation in patients with difficult airways. Anesth Analg 2001;92:1342–6.
21. Reardon RF, Martel M. The intubating laryngeal mask airway: suggestions for use in the emergency department. Acad Emerg Med 2001;8:833–8.
22. Kihara S, Watanabe S, Brimacombe J, et al. Segmental cervical spine movement with the intubating laryngeal mask during manual in-line stabilization in patients with cervical pathology undergoing cervical spine surgery. Anesth Analg 2000;91:195–200.
23. Aziz MF, Healy D, Kheterpal S, et al. Routine clinical practice effectiveness of the Glidescope in difficult airway management: an analysis of 2,004 Glidescope intubations, complications, and failures from two institutions. Anesthesiology 2011;114:34–41.
24. Aziz MF, Dillman D, Fu R, et al. Comparative effectiveness of the C-MAC video laryngoscope versus direct laryngoscopy in the setting of the predicted difficult airway. Anesthesiology 2012;116:629–36.
25. Jungbauer A, Schumann M, Brunkhorst V, et al. Expected difficult tracheal intubation: a prospective comparison of direct laryngoscopy and video laryngoscopy in 200 patients. Br J Anaesth 2009;102:546–50.
26. Maharaj CH, Costello JF, Harte BH, et al. Evaluation of the Airtraq and Macintosh laryngoscopes in patients at increased risk for difficult tracheal intubation. Anaesthesia 2008;63:182–8.
27. Malik MA, Subramaniam R, Maharaj CH, et al. Randomized controlled trial of the Pentax AWS, Glidescope, and Macintosh laryngoscopes in predicted difficult intubation. Br J Anaesth 2009;103:761–8.
28. Malik MA, Subramaniam R, Churasia S, et al. Tracheal intubation in patients with cervical spine immobilization: a comparison of the Airwayscope, LMA CTrach, and the Macintosh laryngoscopes. Br J Anaesth 2009;102:654–61.
29. Serocki G, Bein B, Scholz J, et al. Management of the predicted difficult airway: a comparison of conventional blade laryngoscopy with video-assisted blade laryngoscopy and the GlideScope. Eur J Anaesthesiol 2010;27:24–30.

30. Enomoto Y, Asai T, Arai T, et al. Pentax-AWS, a new videolaryngoscope, is more effective than the Macintosh laryngoscope for tracheal intubation in patients with restricted neck movements: a randomized comparative study. Br J Anaesth 2008;100:544–8.
31. Malik MA, Maharaj CH, Harte BH, et al. Comparison of Macintosh, Truview EVO2, Glidescope, and Airwayscope laryngoscope use in patients with cervical spine immobilization. Br J Anaesth 2008;101:723–30.
32. Maharaj CH, Buckley E, Harte BH, et al. Endotracheal intubation in patients with cervical spine immobilization: a comparison of Macintosh and Airtraq laryngoscopes. Anesthesiology 2007;107:53–9.
33. Smith CE, Pinchak AB, Sidhu TS, et al. Evaluation of tracheal intubation difficulty in patients with cervical spine immobilization: fiberoptic (WuScope) versus conventional laryngoscopy. Anesthesiology 1999;91:1253–9.
34. Adnet F, Borron SW, Racine SX, et al. The intubation difficulty scale (IDS): proposal and evaluation of a new score characterizing the complexity of endotracheal intubation. Anesthesiology 1997;87:1290–7.
35. McElwain J, Laffey JG. Comparison of the C-MAC(R), Airtraq(R), and Macintosh laryngoscopes in patients undergoing tracheal intubation with cervical spine immobilization. Br J Anaesth 2011;107:258–64.
36. Maruyama K, Yamada T, Kawakami R, et al. Upper cervical spine movement during intubation: fluoroscopic comparison of the AirWay Scope, McCoy laryngoscope, and Macintosh laryngoscope. Br J Anaesth 2008;100:120–4.
37. Hirabayashi Y, Fujita A, Seo N, et al. Cervical spine movement during laryngoscopy using the Airway Scope compared with the Macintosh laryngoscope. Anaesthesia 2007;62:1050–5.
38. Hastings RH, Vigil AC, Hanna R, et al. Cervical spine movement during laryngoscopy with the Bullard, Macintosh, and Miller laryngoscopes. Anesthesiology 1995;82:859–69.
39. Maruyama K, Yamada T, Kawakami R, et al. Randomized cross-over comparison of cervical-spine motion with the AirWay Scope or Macintosh laryngoscope with in-line stabilization: a video-fluoroscopic study. Br J Anaesth 2008;101:563–7.
40. Turkstra TP, Craen RA, Pelz DM, et al. Cervical spine motion: a fluoroscopic comparison during intubation with lighted stylet, GlideScope, and Macintosh laryngoscope. Anesth Analg 2005;101:910–5.
41. Turkstra TP, Pelz DM, Jones PM. Cervical spine motion: a fluoroscopic comparison of the AirTraq Laryngoscope versus the Macintosh laryngoscope. Anesthesiology 2009;111:97–101.
42. Robitaille A, Williams SR, Tremblay MH, et al. Cervical spine motion during tracheal intubation with manual in-line stabilization: direct laryngoscopy versus GlideScope videolaryngoscopy. Anesth Analg 2008;106:935–41.
43. Nouruzi-Sedeh P, Schumann M, Groeben H. Laryngoscopy via Macintosh blade versus GlideScope: success rate and time for endotracheal intubation in untrained medical personnel. Anesthesiology 2009;110:32–7.
44. Cavus E, Callies A, Doerges V, et al. The C-MAC videolaryngoscope for prehospital emergency intubation: a prospective, multicentre, observational study. Emerg Med J 2011;28:650–3.
45. Carlson JN, Quintero J, Guyette FX, et al. Variables associated with successful intubation attempts using video laryngoscopy: a preliminary report in a helicopter emergency medical service. Prehosp Emerg Care 2012;16:293–8.
46. Trimmel H, Kreutziger J, Fertsak G, et al. Use of the Airtraq laryngoscope for emergency intubation in the prehospital setting: a randomized control trial. Crit Care Med 2011;39:489–93.

47. Levitan RM, Kush S, Hollander JE. Devices for difficult airway management in academic emergency departments: results of a national survey. Ann Emerg Med 1999;33:694–8.
48. Mlinek EJ Jr, Clinton JE, Plummer D, et al. Fiberoptic intubation in the emergency department. Ann Emerg Med 1990;19:359–62.
49. Bair AE, Filbin MR, Kulkarni RG, et al. The failed intubation attempt in the emergency department: analysis of prevalence, rescue techniques, and personnel. J Emerg Med 2002;23:131–40.
50. Lim HC, Goh SH. Utilization of a Glidescope videolaryngoscope for orotracheal intubations in different emergency airway management settings. Eur J Emerg Med 2009;16:68–73.
51. Choi HJ, Kang HG, Lim TH, et al, Korean Emergency Airway Management Registry (KEAMR) Investigators. Endotracheal intubation using a GlideScope video laryngoscope by emergency physicians: a multicentre analysis of 345 attempts in adult patients. Emerg Med J 2010;27:380–2.
52. Platts-Mills TF, Campagne D, Chinnock B, et al. A comparison of GlideScope video laryngoscopy versus direct laryngoscopy intubation in the emergency department. Acad Emerg Med 2009;16:866–71.
53. Sakles JC, Mosier JM, Chiu S, et al. Tracheal intubation in the emergency department: a comparison of GlideScope((R)) video laryngoscopy to direct laryngoscopy in 822 intubations. J Emerg Med 2012;42:400–5.
54. Sakles JC, Mosier J, Chiu S, et al. A comparison of the C-MAC video laryngoscope to the Macintosh direct laryngoscope for intubation in the emergency department. Ann Emerg Med 2012. [Epub ahead of print].
55. Mosier JM, Stolz U, Chiu S, et al. Difficult airway management in the emergency department: glidescope videolaryngoscopy compared to direct laryngoscopy. J Emerg Med 2012;42:629–34.
56. Liu EH, Goy RW, Tan BH, et al. Tracheal intubation with videolaryngoscopes in patients with cervical spine immobilization: a randomized trial of the Airway Scope and the GlideScope. Br J Anaesth 2009;103:446–51.
57. Watts AD, Gelb AW, Bach DB, et al. Comparison of the Bullard and Macintosh laryngoscopes for endotracheal intubation of patients with a potential cervical spine injury. Anesthesiology 1997;87:1335–42.

Training in Trauma Management

The Role of Simulation-Based Medical Education

Haim Berkenstadt, MD[a,b,d,*],
Erez Ben-Menachem, MBCHB, MBA, FANZCA[b], Daniel Simon, MD[c],
Amitai Ziv, MD, MHA[a,d]

KEYWORDS

• Simulation-based medical education • Trauma management • Trauma training
• Medical simulation

KEY POINTS

- Simulation-based medical education (SBME) offers a safe and "mistake-forgiving" environment to teach and train medical professionals.
- The diverse range of medical-simulation modalities enables trainees to acquire and practice an array of tasks and skills.
- SBME offers the field of trauma training multiple opportunities to enhance the effectiveness of the education provided in this challenging domain.

Trauma management poses a unique challenge to the medical system. Casualties presenting within the first 2 hours of injury represent a population with potentially preventable death, thus medical professionals who are not routinely exposed to treating trauma casualties need to be trained to assess and manage these patients during this definitive period.[1] Moreover, the low incidence of penetrating trauma and reduced resident training hours results in training deficits among surgical residents and fellows.[2] Anesthesiologists drafted from civilian hospitals to military field hospitals face more severe trauma injuries, different injury patterns, unfamiliar blood products administration protocols, and different, increasingly complex, equipment.[3]

Simulation-based medical education (SBME) may be used as part of the interventions aimed at overcoming these, and other gaps in trauma-management training. Important driving forces for the integration of SBME in formal curriculum and evaluation in medicine include training for uncommon medical situations, minimizing risks to patients,[4] avoiding the use of live animals for training,[5] economic considerations that

[a] The Israel Center for Medical Simulation (MSR), Sheba Medical Center, Tel Aviv University, Tel Hashomer, Israel 52621; [b] Department of Anesthesiology, Sheba Medical Center, Tel Aviv University, Tel Hashomer, Israel 52621; [c] Trauma Unit, Sheba Medical Center, Tel Aviv University, Tel Hashomer, Israel 52621; [d] Sackler Faculty of Medicine, Tel Aviv University, Israel
* Corresponding author. The Israel Center for Medical Simulation (MSR), Sheba Medical Center, Tel Aviv University, Tel Hashomer, Israel 52621.
E-mail address: haim.berkenstadt@sheba.health.gov.il

Anesthesiology Clin 31 (2013) 167–177
http://dx.doi.org/10.1016/j.anclin.2012.11.003 **anesthesiology.theclinics.com**
1932-2275/13/$ – see front matter

have reduced patient accessibility for traditional bedside medical teaching,[6] demands for accountability and high safety/quality standards,[4] and the need for objective and reliable performance/competence evaluation. Following on from the aviation industry,[7] the medical-simulation industry is now producing improved and increasingly realistic high-fidelity training devices, which are expanding and opening new horizons for medical training and education.

SBME offers the opportunity for task training in various medical and surgical procedures, and provides a "hands-on" empiric educational modality, enabling controlled proactive exposure of trainees to both routine common and complex uncommon clinical scenarios.[8] SBME training is trainee oriented and conducted in a safe and "mistake-forgiving" environment in which trainees can learn from their errors, and training can be adjusted to the trainees' needs and deficiencies.[9,10] Additionally, SBME offers a unique opportunity for team training, an important contributing factor to enhanced patient safety and outcome, and seldom addressed in traditional medical education.[11,12] Training is performed without the ethically disturbing duality of patient care and medical training associated with traditional bedside teaching. Another important benefit of SBME is the reproducible, standardized, objective setting it provides for formative assessment (debriefing)[13–15] and summative assessment (testing).[16,17]

A major component of SBME, regardless of the simulation modality used, is the ability to observe, record, and debrief the simulation session. During the debriefing session, participants get feedback from peers and trainers on their clinical performance and nontechnical skills. In most simulation centers, video recordings of training are used for debriefing; this tool provides the participants the opportunity to see their personal performance and how it affects team performance. From an educational point of view, the debriefing session may be the most important part of the SBME experience, because it gives the participant the possibility of reflecting on behavior and receiving feedback.[18,19]

As already indicated, these potential benefits of SBME are relevant for the training and evaluation of trauma care in various environments and conditions: prehospital care, in-hospital emergency room, conventional mass casualties scenarios, and in nonconventional warfare conditions. In the course of this article, the use of various simulation modalities, including simulated patients (role-play actors), skills trainers, and computerized patient simulators and their role in trauma care training are reviewed.

SIMULATED PATIENTS

Objective Structured Clinical Examination using standardized simulated patients is a widely used model of medical training and assessment.[20,21] Using this methodology, a participant is trained and evaluated on his or her ability to take a patient history, perform a physical examination, communicate with the patient, and suggest appropriate treatment options. This simulation modality is used widely by medical and nursing schools and by medical boards worldwide.[22] These examinations reflect a major shift in the field of medical accreditation and licensure by acknowledging the crucial role of performance assessment in professional accreditation. This simulation modality was also adopted by the American College of Surgeons as one of the training and evaluation tools used in the Advanced Trauma Life Support (ATLS) course. This course was developed in an effort to standardize and improve trauma care, thereby increasing the consistency of medical treatment to trauma casualties.[23] Several studies have demonstrated the benefit of simulated patient–based evaluation of trauma management skills and the difference between this modality and cognitive knowledge assessment using a written standardized multiple-choice examination.[24,25]

SKILLS TRAINING

The use of task-training simulators for the teaching of technical skills has become common in many fields of medicine, and demonstrates a reasonably good transfer of skills from models to humans.[26,27] Various skills trainers are used for teaching novices trauma-related procedures, such as airway management, chest drain insertion, cricothyroidotomy, and focused abdominal sonography for trauma (FAST).

Manikin-based simulation is widely used for airway management training and for the assessment of new airway devices. Simulation-based training was also demonstrated to significantly improve performance of anesthesiologists in unanticipated difficult airway scenarios[28]; however, the limitations of such devices must realized. Recently published studies raise questions regarding the use of manikins for these purposes. Schebesta and colleagues[29] compared computed tomography (CT) scans of trauma patients with scans of 4 high-fidelity patient simulators and 2 airway trainers. The results demonstrated that the anatomy of the simulators does not reflect the upper airway anatomy of actual patients. Similar results were found with the anatomic features of the SimBaby.[30] Moreover, data from 2 different studies by Russell and colleagues[31,32] demonstrate that forces used during laryngoscopy are different in patients compared with manikins. Despite this information, simulation is still an important tool in airway management training, although a more realistic simulator is needed.

The emergency insertion of a chest drain for tension pneumothorax or hemothorax following trauma is considered to be safe when performed by trained physicians[33]; however, the use of live animals to train novices in the performance of this procedure is prohibited in some countries because of increasing pressure from animal-rights advocates. Therefore, alternative models of thoracic drainage, based on animal cadaveric models[34] or simulation-based training, have been adopted.[35] In a validation study of the TraumaMan simulator, experienced ATLS instructors recommended the simulator to train novice physicians in this procedure. Moreover, novice participants of the ATLS course, who trained with both the animal skills laboratory and the simulator, found the simulator superior to the animal model in teaching anatomic landmarks.[36] Other studies demonstrated that a brief 2-hour-long teaching module using a simulation model (SuperAnnie) is effective in improving confidence and skill in chest tube insertion,[37] and that a simple homemade simulator (wood base with a large rack of ribs secured to simulate the thorax and partially inflated examination gloves and bagels used to simulate the lung and diaphragm, respectively) can be used for this purpose.[38]

In another life-saving procedure, cricothyroidotomy, simulation modalities were used to assess the success rate by novices in performing the procedure, and its learning curve. In one simulation-based evaluation, a 100% success rate in achieving an adequate airway within acceptable time limits was found.[39] Training of at least 5 attempts, or until cricothyroidotomy time was 40 seconds or less, was recommended.[40] In a recent study, incorporating the task of cricothyroidotomy into a "can't intubate/can't ventilate" simulation training session demonstrated that following a single training session performed by senior anesthesiologists, improvements in cricothyroidotomy skills are retained for at least 1 year.[41] Another study found that age affects the learning and performance of emergency percutaneous cricothyroidotomy in a high-fidelity simulated "can't intubate/can't ventilate" scenario.[42] This study demonstrates the value of simulation-based assessment to highlight deficits in performance, establish the limits of performance, and identify practitioner subgroups that may benefit from focused or more regular training. Unfortunately, because emergency cricothyroidotomy is rarely performed, there are no studies assessing the transference of skills from simulation to clinical performance, and conclusions are limited to the skills trainer.

The FAST examination allows for rapid bedside diagnosis of intra-abdominal, pleural, or pericardial hemorrhage in trauma casualties, even in the prehospital setting when radiologists are not available.[43] A training program for the performance of FAST by nonradiologists using the UltraSim simulator (MedSim, Raanana, Israel) has been developed and validated.[44] The simulation-based curriculum improved the correct transducer placement and the quality of images obtained, shortened the time required for obtaining images, and increased the incidence of correct diagnosis. Construct validity, namely the ability of the simulation-training program and the assessment tools to differentiate among participants according to their experience in performing the task, was demonstrated, and participants recommended using this training modality for all trauma physicians. A recent study demonstrated no differences in the skills of image acquisition and interpretation between novices trained using multimedia simulators or human models. The investigators concluded that these data support the premise that skills learned during simulation training can be applied to patients.[45]

COMPUTERIZED PATIENT SIMULATORS

Computerized patient simulators, based on a manikin connected to a physiologic monitor and run by a computerized system, located in the relevant clinical environment (or a mock-up of that environment), can be programmed for diverse clinical scenarios and can permit a safe and reproducible training environment. This type of simulation-based training requires physicians to identify problems and provide solutions, as if it was a real emergency situation (ie, infuse fluids, perform orotracheal intubation or cricothyroidotomy, or insert a chest drain). For example, while using this type of simulator, the treating physician can talk to the manikin and get an answer from the simulator or the operator; check pupils (which in some simulators react to light); feel arterial pulses; listen to cardiac and lung sounds; and collect information on heart rate, blood pressure, respiratory rate, and oxygen saturation. Medications and fluids can be administered to the simulator, which responds appropriately, based on an interaction between the manikin's current underlying physiology and the dose and the pharmacokinetics and pharmacodynamics of the medication.

Advanced medical simulation has been used in several medical fields to improve training, clinical performance, and competence assessment, and in emergency room or operating room crisis resource management training.[46–48] Advanced simulation has also been used for learning about errors made during critical emergency situations, and understanding the patterns of human errors during anesthesia, thus providing recommendations for changes in teaching and education.[49,50] In trauma care, advanced simulation has been incorporated into the training programs of medics, paramedics, physicians, and medical teams worldwide. For example, advanced simulation has been introduced into the training of basic trauma-related skills for military emergency personnel,[51] to evaluate the competence of surgery interns after a standard ATLS course,[52] and to promote pediatric disaster triage performance.[14] Although the face validity (appearance of a model or test to adequately measure/train what is intended to be measured/trained) of such training is high, and there are high expectations and acceptance for this training modality,[53,54] validation of simulation-based training in trauma management is limited. The construct validity (the degree to which an instrument measures the characteristic being investigated) of advanced simulation in the training of emergency medicine scenarios was established by Gordon and colleagues,[55] and the value of advanced simulation in promoting trauma management was demonstrated.[56,57] Ali and colleagues,[58] however, demonstrated that improvement in knowledge and skills is equally enhanced by using either expensive computerized manikin simulators or patient models in trauma teaching. Student feedback demonstrated that students overwhelmingly preferred the computerized manikin model.

Medical simulation was used also to identify deficiencies in the stabilization of children presenting to emergency departments, revealing that mistakes, including estimating a child's weight, preparing for intraosseous needle placement, ordering intravenous fluid boluses, and applying warming measures, are ubiquitous.[59] In another study, the finding of major deviations in airway management, and in the evaluation of secondary respiratory and hemodynamic deterioration in the intubated trauma patient, were followed by changes in the training curriculum and, as a consequence, improvement in performance.[60] These findings of performance improvement after changes in curriculum are not trivial in view of the limited data published supporting the beneficial effects of simulation-based training. The report by Chopra and colleagues[61] demonstrated the positive effect of simulation training on the subsequent management of similar critical incidents, but Olympio and colleagues[62] failed to demonstrate the influence of simulation training on the management of esophageal intubation.

TEAM TRAINING

One of the major applications of SBME in the training of trauma management is its use in team training. Although surgical, anesthesiology, and emergency medicine trainees receive feedback on their technical performance from their trainers, they rarely receive feedback on their nontechnical or team skills. The importance of nontechnical skills is highlighted by data from aviation, demonstrating that 70% of errors have human causes and that a large number of errors are a result of failures in interpersonal communication, decision making, and leadership.[63] Further support for this theory comes from the finding that errors in the operating theater are rarely caused by deficiencies in technical performance,[64] and result more from impaired decision making, an absence of situational awareness, and failures in interpersonal communication. The similarities between surgery, anesthesiology, and trauma management and aviation led to the adoption of the concept of crew resource management from aviation, and courses in crisis management for anesthesiologists and surgical teams based on the crew resource management concept were developed.[65–67]

A recent study described that structured trauma resuscitation team training, augmented by simulation, improved team performance, resulting in improved efficiency of patient care. Training induced significant improvement in all teamwork domains, including leadership, situational awareness, mutual support, and communication. Moreover, times from arrival at the hospital until transfer to the CT scanner, initiation of endotracheal intubation, and entrance to the operating room were decreased significantly after the training.[68] These results of improved team performance are further supported by other studies in adult and pediatric trauma care.[69,70]

One of the reasons for the apparent failure to make nontechnical skills a focus of training among medical specialties has been the difficulty encountered in the objective assessment of these skills to enable structured feedback. Efforts in the direction of nontechnical skills assessment are being made by the authors and by other groups in the fields of surgery and anesthesiology.[71,72] Recently, a modified nontechnical skills (NOTECHS) scale for trauma (T-NOTECHS) aimed to teach and assess teamwork skills of multidisciplinary trauma resuscitation teams was developed and initially validated.[73]

SURGICAL TRAINING

Training of surgical fellows in the management of trauma victims is a major challenge. Because of the limitations of existing surgical simulators, courses like Advanced Trauma Operative Management include cognitive knowledge learning followed by short lectures and training in a full-scale operating room with standardized injuries created in a porcine model.[74] Self-efficacy, trauma knowledge, and skills were reported to improve significantly with training,[75] and a worldwide questionnaire demonstrated that participants perceived the course as worthwhile and helped surgeons improve knowledge, confidence, and skills in penetrating injuries.[2] A similar course, also using a porcine model, demonstrated positive impact on surgical decision making of surgical residents.[76] Another course, the Trauma Exposure Course, uses fresh cadavers for training.[77] Unfortunately, current simulation technology cannot replace the animal models and fresh cadavers and poses a real challenge to the simulation manufacturers.

VIRTUAL REALITY

Virtual reality (VR) is a simulation methodology in which the participant wears eye goggles allowing the experience of being part of an immersive interactive environment that is computer controlled. Although disaster drills using standardized patients and/or simulators are the principal method for mass casualty training,[78] full immersive VR was shown to be an effective tool for triage skills training of emergency medicine trainees.[79]

WEB-BASED TEACHING

In any modality of SBME, it is useful to provide participants with associated theoretical material in advance of their simulation-based training, to achieve a more homogeneous group by triggering prior knowledge, and stressing important learning points.[80] One of the options is to use Web-based teaching tools to facilitate learning of the cognitive knowledge relevant for training.

PRACTICAL ASPECTS

SBME is used increasingly for training medical personnel in trauma care. It is important to recognize the broad spectrum of simulation modalities and devices and to use simulation in a cost-effective manner, while recognizing SBME's limitations and adjusting the training program and the simulation tools to the target population and the educational goals. Each simulation modality should be used in a targeted and thoughtful manner, which accounts for the relevant strengths and weaknesses of each respective modality (**Table 1**). Simulation technologies should supplement, not replace, the traditional methods of teaching cognitive knowledge. For example:

- The cognitive aspects of the teaching module can be taught by the traditional methods of self-guided learning and lectures before participation in the simulation training.
- The acquisition and practice of technical skills, such as chest drain insertion and airway management, can be performed on task trainer simulators. It is important that the model is relevant and validated for the skill being taught.

Table 1
Relevant advantages and disadvantages according to teaching modality

Teaching Modality	Cost	Cognitive Learning	Technical Skills	Nontechnical Skills	Team Training	Complex Assessment and Management
Task trainers	+	++	+++	+	–	–
Simulated patients	++	+	+	++	+	++
Simple manikins	++	++	++	++	++	++
Computerized patient simulators	+++	++	++	++	+++	+++
Virtual reality	++	+	+	++	+	++
Web-based learning	+	+++	+	+	–	+

The strength of each simulation modality in each criteria is presented by (–) not at all, (+) low, (++) medium, (+++) high.

- Following the acquisition of task performance, the task should be incorporated into a scenario in which the trainee needs to assess the patient situation, decide on task performance, and perform the task within the context of whole-patient management.
- Computerized simulators can be used for full-scale, high-fidelity simulation scenarios, and video recordings of the training can be used for debriefing teamwork, exploring nontechnical skills, and other aspects of performance.

SUMMARY

Simulation-based medical education offers a safe and "mistake-forgiving" environment to teach and train medical professionals. The diverse range of medical simulation modalities enables trainees to acquire and practice an array of tasks and skills. SBME offers the field of trauma training multiple opportunities to enhance the effectiveness of the education provided in this challenging domain. Further research is needed to better learn the role of simulation-based learning in trauma management and education.

REFERENCES

1. Hogan MP, Boone DC. Trauma education and assessment. Injury 2008;39(6):681–5.
2. Jacobs L, Burns K, Luk S, et al. Advanced trauma operative management course: participant survey. World J Surg 2010;34(1):164–8.
3. Mercer SJ, Whittle CL, Mahoney PF. Lessons from the battlefield: human factors in defence anaesthesia. Br J Anaesth 2010;105(1):9–20.
4. Kohn LT, Corrigan JM, Donaldson MS, editors. Committee on Quality of Health Care in America, Institute of Medicine. To err is human: building a safer health system. Washington, DC: Institute of Medicine, National Academy Press; 2000. p. 312.
5. Cohen C. The case for the use of animals in biomedical research. N Engl J Med 1986;315:865–70.
6. The Israel National Institute for Health Policy and Health Services Research. Curriculum for medical schools towards the 21st century. Jerusalem (Israel): The Israel National Institute for Health Policy and Health Services Research; 2002.

7. Helmreich RL, Davies JM. Anaesthetic simulation and lessons to be learned from aviation. Can J Anaesth 1997;44(9):907–12.
8. Nestel D, Groom J, Eikeland-Husebø S, et al. Simulation for learning and teaching procedural skills: the state of the science. Simul Healthc 2011;6(Suppl):S10–3.
9. Issenberg SB, McGaghie WC, Hart IR, et al. Simulation technology for health care professional skills training and assessment. JAMA 1999;282(9):861–6.
10. Kolozsvari NO, Feldman LS, Vassiliou MC, et al. Sim one, do one, teach one: considerations in designing training curricula for surgical simulation. J Surg Educ 2011;68(5):421–7.
11. Yeung JH, Ong GJ, Davies RP, et al. Factors affecting team leadership skills and their relationship with quality of cardiopulmonary resuscitation. Crit Care Med 2012;40(9):2617–21.
12. Theilen U, Leonard P, Jones P, et al. Regular in situ simulation training of paediatric Medical Emergency Team improves hospital response to deteriorating patients. Resuscitation 2012. [Epub ahead of print].
13. Ende J. Feedback in clinical medical education. JAMA 1983;250(6):777–81.
14. Cicero MX, Auerbach MA, Zigmont J, et al. Simulation training with structured debriefing improves residents' pediatric disaster triage performance. Prehosp Disaster Med 2012;27(3):239–44.
15. Sawyer T, Sierocka-Castaneda A, Chan D, et al. The effectiveness of video-assisted debriefing versus oral debriefing alone at improving neonatal resuscitation performance: a randomized trial. Simul Healthc 2012;7(4):213–21.
16. Ben-Menachem E, Ezri T, Ziv A, et al. Objective Structured Clinical Examination-based assessment of regional anesthesia skills: the Israeli National Board Examination in Anesthesiology experience. Anesth Analg 2011;112(1):242–5.
17. Ziv A, Rubin O, Sidi A, et al. Credentialing and certifying with simulation. Anesthesiol Clin 2007;25(2):261–9.
18. Dieckmann P. Debriefing Olympics—a workshop concept to stimulate the adaptation of debriefings to learning contexts. Simul Healthc 2012;7(3):176–82.
19. Raemer D, Anderson M, Cheng A, et al. Research regarding debriefing as part of the learning process. Simul Healthc 2011;6(Suppl):S52–7.
20. Griesser MJ, Beran MC, Flanigan DC, et al. Implementation of an objective structured clinical exam (OSCE) into orthopedic surgery residency training. J Surg Educ 2012;69(2):180–9.
21. Shah B, Miler R, Poles M, et al. Informed consent in the older adult: OSCEs for assessing fellows' ACGME and geriatric gastroenterology competencies. Am J Gastroenterol 2011;106(9):1575–9.
22. Papadakos MA. The step 2 clinical skills examination. N Engl J Med 2004;350(17):1703–5.
23. van Olden GD, Meeuwis JD, Bolhuis HW, et al. Clinical impact of advanced trauma life support. Am J Emerg Med 2004;22(7):522–5.
24. Ali J, Adam R, Pierre I, et al. Comparison of performance two years after the old and new (interactive) ATLS courses. J Surg Res 2001;97(1):71–5.
25. Ali J, Adam RU, Josa D, et al. Comparison of performance of interns completing the old (1993) and new interactive (1997) Advanced Trauma Life Support courses. J Trauma 1999;46(1):80–6.
26. Perrenot C, Perez M, Tran N, et al. The virtual reality simulator dV-Trainer (®) is a valid assessment tool for robotic surgical skills. Surg Endosc 2012;26(9):2587–93.
27. Hseino H, Nugent E, Lee MJ, et al. Skills transfer after proficiency-based simulation training in superficial femoral artery angioplasty. Simul Healthc 2012;7(5):274–81.

28. Kuduvalli PM, Jervis A, Tighe SQ, et al. Unanticipated difficult airway management in anaesthetised patients: a prospective study of the effect of mannequin training on management strategies and skill retention. Anaesthesia 2008;63(4):364–9.
29. Schebesta K, Hüpfl M, Rössler B, et al. Degrees of reality: airway anatomy of high-fidelity human patient simulators and airway trainers. Anesthesiology 2012; 116(6):1204–9.
30. Schebesta K, Hüpfl M, Ringl H, et al. A comparison of paediatric airway anatomy with the SimBaby high-fidelity patient simulator. Resuscitation 2011;82(4):468–72.
31. Russell T, Khan S, Elman J, et al. Measurement of forces applied during Macintosh direct laryngoscopy compared with GlideScope® videolaryngoscopy. Anaesthesia 2012;67(6):626–31.
32. Russell T, Lee C, Firat M, et al. A comparison of the forces applied to a manikin during laryngoscopy with the GlideScope and Macintosh laryngoscopes. Anaesth Intensive Care 2011;39(6):1098–102.
33. Collop NA, Kim S, Sahn SA. Analysis of tube thoracostomy performed by pulmonologists at a teaching hospital. Chest 1997;112(3):709–13.
34. Eaton BD, Messent DO, Haywood IR. Animal cadaveric models for advanced trauma life support training. Ann R Coll Surg Engl 1990;72(2):135–9.
35. Simulab Corporation. Available at: http://www.simulab.com/. Accessed January, 2013.
36. Berkenstadt H, Munz Y, Trodler G, et al. Evaluation of the trauma-man® simulator for training in chest drain insertion. Eur J Trauma 2006;32:523–6.
37. Hutton IA, Kenealy H, Wong C. Using simulation models to teach junior doctors how to insert chest tubes: a brief and effective teaching module. Intern Med J 2008;38(12):887–91.
38. Ching JA, Wachtel TL. A simple device to teach tube thoracostomy. J Trauma 2011;70(6):1564–7.
39. Vadodaria BS, Gandhi SD, McIndoe AK. Comparison of four different emergency airway access equipment sets on a human patient simulator. Anaesthesia 2004; 59(1):73–9.
40. Wong DT, Prabhu AJ, Coloma M, et al. What is the minimum training required for successful cricothyroidotomy? A study in mannequins. Anesthesiology 2003; 98(2):349–53.
41. Boet S, Borges BC, Naik VN, et al. Complex procedural skills are retained for a minimum of 1 yr after a single high-fidelity simulation training session. Br J Anaesth 2011;107(4):533–9.
42. Siu LW, Boet S, Borges BC, et al. High-fidelity simulation demonstrates the influence of anesthesiologists' age and years from residency on emergency cricothyroidotomy skills. Anesth Analg 2010;111(4):955–60.
43. Walcher F, Weinlich M, Conrad G, et al. Prehospital ultrasound imaging improves management of abdominal trauma. Br J Surg 2006;93(2):238–42.
44. Kapelian I, Simon D, Ziv A, et al. The use of simulation for focused abdominal sonography in trauma (FAST) training. Presented at the 17th Annual Meeting of the Israeli Trauma Society. Herzelia (Israel), September, 2005.
45. Damewood S, Jeanmonod D, Cadigan B. Comparison of a multimedia simulator to a human model for teaching FAST exam image interpretation and image acquisition. Acad Emerg Med 2011;18(4):413–9. http://dx.doi.org/10.1111/j.1553-2712.2011.01037.x.
46. Steadman RH, Huang YM. Simulation for quality assurance in training, credentialing and maintenance of certification. Best Pract Res Clin Anaesthesiol 2012; 26(1):3–15.

47. Levine AI, Flynn BC, Bryson EO, et al. Simulation-based Maintenance of Certification in Anesthesiology (MOCA) course optimization: use of multi-modality educational activities. J Clin Anesth 2012;24(1):68–74.
48. Batchelder AJ, Steel A, Mackenzie R, et al. Simulation as a tool to improve the safety of pre-hospital anaesthesia—a pilot study. Anaesthesia 2009;64(9):978–83.
49. Berkenstadt H, Ben-Menachem E, Dach R, et al. Deficits in the provision of cardiopulmonary resuscitation during simulated obstetric crises: results from the Israeli Board of Anesthesiologists. Anesth Analg 2012;115(5):1122–6.
50. Berkenstadt H, Haviv Y, Tuval A, et al. Improving handoff communications in critical care: utilizing simulation-based training toward process improvement in managing patient risk. Chest 2008;134(1):158–62.
51. Treloar D, Hawayek J, Montgomery JR, et al. On site and distance education of emergency personnel with a human patient simulator. Mil Med 2001;166(1):103–6.
52. Ali J, Gana TJ, Howard M. Trauma mannequin assessment of management skills of surgical residents after advanced trauma life support training. J Surg Res 2000;93(1):197–200.
53. Barsuk D, Berkenstadt H, Stein M, et al. [Advanced patient simulators in pre-hospital trauma management training—the trainees' perspective]. Harefuah 2003;142(2):87–90 [in Hebrew].
54. Kim TE, Reibling ET, Denmark KT. Student perception of high fidelity medical simulation for an international trauma life support course. Prehosp Disaster Med 2012;27(1):27–30.
55. Gordon JA, Tancredi D, Binder W, et al. Assessing global performance in emergency medicine using high fidelity patient simulator: a pilot study. Acad Emerg Med 2003;78(Suppl 10):S45–7.
56. Marshall RL, Smith JS, Gorman P, et al. Use of a human patient simulator in the development of resident trauma management skills. J Trauma 2001;51(1):17–21.
57. Lee SK, Pardo M, Gaba D, et al. Trauma assessment training with a patient simulator: a prospective, randomized study. J Trauma 2003;55(4):651–7.
58. Ali J, Al Ahmadi K, Williams JI, et al. The standardized live patient and mechanical patient models—their roles in trauma teaching. J Trauma 2009;66(1):98–102.
59. Hunt EA, Hohenhaus SM, Luo X, et al. Simulation of pediatric trauma stabilization in 35 North Carolina emergency departments: identification of targets for performance improvement. Pediatrics 2006;117(3):641–8.
60. Barsuk D, Ziv A, Lin G, et al. Using advanced simulation for recognition and correction of gaps in airway and breathing management skills in prehospital trauma care. Anesth Analg 2005;100(3):803–9.
61. Chopra V, Gesink BJ, de Jong J, et al. Does training on an anaesthesia simulator lead to improvement in performance? Br J Anaesth 1994;73(3):293–7.
62. Olympio MA, Whelan R, Ford RP, et al. Failure of simulation training to change residents' management of oesophageal intubation. Br J Anaesth 2003;91(3):312–8.
63. Helmreich RL, Merritt AC, Wilhelm JA. The evolution of crew resource management training in commercial aviation. Int J Aviat Psychol 1999;9:19–32.
64. Chopra V, Bovill JG, Spierdijk J, et al. Reported significant observations during anaesthesia: a prospective analysis over an 18-month period. Br J Anaesth 1992;68:13–7.
65. Howard SK, Gaba DM, Fish KJ, et al. Anesthesia crisis resource management training: teaching anesthesiologists to handle critical incidents. Aviat Space Environ Med 1992;63(9):763–70.

66. Holzman RS, Cooper JB, Gaba DM, et al. Anesthesia crisis resource management: real-life simulation training in operating room crises. J Clin Anesth 1995; 7:675–87.
67. Shapiro MJ, Morey JC, Small SD, et al. Simulation based teamwork training for emergency department staff: does it improve clinical team performance when added to an existing didactic teamwork curriculum? Qual Saf Health Care 2004;13(6):417–21.
68. Capella J, Smith S, Philp A, et al. Teamwork training improves the clinical care of trauma patients. J Surg Educ 2010;67(6):439–43.
69. Steinemann S, Berg B, Skinner A, et al. In situ, multidisciplinary, simulation-based teamwork training improves early trauma care. J Surg Educ 2011;68(6):472–7.
70. Hunt EA, Heine M, Hohenhaus SM, et al. Simulated pediatric trauma team management: assessment of an educational intervention. Pediatr Emerg Care 2007;23(11):796–804.
71. Moorthy K, Munz Y, Adams S, et al. A human factors analysis of technical and team skills among surgical trainees during procedural simulations in a simulated operating theatre. Ann Surg 2005;242(5):631–9.
72. Fletcher G, Flin R, McGeorge P, et al. Anaesthetists' Non-Technical Skills (ANTS): evaluation of a behavioural marker system. Br J Anaesth 2003;90:580–8.
73. Steinemann S, Berg B, DiTullio A, et al. Assessing teamwork in the trauma bay: introduction of a modified "NOTECHS" scale for trauma. Am J Surg 2012; 203(1):69–75.
74. Jacobs LM, Burns KJ, Kaban JM, et al. Development and evaluation of the advanced trauma operative management course. J Trauma 2003;55(3):471–9 [discussion: 479].
75. Ali J, Ahmed N, Jacobs LM, et al. The advanced trauma operative management course in a Canadian residency program. Can J Surg 2008;51(3):185–9.
76. Scott TM, Hameed SM, Evans DC, et al. Objective assessment of surgical decision making in trauma after a laboratory-based course: durability of cognitive skills. Am J Surg 2008;195(5):599–602 [discussion: 602–3].
77. Gunst M, O'Keeffe T, Hollett L, et al. Trauma operative skills in the era of nonoperative management: the trauma exposure course (TEC). J Trauma 2009;67(5): 1091–6.
78. Gillett B, Peckler B, Sinert R, et al. Simulation in a disaster drill: comparison of high-fidelity simulators versus trained actors. Acad Emerg Med 2008;15(11): 1144–51.
79. Andreatta PB, Maslowski E, Petty S, et al. Virtual reality triage training provides a viable solution for disaster-preparedness. Acad Emerg Med 2010;17(8):870–6.
80. Østergaard HT, Østergaard D, Lippert A. Implementation of team training in medical education in Denmark. Qual Saf Health Care 2004;13(Suppl):i91–5.

Pitfalls of Hemodynamic Monitoring in Patients with Trauma

Richard R. McNeer, MD, PhD[a,b,*], Albert J. Varon, MD, MHPE, FCCM[a,c]

KEYWORDS

- Trauma • Hemodynamic monitoring • Hemorrhagic shock
- Blood pressure measurement • Dynamic response • Natural frequency
- End-tidal carbon dioxide • Assessment of cardiac output

KEY POINTS

- Hypotensive resuscitation imposes additional burdens on the anesthesiologist to maintain adequate blood pressure while also avoiding blood pressure overshoots or sustained hypertension.
- Accuracy and interpretation of blood pressure monitoring in trauma depend on complex interactions between patient physiology and factors intrinsic to measurement devices.
- Oscillometry overestimates systolic blood pressure in hypotensive patients.
- The impact of hemorrhagic shock on reflection wave behavior may limit the reliability or confound interpretation of both noninvasive and invasive blood pressure measurements.
- Adequate dynamic response is required for proper recording of an arterial waveform, and dynamic response requirements increase with tachycardia.
- The only way to determine dynamic response is to conduct a flush test.
- End-tidal CO_2 is correlated with cardiac output; however, this correlation is affected following cardiac or respiratory arrest.

INTRODUCTION

Resuscitation of the patient with trauma with ongoing blood loss has historically been geared toward maintaining normal or higher than normal blood pressure. Investigations of the role of hypotensive resuscitation have been conducted with mixed results.

Funding sources: None.
Conflict of interest: None.

[a] Division of Trauma Anesthesiology, Department of Anesthesiology, University of Miami Miller School of Medicine, PO Box 016370-M820, Miami, FL 33101, USA; [b] Department of Biomedical Engineering, College of Engineering, University of Miami, PO Box 248294, Coral Gables, FL 33146, USA; [c] Ryder Trauma Center at Jackson Memorial Hospital, 1800 NW 10th Avenue, Miami, FL 33136, USA

* Corresponding author. Division of Trauma Anesthesiology, University of Miami Miller School of Medicine, PO Box 016370-M820, Miami, FL 33101.
E-mail address: mcneer@miami.edu

Anesthesiology Clin 31 (2013) 179–194
http://dx.doi.org/10.1016/j.anclin.2012.11.005 **anesthesiology.theclinics.com**

A review of 52 animal studies of mortality during induced hemorrhage found that hypotensive resuscitation reduced the risk of death.[1] However, in human studies, decreased blood loss and transfusion requirements have only been confirmed in penetrating injury.[2] Other studies[3] are currently in progress and may add evidence to support a paradigm shift in the management of blood pressure in the patient with trauma. It may no longer be sufficient to maintain blood pressure at an adequate level, and added vigilance may be needed to prevent sustained overshoots in blood pressure. It is therefore ironic that the monitoring strategies meant to inform the anesthesiologist of a patient's hemodynamic status are limited in the context of hypotension and the deranged physiology associated with hemorrhagic shock.

This article discusses the complex interplay between alterations in the physiology of a patient with trauma, the monitoring devices engineered to measure these alterations, and interpretation of these data by the anesthesiologist. Focus is placed on the early stages of caring for the patient with trauma before surgical hemostasis is obtained, when hemodynamic assessment must be made quickly and accurately to maintain sufficient cardiac output and blood pressure without exceeding levels that may worsen outcome. Hemodynamic monitoring and resuscitation end points of patients in the period after surgical hemostasis have been reviewed elsewhere[4] and are only mentioned here. For example, monitoring strategies based on arterial pressure waveform variation, venous oxygen saturation ($S\bar{v}O_2$) and central venous oxygen saturation ($ScvO_2$), and laboratory parameters such as base excess and lactate have been, or are increasingly becoming, a part of the trauma anesthesiologist's armamentarium, but it is often not feasible to implement these strategies during the initial, frenetic stages of care. The 3 bread-and-butter monitors heavily relied on during the initial assessment and resuscitation of the unstable patient with trauma are arguably the end-tidal pressure of CO_2 ($PETCO_2$), noninvasive blood pressure (NIBP), and invasive arterial blood pressure (IABP). The underpinnings and limitations of these monitors in the patient with trauma are discussed in reverse order starting with invasive blood pressure, acknowledging that the other two may be the only hemodynamic monitors available before an arterial catheter can be inserted. Wherever possible, figures are included to illustrate important points from the text.

Invasive Blood Pressure Monitoring

When using IABP to guide the management of patients with trauma, it is incumbent on the physician to discern true signal (the physiologic waveform) from artifact (a distorted waveform). The physiologic waveform should be processed with high fidelity to obtain an accurate recording. Several characteristics of the patient with trauma and of the recording device can lead to the generation of distorted (or what appears to be distorted) waveform morphology. Patients with trauma are likely to exhibit tachycardia, hypotension, decreased cardiac output, and high (or occasionally low) systemic vascular resistance (SVR). These derangements in patient physiology can exceed the processing capability of the catheter-tube-transducer (CTT) system used to invasively measure blood pressure. Factors that affect waveform morphology can lead to the display of inaccurate blood pressure values and potentially confound clinical interpretation. Two of the main factors are pulse wave reflection within arterial vasculature and the dynamic response characteristics inherent to the CTT system.

To understand why these factors are important, it is useful to recall that any physiologic waveform is decomposable into several sine waves of varying amplitude, frequency, and phase (**Fig. 1**). The reverse process is also true, and sign waves can be selected and summed to generate a simulated waveform. It takes just 3 sine waves to give a persuasive approximation of the typical arterial waveform.[5] Of the 3 sine waves

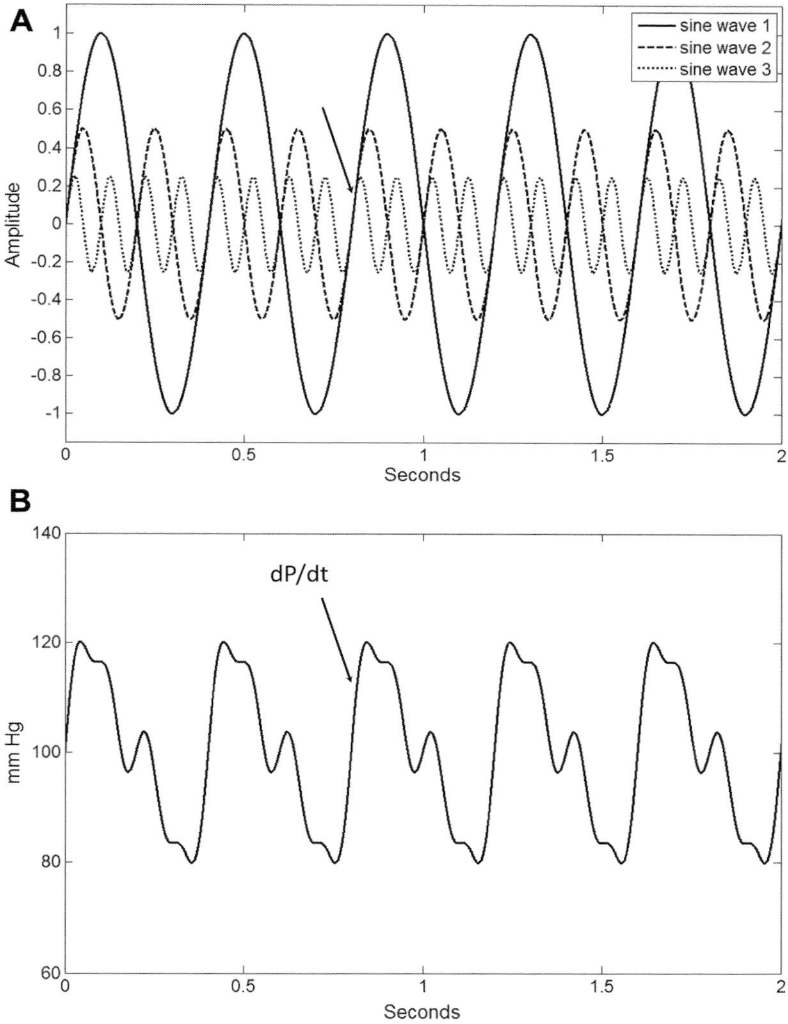

Fig. 1. Generation of simulated arterial waveform from sine waves. Summation of 3 sine waves (*A*), 1 fundamental (sine wave 1) with frequency equal to pulse rate and 2 harmonics (sine waves 2 and 3) produces a good approximation of an arterial waveform at a pulse rate of 150 beats per minute (*B*). Sine waves of higher frequency relative to pulse rate are required to produce detailed features in the waveform such as the dicrotic notch and steep systolic upstroke; change in pressure (dP)/change in time (dt) (*arrows*). The simulation was performed using custom scripts written in MATLAB, and sine wave frequencies and amplitudes from Szockik and colleagues[5] (2000). (*Data from* Szockik JF, Barker SJ, Tremper KK. Fundamental principles of monitoring instrumentation. In: Miller RD, editor. Anesthesia. 5th edition. Philadelphia: Churchill Livingstone; 2000. p. 1053.)

(see **Fig. 1**A), the first has the lowest frequency, which corresponds with the heart rate. The second and third sine waves have successively higher frequencies and lower amplitudes, which give the simulated waveform finer features such as the dicrotic notch. The second and third sine waves are required to simulate the systolic upstroke (see **Fig. 1**B).

Steeper upstrokes require the summation of sine waves of even higher frequencies. The CTT system must be able to process these higher frequencies to avoid waveform distortion (discussed later). The concept of waveform summation is also applicable to the morphology of the physiologic arterial waveform, which is determined by the overlap of pulse waves generated by the heart and waves reflected from the arterioles.

Pulse wave reflection

Reflection waves are not abnormal, but are important contributors to the arterial waveform in most animals.[6] When blood is ejected from the heart, pulse pressure waves generated in the ascending aorta propagate toward the periphery at a velocity that is faster than the flow wave. On reaching distal arteriolar beds, the incident pulse wave is reflected, generating a retrograde pulse wave.[6] The incident and reflected pulse waves overlap (summate) to form a new composite waveform (**Fig. 2**). However,

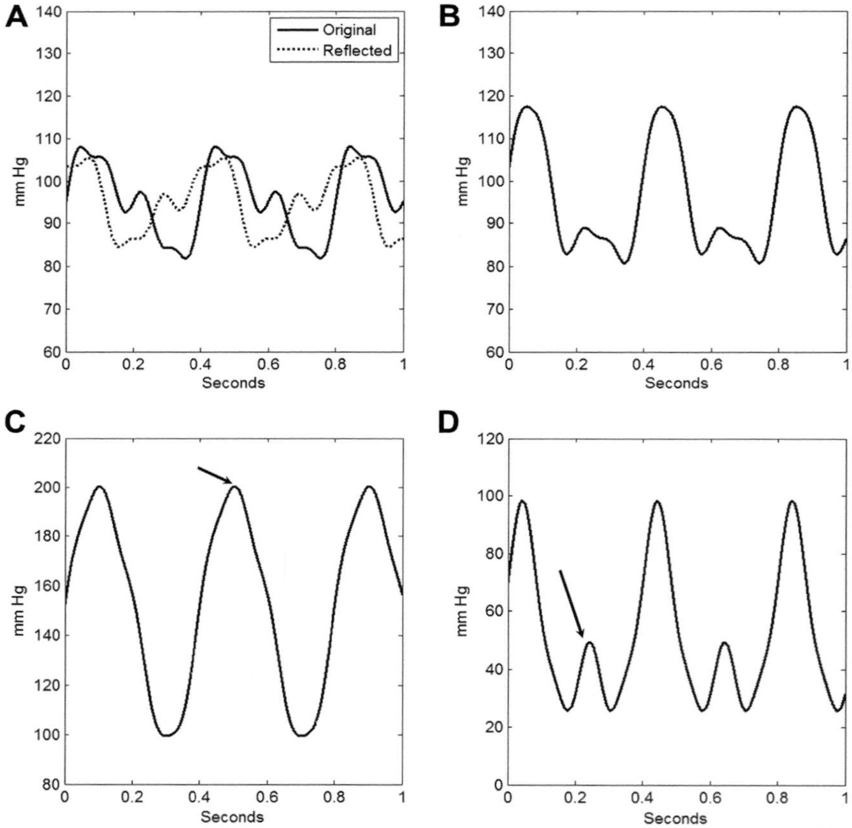

Fig. 2. Demonstration of the effect of pulse wave reflection on arterial waveform morphology. The simulated arterial waveform from **Fig. 1** is shown with its reflection (*A*). Summation of the incident and reflected wave produces a composite arterial waveform with systolic and diastolic waves (*B*). When pulse wave velocity is increased, as in hypertension, the reflected wave overlaps sooner (*C*) yielding a characteristic late systolic peak (*arrow*) and diminished diastolic wave. Hypotension is associated with slower pulse wave velocities, which leads to overlap of reflected waves later in the cardiac cycle (*D*), and large diastolic waves are seen (*arrow*). These simulations were performed using custom scripts written in MATLAB.

in the vasculature, the final arterial waveform is the summation of reflected waves from all arteriolar beds, with reflected waves sometimes being rereflected several times. Wave reflection is important in maintaining normal blood pressure and organ perfusion. Three factors influence the effect of wave reflection on the final arterial waveform: distance to reflection points (arteriolar beds), pulse wave velocity, and degree of vasoconstriction. The typical distance a pulse wave has to travel before it is reflected depends on the location of the arteriolar bed. For example, the distance from the heart to the brachial bed is about 0.5 m. In a normal adult, pulse waves travel about 10 m/s, with the velocity varying directly with the arterial blood pressure.[7] Reflected waves typically have amplitudes of 80% of the originating waveform amplitude.[8] In young patients, diastolic blood pressure (DBP) is increased by reflected waves overlapping during diastole, and this helps maintain coronary perfusion. However, in elderly and hypertensive patients, pulse wave velocity is increased because of blood pressure and decreased arterial distensibility.[6,9] This increased velocity allows the reflected wave to arrive sooner and overlap with the incident wave, leading to increased systolic blood pressure (SBP), decreased DBP, and the formation of a characteristic late systolic peak in the arterial waveform (see **Fig. 2**C, arrow).[6]

Pulse wave reflection is particularly important in explaining the arterial waveform in the setting of hemorrhagic shock, which is associated with hypotension, tachycardia, and increased arteriolar vasoconstriction. At low blood pressures, pulse wave velocity can be significantly decreased, whereas the duration of systole is decreased in tachycardia. Vasoconstriction is a common physiologic response to shock and is often manipulated with pharmacotherapy by the anesthesiologist. Conditions that decrease SVR, such as sepsis or pharmacologic vasodilation, minimize the degree of wave reflection. However, as noted earlier, increased vasoconstriction in response to shock or administration of peripheral vasoconstrictors maximizes wave reflection.[6] The net effect of hypotension, tachycardia, and vasoconstriction contributes to the generation of a composite arterial waveform with a characteristic large diastolic wave (see arrow in **Fig. 2**D and waveform in **Fig. 3**B), and, at times, a slowed systolic upstroke.[6]

Central aortic pressure may be overestimated by up to 20% if SBP is measured with a peripheral catheter.[10] This is because, in addition to the factors already discussed, waveform morphology depends strongly on the location of measurement, as shown by the observed differences in waveform appearance at the dorsalis pedis relative to the radial artery catheter site. These differences are attributed to overlap of incident, reflected, and rereflected waves from various arteriolar beds, and to the contribution of reflected waves to systolic pressure occurring earlier as measurements are recorded further from the heart.[8] Therefore, many factors contribute to the morphology of the arterial waveform (**Table 1**), and the anesthesiologist must be careful to consider these factors when interpreting information obtained from arterial CTT systems. In particular, SBP overestimation should be avoided by considering SBP in conjunction with mean arterial pressure (MAP), because MAP is not significantly affected by reflection waves[6] and measurement site.

The impact of trauma pathophysiology on the contribution of reflected waves to the arterial waveform can lead to incorrect identification of waveform distortion. Contrary to popular opinion, it is not possible to determine whether a recorded arterial waveform is overdamped or underdamped simply by casually observing waveform morphology (see **Fig. 3**).[11] The only way to determine whether a recorded waveform is distorted is to assess the dynamic response of the CTT system.[11,12] This assessment can be accomplished at the bedside by performing a flush test,[13] or in simulations by introducing a square wave[11] and analyzing the resulting oscillating waves.[13]

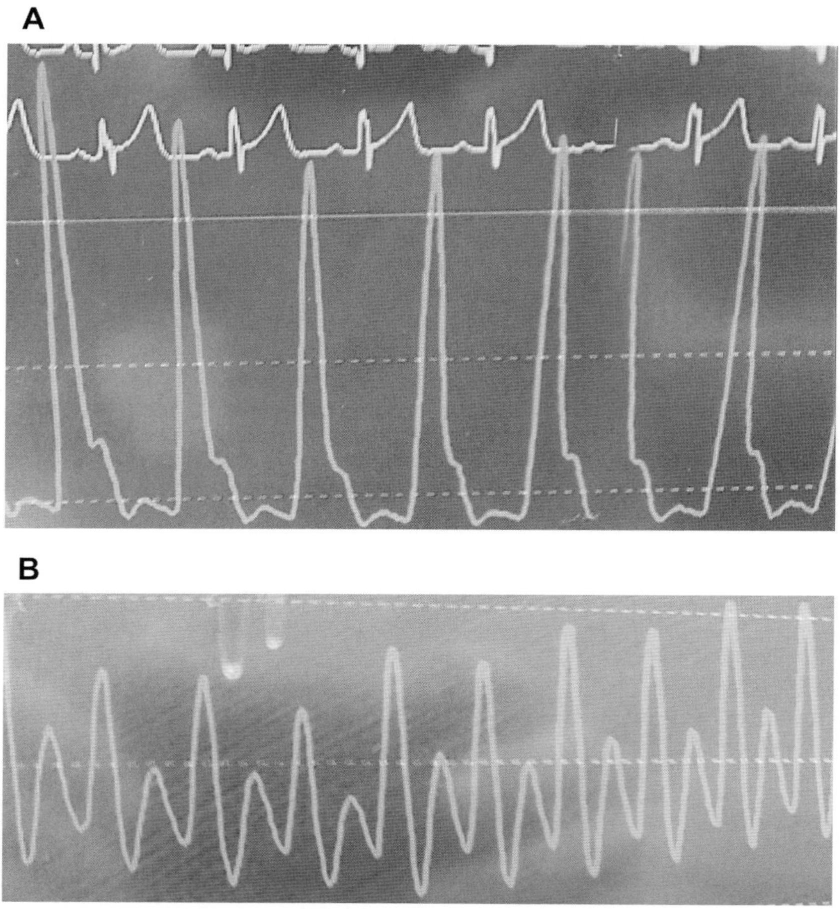

Fig. 3. Two arterial waveform recordings typically seen in trauma. The first waveform could be incorrectly considered to be underdamped (*A*), whereas the second might be considered to be overdamped (*B*). However, the dynamic response characteristics underlying each recording were satisfactory.

Table 1
Factors affecting invasive and NIBP measurement

	CTT		Oscillometry	
	Systolic	Mean	Systolic	Mean
Distal measurement site	O	—	—	—
Hypotensive (shock)	V	—	O	V[a]
Wave reflection	V	—	V[b]	V[b]
Overdamped	U	—	n/a	n/a
Underdamped	O	—	n/a	n/a

Abbreviations: n/a, not applicable; O, overestimated; U, underestimated; V, variable effect.
[a] Possible unreliability caused by group-specific differences in amplitude envelope.
[b] The algorithm used in oscillometry to calculate blood pressures is affected in part by arterial waveform morphology and pulse rate.

Dynamic response of the IABP monitoring system

CTT systems have been shown to behave like underdamped second-order systems.[14] As such, the dynamic response of the CTT can be characterized in terms of its natural frequency and damping coefficient. This dynamic response depends on the mass of fluid in the tubing, the compliance of the tubing, and friction to fluid movement in the tubing. Clinical CTT systems are designed with short, thin, noncompliant tubing with the goal of obtaining an optimal dynamic response. The anesthesiologist can determine these values for a particular CTT system by performing a flush test. The resulting oscillating waveform is then analyzed to obtain the natural frequency of oscillation and the amplitude ratio of the first 2 oscillation peaks (for details see Mark[13] [1998]). Next, a plot of natural frequency versus damping coefficient (**Fig. 4**) is referenced to determine whether the dynamic response is adequate to allow proper processing of the physiologic waveform.[11] If the dynamic response is not adequate, the measured waveform may be distorted. The fallacy in attempting to determine dynamic response by casual observation of the waveform was shown by Gardner[11] (1981) on analysis of waveforms from 37 patients. He showed that it is possible to have a waveform that appears to be underdamped when its dynamic response is determined to be overdamped, and vice versa.[11]

Introduction of a bubble into the tubing or the use of a resonance overshoot eliminator (ROSE) damping device (Spectramed, Oxnard, CA) are strategies commonly used to correct an underdamped CTT system. However, introduction of an air bubble increases damping and simultaneously decreases natural frequency,[11,15] which may do little to improve, or may even worsen, the dynamic response of an underdamped system (see *a* in **Fig. 4**). Furthermore, an optimal dynamic response can inadvertently be made suboptimal (see *b* in **Fig. 4**), increasing the likelihood that the SBP measurement will be inaccurate. The ROSE damping device has been shown to increase the

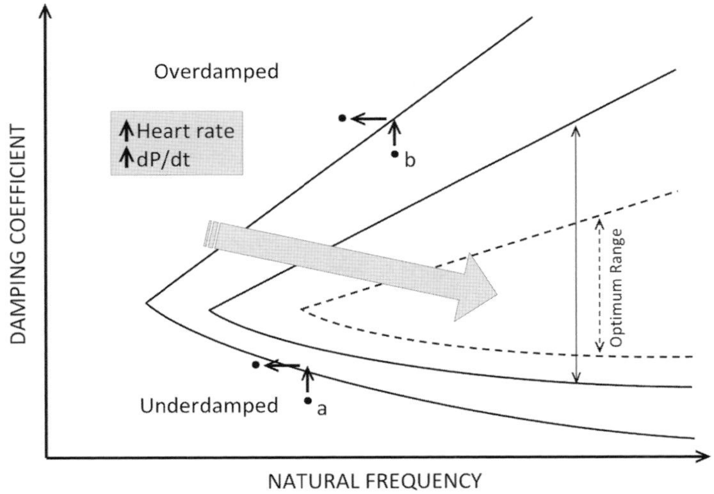

Fig. 4. How natural frequency, damping coefficient, and patient physiology interact to define optimum dynamic response requirement. As either heart rate or the slope of the systolic upstroke (dP/dt) increases, the natural frequency necessary to allow proper processing of the arterial waveform increases and the range of damping coefficient associated with optimum dynamic response decreases (compare vertical arrow bars). Presence of a bubble increases damping coefficient and decreases natural frequency (*a* and *b*).

damping coefficient while having little effect on natural frequency, and therefore may improve measurement accuracy of an underdamped system. However, resonance may still occur at high heart rates (a common occurrence in patients with trauma) and with steep systolic upstroke.[15]

In the case in which dynamic response is suboptimal because of low natural frequency, the recorded waveform may become distorted because of resonance and appear to be underdamped. A recorded waveform appears to resonate when the frequencies of sine waves that compose the physiologic waveform approach the natural frequency of the CTT system. The effect is increased in an underdamped system. A simple demonstration helps to explain the interaction between the natural frequency of the CTT system and the sine waves that make up the arterial waveform. **Fig. 5** shows the effect of resonance on the simulated arterial waveform constructed from 3 sine waves from **Fig. 1**. The frequencies of these sine waves increase with heart rate. For example, at a heart rate of 60 beats per minute (bpm), sine waves 1, 2, and 3, have frequencies of 1, 2, and 4 Hz, respectively. These frequencies are increased to 2.5, 5.0, and 10 Hz, respectively, when the heart rate is 150 bpm. At the higher heart rate, sine waves 2 and 3 resonate in a CTT system with natural frequencies of 5 (see **Fig. 5**A) and 10 Hz (see **Fig. 5**B), respectively. The effect of resonance is to distort the recorded waveform such that SBP is overestimated by 10 to 30 mm Hg and the diastolic pressure is underestimated, whereas the effect on MAP is not significant.[11]

The dynamic response plot published by Gardner[11] (1981) (see **Fig. 4**) was derived from analysis of only 2 physiologic waveforms. One waveform was thought to represent the general patient population and had a heart rate of 94 bpm. The other waveform (118 bpm) was chosen because it required the greatest dynamic response attributed to its steep systolic upstroke. Although there are no experiments that address this in the literature, it is feasible that physiologic waveforms obtained from patients with trauma in hemorrhagic shock with heart rates of 150 bpm or more and increased ventricular contractility may exceed the capability of the CTT system. Future research may help to determine whether this is the case and, if so, consideration for the design of CTT systems with natural frequencies more relevant to the trauma setting may be warranted. This possibility is especially germane when considering the potential role of hypotensive resuscitation in the management of patients with trauma. In the meantime, anesthesiologists should rely more on monitoring MAP than SBP, because MAP measurements are the least affected by the dynamic response characteristics of the CTT system.

Current CTT systems are claimed to have natural frequency between 10 and 20 Hz.[5] At our institution, we have taken steps to optimize the dynamic response of our CTT systems. We now perform flush tests on the CTT system when we use invasive monitoring. We have found that the natural frequency is usually between 10 and 20 Hz, as advertised (**Fig. 6**). When extension tubing is used (eg, dorsalis pedis site), the natural frequency is reduced about 50% (on occasion, we have observed natural frequencies of less than 5 Hz). Based on our observations, we now instruct residents not to use extension tubing, but instead to place the CTT transducer close to the catheter site. However, in considering that the pulse waveform of unstable patients with trauma may demand higher dynamic response than is advertised on out-of-the-box CTT systems, we have changed our practice further by removing any unnecessary tubing between the transducer and the catheter insertion site. By performing this modification, the natural frequency is usually doubled (see **Fig. 6**). We are currently investigating whether these modifications improve the fidelity of recorded waveforms in the setting of hemorrhagic shock.

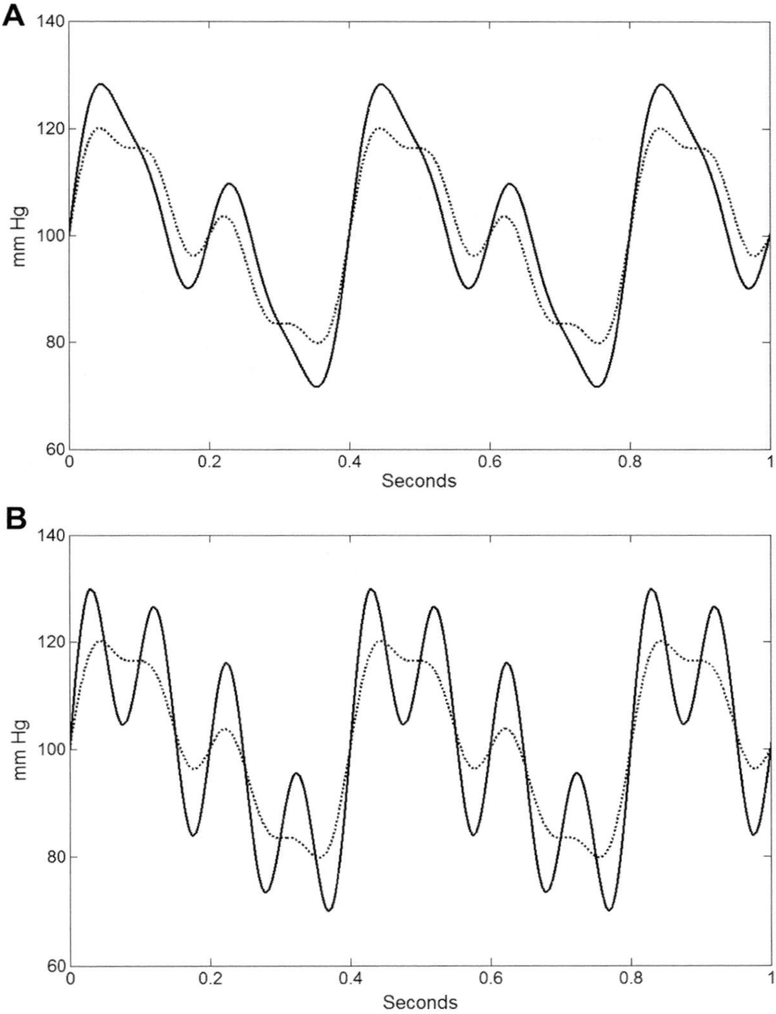

Fig. 5. The effect of resonance on arterial waveform morphology. Resonance occurs when a harmonic frequency of the physiologic waveform approaches the natural frequency of a particular CTT system. Two examples are shown using the first (*A*) and second (*B*) harmonics from **Fig. 1**. In both cases, amplification of the harmonic wave is observed in the recorded waveform, and SBPs and DBPs are overestimated and underestimated, respectively.

NIBP Monitoring

NIBP monitoring is likely to be relied on to manage the patient with acute trauma in prehospital and emergency room settings. In the operating room, NIBP can be valuable in assessing hemodynamic status and effects of fluid and pharmacologic treatments until invasive monitoring is established. NIBP is easy to implement as long as an extremity is available for cuff placement. It is common for a patient with trauma to sustain injury in both upper extremities and, in such cases, cuff placement at the thigh or ankle provides MAP values that correlate well with values obtained at the

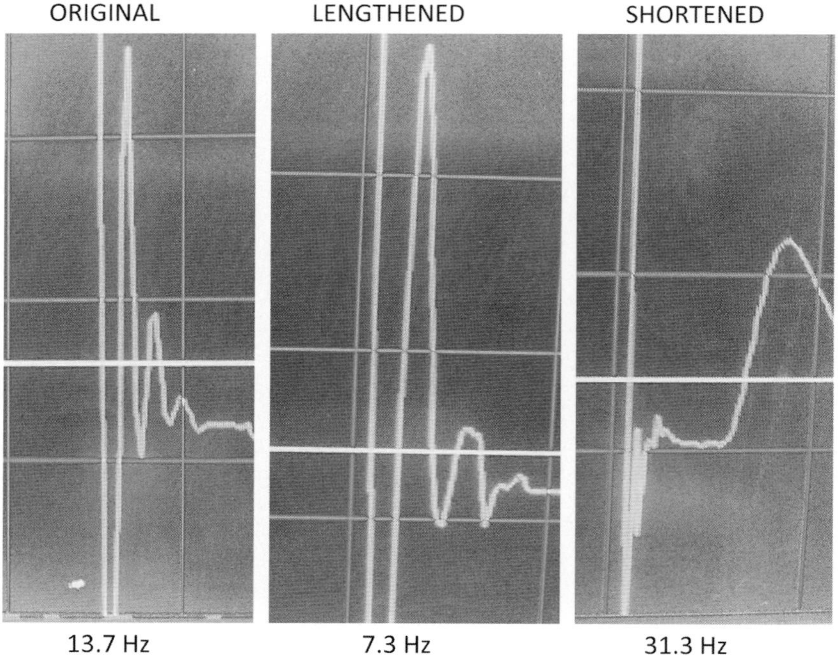

Fig. 6. The effect of tube length on CTT system natural frequency. At our institution, natural frequency is typically between 10 and 20 Hz (*ORIGINAL*). The effect of adding extension tubing (*LENGTHENED*) or removing unnecessary tubing (*SHORTENED*) can significantly affect CTT natural frequency (unpublished data, McNeer RR, 2013).

arm, although measurements with thigh cuff placement take the longest to complete.[16] NIBP has been reported as an effective means of tracking blood pressure changes and hypotension in unstable patients.[17] However, it is usually desirable to establish an arterial line as soon as other procedures have been performed, such as securing the airway and obtaining large-bore intravenous access. Limitations to the use of NIBP include placing an inappropriately sized cuff,[18,19] presence of dysrhythmias,[20] and patient movement or movement associated with the surgical procedure (including surgeons). However, more relevant for the patient with trauma is the limitation of obtaining accurate blood pressure values during hypotension.[21]

Most intraoperative NIBP measurements are performed with automated devices, which use the principle of oscillometry.[20] In this technique, the amplitude of oscillations in an air-filled occlusive cuff is measured at cuff pressures that start at more than SBP and extend to less than DBP. A plot of oscillation amplitude versus cuff pressure generates the oscillation amplitude envelope (**Fig. 7**). The maximum amplitude algorithm (MAA) is used by most devices to estimate MAP, which is considered to be the pressure in the cuff at maximum oscillation amplitude.[22] The SBP and DBP are calculated based on the shape of the amplitude envelope. However, the algorithm used is proprietary, not standardized, and varies with manufacturer.[18,20] Clinical studies have shown that NIBP correlates well with IABP for pressure values in the normal range, whereas it has been shown to be less accurate at extremes of blood pressure. When compared with sphygmomanometry, oscillometric SBP values between 90 and 110 mm Hg

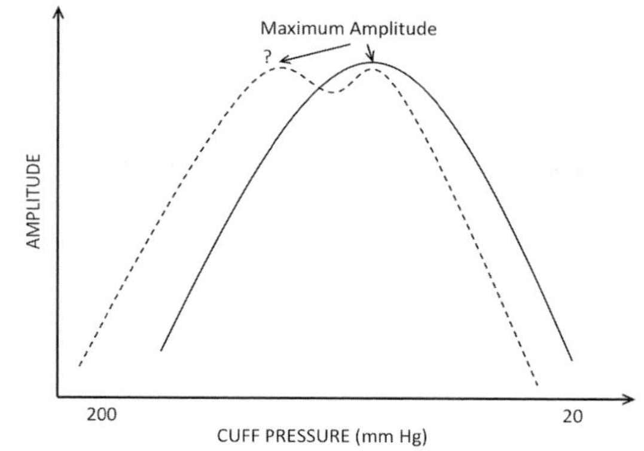

Fig. 7. The maximum amplitude algorithm for measuring MAP. The pressure in the occlusive cuff at maximum oscillation amplitude is considered to be the MAP (*solid line curve*). Factors such as arterial waveform morphology and pulse rate can affect the shape of the amplitude envelope such that the pressure corresponding with maximum oscillation amplitude is not easy to identify.[31] For example, the ambiguous amplitude envelope illustrated by the dashed curve has been observed in hypertensive patients, where the maximum amplitude cannot be identified (?).

overestimate SBP (119 $\pm$ 6 mm Hg vs 103 $\pm$ 4 mm Hg). The overestimation is more significant for SBP values less than 90 mm Hg (106 $\pm$ 6 mm Hg vs 80 $\pm$ 2 mm Hg)[21] In contrast, oscillometric MAP has been shown to be consistent with IABP MAP for values less than 65 mm Hg,[16] which may seem appropriate because MAP is considered to be a directly measured parameter in oscillometry.

Although it is commonly assumed that the MAP as measured by the MAA algorithm is more accurate than SBP and DBP, all 3 parameters have been shown in simulation studies to be influenced by other factors independent of MAA, such as pulse pressure, arterial pressure/volume relationship, and pulse wave morphology and heart rate.[22–25] In addition, errors in estimates of SBP, DBP, and MAP have been shown in simulation studies to depend on interactions between the arterial waveform amplitude, waveform morphology, and arterial wall mechanical characteristics.[23] Furthermore, there may be twice as much error associated with MAP than with SBP and DBP measurements.[26] Another simulation study suggested that there is no direct relationship between the MAP estimate obtained with MAA and the actual MAP.[22]

There is no standardization of the oscillometric algorithm used by manufacturers, and most validation studies have been conducted in healthy patients with hypertensive and hypotensive conditions being absent or underrepresented. These facts may add an additional layer of error to oscillometric measurements in certain patient populations. Group-specific differences between oscillometry and the auscultatory method have been reported in pregnant women,[27,28] diabetics,[29] and patients with decreased arterial elasticity.[30] For example, hypertensive patients have been observed to display an oscillation amplitude envelope with an ambiguous maximum amplitude[31] (see **Fig. 7**) leading to significant errors in estimated MAP. Although the effect of hypotension on the oscillation amplitude envelope has not been investigated in the setting of hemorrhagic shock, patient physiology and device factors may explain the unreliability of oscillometric measurements in unstable patients with trauma.

Given the many factors (see **Table 1**) that contribute to the unreliability of oscillometric monitoring, it is sobering to acknowledge that patients being managed with a hypotensive resuscitation strategy are sometimes monitored with these devices. Future investigations on hypotensive resuscitation should indicate the methods used for blood pressure measurement to allow clinical interpretation of study results.

PETco_2 as a Measure of Cardiac Output

Initial hemodynamic assessment and monitoring of patients with acute trauma can be difficult because of the frenetic and at times chaotic operating room environment in these cases. The act of placing monitors on the patient can be challenging, especially because many of the standard monitors are either inaccurate or do not function during low-flow circulatory and hypotensive states. Initial intraoperative hemodynamic assessment of the patient needs to be attained in a timely and efficient manner. A simple way to assess whether a patient has cardiac output on arrival to the operating room is to ventilate the patient and observe the end-tidal CO_2 level (PETco_2).[4] Although this can be accomplished with a colorimetric CO_2 detector (eg, in the emergency room or bay), capnography provides numerical values for PETco_2 and is easily established on attaching the patient to the ventilator. However, special considerations must be taken into account when using this approach in the patient with trauma to avoid misdiagnosis or missed detection of severe hemodynamic instability.

The relationship between PETco_2 and cardiac output has been investigated in animals[32–36] and humans.[37–39] Cardiac output and PETco_2 have been shown to correlate during low-flow circulatory states including cardiogenic, septic, and hemorrhagic shock.[32] The relationship between PETco_2 and cardiac output has been shown to be a logarithmic curve.[34] A study in patients being weaned from cardiopulmonary bypass reported that when PETco_2 was more than 30 mm Hg, the cardiac output was greater than 4 L/min. However, at PETco_2 levels of more than 34 mm Hg, further increases in cardiac output did not correlate with comparable changes in PETco_2.[37]

The correlation between PETco_2 and cardiac output in low-flow states can be explained based on the pathophysiology of shock. As cardiac output to the lungs decreases, less CO_2 is available for transfer into alveoli, there is an increase in the West zone 1, which contributes to dead space–like ventilation (ie, VQ mismatch), and absolute dead space secondary to pulmonary vessel collapse can occur.

An additional explanation can be obtained by considering 2 fundamental expressions from respiratory physiology that describe the relationship between alveolar ventilation (VA), CO_2 elimination (Vco_2), and partial pressure of alveolar CO_2 (PAco_2), (VA = Vco_2/PAco_2 $\times$ K), and the relationship between CO_2 elimination, cardiac output, and arterial and venous CO_2 content (C$\bar{v}co_2$) or Fick principle (Vco_2 = Q $\times$ (Caco_2 − C$\bar{v}co_2$)).[40] After assuming normal lung function and that PETco_2, PAco_2, and partial pressure of arterial CO_2 (Paco_2) are equal, Maslow and colleagues[37] (2001) rearranged these expressions to obtain the following:

$$PETco_2 \cong \frac{A\dot{Q}_P P_{\bar{v}}co_2}{\dot{V}_A + A\dot{Q}_P}$$

where Q_p is pulmonary blood flow (ie, cardiac output), *P$\bar{v}co_2$* is partial pressure of mixed venous CO_2, and *A* is CO_2 solubility in blood. A limitation of this equation is the assumption that lungs are homogeneous; however, in the setting of shock, VQ mismatch and absolute dead space are likely to be present. Nonetheless, the equation is useful in showing that PETco_2 is affected by several interdependent factors.

During periods of apnea or hypoventilation, P$\bar{v}co_2$ (as well as Paco_2) increases because of decreased or absent pulmonary elimination of CO_2.[40] Reestablishment of ventilation in this circumstance reveals a PETco_2 that is normal or greater than normal even if cardiac output is unchanged. In contrast, in cardiac arrest or low cardiac output states $P\bar{v}CO_2$ increases because less CO_2 is delivered to the lungs. In this situation, $PaCO_2$ does not increase as much as $P\bar{v}CO_2$ and may decrease,[12] whereas the $P\bar{v}CO_2$-$PaCO_2$ difference increases.

Restoration of cardiac output after cardiac arrest or low-flow state results in increased $PETCO_2$ level. However, in this circumstance, increased $PETCO_2$ does not necessarily reflect adequate cardiac output. Experimental evidence in support of this phenomenon was shown in a study in which hemorrhagic shock was induced in sheep while mechanical ventilation rate was held constant.[12] Arterial and venous CO_2 were measured during baseline, hemorrhagic shock, and postresuscitation periods. During the shock period, cardiac output decreased (from 2.3 to 0.6 L/min), resulting in significant increase in $P\bar{v}CO_2$, modest decrease in $PaCO_2$, and decrease in $PETCO_2$. The decrease in $PETCO_2$ was predominantly caused by the decreased cardiac output. After resuscitation and return of normal cardiac output, $PaCO_2$ increased to more than baseline levels and the $P\bar{v}CO_2$-$PaCO_2$ difference decreased. Although $PETCO_2$ was not measured in the postresuscitation period, it is possible to infer that it would have been increased to more than the baseline, assuming that the $PaCO_2$-$PETCO_2$ difference remained the same between baseline and postresuscitation periods.

Applying this analysis to patients with trauma, there is the prospect that $PETCO_2$ can reach near-normal levels with small increases in cardiac output after a period of shock or cardiac arrest. These relationships have not yet been quantified experimentally in patients with trauma. Nonetheless, it is prudent to consider prehospital events (ie, cardiac or respiratory arrest) that increase $P\bar{v}CO_2$ when using $PETCO_2$ to assess hemodynamic status.

SUMMARY

The ultimate goal of resuscitation in the setting of uncontrolled hemorrhagic shock is to ensure adequate organ perfusion until surgical hemostasis is obtained. Tissue perfusion in this setting is usually indirectly assessed by monitoring blood pressure with either NIBP or IABP and cardiac output by monitoring $PETCO_2$ level. A general theme of this article is that factors common in the trauma setting and characteristics of current monitoring devices can often interfere with accurate assessment of hemodynamic status. Overestimation of SBP as can occur with oscillometry and IABP is arguably one of the most important monitoring pitfalls to be avoided. More accurate assessment can be accomplished by considering SBP in conjunction with MAP measurements. However, oscillometric MAP has potential limitations in trauma, especially considering that the amplitude envelope is affected by factors such as arterial waveform shape and heart rate. Research and development need to be applied toward improving algorithms such that oscillometry is more reliable in patient subpopulations including trauma. However, the current lack of standardization is not aligned with this goal. It may be easier to improve the reliability of IABP monitoring, because improving the dynamic response of the CTT system can ensure that the arterial waveform is properly processed and not distorted. However, the extent to which the natural frequency should be increased to provide adequate dynamic response in the setting of trauma is unknown. We are currently conducting studies to address this question.

The unreliability of blood pressure monitoring is likely to be a significant confounding variable in studies investigating the role of hypotensive resuscitation. The most reliably measured blood pressure parameter is currently MAP, and the most reliable method for MAP measurement is invasively with a CTT system independent of dynamic response (see **Table 1**). The reliability of oscillometric MAP measurements is unclear, because most evidence suggesting its unreliability comes from theoretic and simulation studies. Nonetheless, it is prudent to control for the methods used to monitor MAP in future studies.

REFERENCES

1. Mapstone J, Roberts I, Evans P. Fluid resuscitation strategies: a systematic review of animal trials. J Trauma 2003;55(3):571–89.
2. Bickell WH, Wall MJ Jr, Pepe PE, et al. Immediate versus delayed fluid resuscitation for hypotensive patients with penetrating torso injuries. N Engl J Med 1994; 331(17):1105–9.
3. Morrison CA, Carrick MM, Norman MA, et al. Hypotensive resuscitation strategy reduces transfusion requirements and severe postoperative coagulopathy in trauma patients with hemorrhagic shock: preliminary results of a randomized controlled trial. J Trauma 2011;70(3):652–63.
4. McNeer RR, Varon AJ. Monitoring the trauma patient. In: Varon AJ, Smith CE, editors. Essentials of trauma anesthesia. 1st edition. New York: Cambridge University Press; 2012. p. 116–29.
5. Szockik JF, Barker SJ, Tremper KK. Fundamental principles of monitoring instrumentation. In: Miller RD, editor. Anesthesia. 5th edition. Philadelphia: Churchill Livingstone; 2000. p. 1053.
6. O'Rourke MF, Yaginuma T. Wave reflections and the arterial pulse. Arch Intern Med 1984;144(2):366–71.
7. O'Rourke MF. Vascular impedance in studies of arterial and cardiac function. Physiol Rev 1982;62(2):570–623.
8. Henneman EA, Henneman PL. Intricacies of blood pressure measurement: reexamining the rituals. Heart Lung 1989;18(3):263–71.
9. Weber T, O'Rourke MF, Ammer M, et al. Arterial stiffness and arterial wave reflections are associated with systolic and diastolic function in patients with normal ejection fraction. Am J Hypertens 2008;21(11):1194–202.
10. Bridges ME, Middleton R. Direct arterial vs oscillometric monitoring of blood pressure: stop comparing and pick one (a decision-making algorithm). Crit Care Nurse 1997;17(3):58–66, 68–72.
11. Gardner RM. Direct blood pressure measurement–dynamic response requirements. Anesthesiology 1981;54(3):227–36.
12. Garnett AR, Glauser FL, Ornato JP. Hypercarbic arterial acidemia following resuscitation from severe hemorrhagic shock. Resuscitation 1989;17(1):55–61.
13. Mark JB. Atlas of cardiovascular monitoring. New York: Churchill Livingstone; 1998.
14. Shapiro GG, Krovetz LJ. Damped and undamped frequency responses of underdamped catheter manometer systems. Am Heart J 1970;80(2):226–36.
15. Kleinman B, Powell S. Dynamic response of the ROSE damping device. J Clin Monit 1989;5(2):111–5.
16. Lakhal K, Macq C, Ehrmann S, et al. Noninvasive monitoring of blood pressure in the critically ill: reliability according to the cuff site (arm, thigh, or ankle). Crit Care Med 2012;40(4):1207–13.
17. Lakhal K, Ehrmann S, Runge I, et al. Tracking hypotension and dynamic changes in arterial blood pressure with brachial cuff measurements. Anesth Analg 2009; 109(2):494–501.

18. Ng KG, Small CF. Changes in oscillometric pulse amplitude envelope with cuff size: implications for blood pressure measurement criteria and cuff size selection. J Biomed Eng 1993;15(4):279–82.
19. Jilek J, Stork M. Cuff width alters the amplitude envelope of wrist cuff pressure pulse waveforms. Physiol Meas 2010;31(7):N43–9.
20. Smulyan H, Safar ME. Blood pressure measurement: retrospective and prospective views. Am J Hypertens 2011;24(6):628–34.
21. Davis JW, Davis IC, Bennink LD, et al. Are automated blood pressure measurements accurate in trauma patients? J Trauma 2003;55(5):860–3.
22. Baker PD, Westenskow DR, Kuck K. Theoretical analysis of non-invasive oscillometric maximum amplitude algorithm for estimating mean blood pressure. Med Biol Eng Comput 1997;35(3):271–8.
23. Forster FK, Turney D. Oscillometric determination of diastolic, mean and systolic blood pressure–a numerical model. J Biomech Eng 1986;108(4):359–64.
24. Ursino M, Cristalli C. A mathematical study of some biomechanical factors affecting the oscillometric blood pressure measurement. IEEE Trans Biomed Eng 1996;43(8):761–78.
25. Raamat R, Talts J, Jagomagi K, et al. Mathematical modelling of non-invasive oscillometric finger mean blood pressure measurement by maximum oscillation criterion. Med Biol Eng Comput 1999;37(6):784–8.
26. Raamat R, Talts J, Jagomagi K, et al. Errors of oscillometric blood pressure measurement as predicted by simulation. Blood Press Monit 2011;16(5):238–45.
27. Arfeen ZU, Maran NJ, Simon EJ, et al. A comparison of non-invasive methods of blood pressure measurement in normotensive and hypertensive pregnant women. Int J Obstet Anesth 1996;5(3):168–71.
28. Penny JA, Shennan AH, Halligan AW, et al. Blood pressure measurement in severe pre-eclampsia. Lancet 1997;349(9064):1518.
29. van Ittersum FJ, Wijering RM, Lambert J, et al. Determinants of the limits of agreement between the sphygmomanometer and the SpaceLabs 90207 device for blood pressure measurement in health volunteers and insulin-dependent diabetic patients. J Hypertens 1998;16(8):1125–30.
30. van Popele NM, Bos WJ, de Beer NA, et al. Arterial stiffness as underlying mechanism of disagreement between an oscillometric blood pressure monitor and a sphygmomanometer. Hypertension 2000;36(4):484–8.
31. SunTech Medical: the rationale for clinical monitors and validation of the oscillometric method. Available at: http://www.suntechmed.com/downloads/OEM/white_papers/OEM_Whitepaper_0002.pdf. Accessed October 23, 2012.
32. Jin X, Weil MH, Tang W, et al. End-tidal carbon dioxide as a noninvasive indicator of cardiac index during circulatory shock. Crit Care Med 2000;28(7):2415–9.
33. Weil MH, Bisera J, Trevino RP, et al. Cardiac output and end-tidal carbon dioxide. Crit Care Med 1985;13(11):907–9.
34. Ornato JP, Garnett AR, Glauser FL. Relationship between cardiac output and the end-tidal carbon dioxide tension. Ann Emerg Med 1990;19(10):1104–6.
35. Isserles SA, Breen PH. Can changes in end-tidal P_{CO_2} measure changes in cardiac output? Anesth Analg 1991;73(6):808–14.
36. Dubin A, Murias G, Estenssoro E, et al. End-tidal CO_2 pressure determinants during hemorrhagic shock. Intensive Care Med 2000;26(11):1619–23.
37. Maslow A, Stearns G, Bert A, et al. Monitoring end-tidal carbon dioxide during weaning from cardiopulmonary bypass in patients without significant lung disease. Anesth Analg 2001;92(2):306–13.

38. Shibutani K, Muraoka M, Shirasaki S, et al. Do changes in end-tidal P_{CO_2} quantitatively reflect changes in cardiac output? Anesth Analg 1994;79(5):829–33.
39. McManus JG, Ryan KL, Morton MJ, et al. Limitations of end-tidal CO_2 as an early indicator of central hypovolemia in humans. Prehosp Emerg Care 2008;12(2):199–205.
40. West JB. Respiratory physiology: the essentials. 7th edition. Philadelphia: Lippincott Williams & Wilkins; 2005.

Index

Note: Page numbers of article titles are in **boldface** type.

Anesthesiology Clin 31 (2013) 195–205
http://dx.doi.org/10.1016/S1932-2275(12)00167-X anesthesiology.theclinics.com
1932-2275/13/$ – see front matter